Obstetric and Intrapartum Emergencies

A Practical Guide to Management

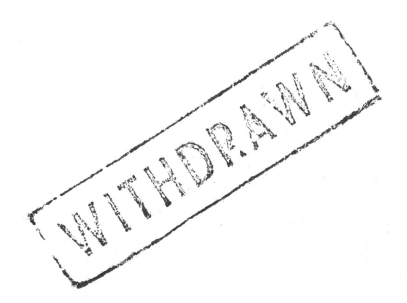

Obstetric and Intrapartum Emergencies

A Practical Guide to Management

Edwin Chandraharan MBBS MS (Obs & Gyn) DFFP MRCOG
Lead Consultant, Labour Ward and Clinical Director for Women's Services
St George's Healthcare NHS Trust, London, UK

Sir Sabaratnam Arulkumaran MBBS MD PhD FRCOG
Professor and Head, Division of Obstetrics and Gynaecology
St George's Hospital Medical School, London, UK

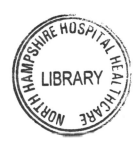

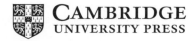

CAMBRIDGE
UNIVERSITY PRESS

CAMBRIDGE UNIVERSITY PRESS
Cambridge, New York, Melbourne, Madrid, Cape Town, Singapore,
São Paulo, Delhi, Mexico City

Cambridge University Press
The Edinburgh Building, Cambridge CB2 8RU, UK

Published in the United States of America by Cambridge University
Press, New York

www.cambridge.org
Information on this title: www.cambridge.org/9780521268271

© Cambridge University Press 2013

First published 2012

Printed and bound in the United Kingdom by the MPG Books
Group

*A catalogue record for this publication is available from the British
Library*

Library of Congress Cataloguing in Publication data
Obstetric and intrapartum emergencies : a practical guide to
management / [edited by] Edwin Chandraharan, Sabaratnam
Arulkumaran.
    p.   ;   cm.
Includes bibliographical references and index.
ISBN 978-0-521-26827-1 (pbk.)
I. Chandraharan, Edwin.   II. Arulkumaran, Sabaratnam.
[DNLM: 1. Pregnancy Complications – therapy.   2. Delivery,
Obstetric – methods.   3. Emergencies.   4. Emergency
Treatment – methods.   5. Obstetrics – methods. WQ 240]
618.3 – dc23   2012019945

ISBN 978-0-521-26827-1 Paperback

Contents

Preface

Pregnancy and childbirth should be a safe and rewarding experience for women and their families, as well as for maternity healthcare providers. However, it is estimated that globally over 300 000 women die during pregnancy and childbirth every year, largely due to substandard care. Even in the United Kingdom, the latest Confidential Enquiries into Maternal Deaths Report suggests that substandard care may contribute to approximately 70% of all maternal deaths.

Substandard care is often due to 'too little being done too late', especially whilst managing emergencies during antepartum, intrapartum and postpartum periods. Failure to recognise warning symptoms and signs of complications, lack of knowledge and skills, failure to seek appropriate experienced or multi-disciplinary input, as well as failures in team working and effective communication, contribute to maternal and perinatal morbidity and mortality.

The book aims to promote evidence-based emergency obstetric and neonatal care both in well-resourced and less well-resourced countries. We have attempted to include 'practical algorithms' for quick reference, a scientific basis for proposed actions for obstetric and intrapartum emergencies and illustrations, where appropriate. In recognition of the fact that over 90% of women die in less well-resourced countries with limited resources, we have included a section on 'Suggested management in low resource settings'. In addition, 'Key facts', 'Pearls' and 'Pitfalls' are included for easy reference.

We are greatly indebted to the authors who come from diverse backgrounds and experience, for not only sacrificing their time, but also for sharing their knowledge and expertise. There has been a collective effort from midwives, trainee obstetricians and gynaecologists, senior obstetricians, anaesthetists, neonatologists, perinatal psychiatrists, toxicologists, physicians and surgeons, from both well-resourced and less well-resourced countries to make pregnancy and childbirth safer for women and their babies. We are indeed delighted to edit this textbook with contributions from such a diverse group of authors that truly reflect the multi-professional and multi-disciplinary care that every pregnant woman and her baby fully deserve.

We have attempted to structure the sections for easy reference, starting with anatomical and physiological changes during pregnancy and their implications on clinical practice, followed by algorithms for the management of the 'Top five killers'. In addition to common antepartum, intrapartum and postpartum emergencies, we have also included management of uncommon but potentially life-threatening emergencies such as drug overdose, road traffic accidents and endocrine and musculo-skeletal emergencies.

We wish to thank our Section Editor for Anaesthetic Emergencies, Dr Anthony Addei for ensuring that common anaesthetic emergencies such as failed intubation, fluid underload and overload and transfusion reactions are addressed.

Effective management of obstetric and intrapartum emergencies involves continuous multi-disciplinary training and education. The Section on 'Setting up skills and drills in maternity services' is aimed at aiding continuously improving care and outcomes for women and their babies.

We hope this textbook will be useful for midwives, medical students, trainee as well as senior obstetricians, anaesthetists and neonatologists both in the well-resourced and less well-resourced countries.

Let us work together to ensure that no woman or her baby should die due to substandard care by optimising management of obstetric and intrapartum emergencies.

Edwin Chandraharan
Professor Sir Sabaratnam Arulkumaran

Acknowledgements

The editors would like to sincerely thank each and every author for their generous contributions of their time, knowledge and expertise. We would like to acknowledge the hard work of Ms Sue Cunningham of St George's University of London, who provided admin support. We are very grateful to Mr Nick Dunton, Ms Katie Hickling, Ms Nisha Doshi, Mr Robert Sykes and Ms Lucy Edwards from Cambridge University Press for their invaluable support and professionalism.

We are greatly indebted to our family, Anomi, Ashane and Avindri Chandraharan, and Gayatri, Shankari, Nishkantha and Kailash Arulkumaran for their patience, tolerance and understanding.

Last but not least, we wish to thank all our patients and their babies, who have taught us what we know and for inspiring us to write this book.

Contributors

Osama Abu-Ghazza
Clinical Fellow in Obstetrics and Gynaecology,
St George's Healthcare NHS Trust, London, UK

Anthony Addei
Consultant Anaesthesist & Lead for Obstetric
Anaesthesia, St George's Healthcare NHS Trust,
London, UK

Karolina Afors
Department of Obstetrics and Gynecology,
St George's Healthcare NHS Trust, London,
UK

Nilesh Agarwal
Clinical Fellow in Fetal Medicine, St George's
Healthcare NHS Trust, London, UK

Hiran Amarasekera
Orthopaedic Research Fellow, University of Warwick
Medical School, Coventry, UK

Sabaratnam Arulkumaran
Professor and Head, Division of Obstetrics and
Gynaecology, St George's Hospital Medical School,
London, UK

Cheron Bailey
Consultant Obstetric Anaesthetist, Department of
Anaesthesiology, Maidstone and Tunbridge Wells
NHS Trust, Maidstone, UK

Amarnath Bhide
Consultant, Fetal Medicine Unit, St George's
Healthcare NHS Trust, London, UK

Edwin Chandraharan
Consultant Obstetrician and Gynecologist and Lead
Clinician for Labour Ward, St George's Healthcare
NHS Trust, London, UK

Hlupekile Chipeta
Specialist Registrar, Bradford Hospital NHS
Foundation Trust, Bradford, UK

Lorraine Cleghorn
Specialist Midwife in Perinatal Mental Health,
St George's Healthcare NHS Trust, London, UK

Kirsty Crocker
Consultant Anaesthetist with Special Interest in
Obstetrics, St George's Healthcare NHS Trust,
London, UK

Stergios K. Doumouchtsis
Consultant Obstetrician and Gynaecologist,
St George's Healthcare NHS Trust, London, UK

Michael Egbor
Consultant Obstetrician, St Helier Hospital NHS
Trust, London, UK

Emma Evans
Consultant Anaesthetist and Lead for Simulation
Training, St George's Healthcare NHS Trust, London,
UK

Inidika Gawarammana
Senior Lecturer, Faculty of Medicine, University of
Peradeniya, Sri Lanka

Malik Goonewardene
Senior Professor and Head, Department of Obstetrics
and Gynaecology, University of Ruhuna, Faculty of
Medicine, Galle, Sri Lanka

Siromi Gunaratne
Consultant Paediatrician and Neonatologist,
Durdan's Hospital, Colombo, Sri Lanka

Kapila Gunawardane
Obstetrician and Gynaecologist, Teaching Hospital
Kandy, Kandy, Sri Lanka

Sarah Hammond
Consultant Anaesthetist, St George's Healthcare NHS Trust, London, UK

Richard Hartopp
Consultant Anaesthetist, St George's Healthcare NHS Trust, London, UK

Adnan Hasan
Specialist Obstetrician and Gynaecologist, Victoria Hospital, Kirkcaldy, UK

Alexander Heazell
Clinical Lecturer in Obstetrics, Maternal and Fetal Health Research Centre, University of Manchester, UK

Lucy Higgins
Academic Clinical Fellow, Maternal and Fetal Health Research Centre, University of Manchester, UK

Polly Hughes
Locum Consultant Obstetrician and Gynaecologist, St George's Healthcare NHS Trust, London, UK

Rehana Iqbal
Consultant Obstetric Anaesthetist, St George's Healthcare NHS Trust, London, UK

Priyantha Kandanearachchi
Speciality Doctor, Royal Shrewsbury Hospital, Shrewsbury, UK

Lakshman Karalliedde
Toxicologist, Guy's and St Thomas' Hospital, London, UK

Nigel Kennea
Consultant Neonatologist, St George's Healthcare NHS Trust, London, UK

Andrew Kent
Consultant, Population Health Sciences and Education Department, St George's, University of London, London, UK

Julia Kopeika
Academic Clinical Fellow, Guy's and St Thomas' NHS Trust, London, UK

Archana Krishna
Specialist Registrar, Guy's and St Thomas' NHS Trust, London, UK

Anay Kulkarni
Specialist Registrar in Neonatology, St George's Healthcare NHS Trust, London, UK

Nicola Lack
Consultant Obstetrician, University College London Hospital, London, UK

Tahir A. Mahmood
Consultant Obstetrician and Gynaecologist, Victoria Hospital, Kirkcaldy, UK

Jessica Moore
Consultant Obstetrician, St George's Healthcare NHS Trust, London, UK

Vivek Nama
Specialist Registrar, St George's Healthcare NHS Trust, London, UK

Anomi Panditharatne
Speciality Doctor in Ophthalmology, University College London Hospital, London, UK

Tim Patel
Consultant in Accident & Emergency, Kingston Hospital NHS Trust, Kingston

Leonie Penna
Consultant Obstetrician, Clinical Director, Kings College Hospital, London, UK

Chitra Ramanathan
Senior Registrar, Obstetrics and Gynaecology, Kings College Hospital, London, UK

M. F. M. Rameez
Senior Lecturer in Obstetrics and Gynaecology, University of Ruhuna, Faculty of Medicine, Galle, Sri Lanka

Probhodana Ranaweera
Senior Registrar in Obstetrics and Gynaecology, Professorial Obstetric Unit, De Soysa Maternity Home, Colombo, Sri Lanka

Justin Richards
Consultant Neonatologist, St George's Healthcare NHS Trust, London, UK

Mohamed Rishard
Senior Registrar in Obstetrics and Gynaecology, Professorial Obstetric Unit, De Soysa Maternity Home, Colombo, Sri Lanka

Hemantha Senanayake
Professor and Head, Department of Obstetrics and
Gynaecology, Faculty of Medicine, University of
Colombo, Colombo, Sri Lanka

Hassan Shehata
Consultant Obstetrician, Maternal Medicine Unit, St
Helier's Hospital, London, UK

Manilka Sumanatilleke
Specialist Registrar in Endocrinology,
St Bartholomew's Hospital, London, UK

Vikram Sinai Talaulikar
Clinical Research Fellow, Department of Obstetrics
and Gynaecology, St George's Hospital Medical
School, London, UK

Derek Tuffnell
Consultant Obstetrician and Gynaecologist, Bradford
Hospital NHS Foundation Trust, Bradford, UK

Austin Ugwumadu
Consultant Obstetrician and Gynaecologist and Lead
for Perinatal Infections, Department of Obstetrics
and Gynaecology, St George's Healthcare NHS Trust,
London, UK

Ingrid Watt-Coote
Consultant in Obstetrics and Gynaecology,
St George's Healthcare NHS Trust, London, UK

Deepal S. Weerasekera
Clinical Director and Consultant Obstetrician and
Gynaecologist, Prarthana Centre for ART, Golden
Key Hospital, Colombo, Sri Lanka

Renate Wendler
Consultant Obstetric Anaesthetist, St George's
Healthcare NHS Trust, London, UK

Christina Wood
Consultant Obstetric Anaesthetist, St George's
Healthcare NHS Trust, London, UK

Niraj Yanamandra
Consultant Obstetrician and Gynaecologist,
Fernandez Hospital, Hyderabad, India

Chapter

1

Anatomical and physiological changes in pregnancy and their implications in clinical practice

Niraj Yanamandra and Edwin Chandraharan

Key facts

Pregnancy is associated with profound anatomical, physiological, biochemical and endocrine changes that affect multiple organs and systems. These changes are essential to help the woman to adapt to the pregnant state and to aid fetal growth and survival. However, such anatomical and physiological changes may cause confusion during clinical examination of a pregnant woman. Similarly, changes in blood biochemistry during pregnancy may create difficulties in interpretation of results. Conversely, clinicians also need to recognise pathological deviations in these normal anatomical and physiological changes during pregnancy to institute appropriate action to improve maternal and fetal outcome.

Haematology

Blood volume

There is an overall increase in plasma, red blood cell (RBC) and total blood volume. Plasma volume increases by 15% during the first trimester, accelerates in the second trimester, peaks at around 32 weeks reaching up to 50% above non-pregnant levels, and stays elevated until term. It returns to non-pregnant levels by 6 days post-delivery. There is often a sharp rise of up to 1 litre in plasma volume, within maternal circulation, 24 hours after delivery.

Red blood cell volume

RBC volume falls during the first 8 weeks of pregnancy, increasing back to non-pregnant levels by 16 weeks

and then rising to 30% above non-pregnant levels by term. The relatively smaller increase in RBC compared with plasma results in haemodilution and 'physiological anaemia' of pregnancy.

Coagulation and fibrinolysis in pregnancy

Plasma levels of factors VII, VIII, IX, XII, together with fibrinogen and fibrin degradation products, increase during pregnancy (fibrinogen from 2.5 to 4 g/l). Factor XI and III decrease. These changes overall increase coagulability and make pregnancy a 'hyper coagulable' state.

Platelets

Pregnancy is associated with enhanced platelet turnover. Thrombocytopenia (platelets $< 100 \times 10^9/l$) occurs in 0.8–0.9% of normal pregnant women, while increases in platelet factor and β thromboglobulin suggest elevated platelet activation and consumption. Since there is no change in platelet count in the majority of pregnant women, there is probably an increase in platelet production to compensate for the increased consumption.

Cardiovascular system

Heart

The heart is pushed upwards and rotated forwards, with lateral displacement of the left border. All heart sounds are louder and the first sound is split. A systolic ejection murmur is normal and is due to turbulence secondary to increased blood flow through normal heart valves. A diastolic murmur is heard occasionally. Cardiac output is increased as a result of increased

Obstetric and Intrapartum Emergencies, ed. Edwin Chandraharan and Sabaratnam Arulkumaran. Published by Cambridge University Press. © Cambridge University Press 2012.

heart rate, reduced systemic vascular resistance and increased stroke volume. Heart rate is increased above non-pregnant values by 15% at the end of the first trimester. This increases to 25% by the end of the second trimester, but there is no further change in the third trimester.

Stroke volume is increased by about 20% at 8 weeks and up to 30% by the end of the second trimester, then remains level until term.

Blood pressure

Systolic blood pressure does not show a significant drop in pregnancy. It may drop slightly by 6–8%. However, there is a marked drop in diastolic pressure. It is reduced in the first two trimesters by up to 20–25% and returns to the non-pregnant level at term. This is due to the placenta acting as an arteriovenous shunt, together with peripheral vasodilating factors such as oestrogen, progesterone and increased endothelial synthesis of prostaglandin E2 and prostacyclins. Both blood pressure and cardiac output are reduced during epidural analgesia. In a supine position, 70% of mothers have a fall in blood pressure of at least 10%, and 8% have decreases between 30 and 50%.

ECG changes during pregnancy

These changes are of no clinical significance:

- Sinus tachycardia, atrial and ventricular ectopics.
- Rotation of the electrical axis of the heart to the left.
- ST segment depression and T-wave inversion in inferior and lateral leads.

Changes in echocardiograph during pregnancy:

- Left ventricular hypertrophy by 12 weeks.
- 50% increase in left ventricular mass at term.
- 12–14% increase in aortic, pulmonary and mitral valve sizes.

Respiratory system

Anatomical changes

Capillary engorgement of the nasal and pharyngeal mucosa and larynx begins early in the first trimester. This may explain why many pregnant women complain of difficulty in nasal breathing, experience more episodes of epistaxis and experience voice changes. The thoracic cage increases in circumference by 5–7 cm because of the increase in both the anteroposterior and transverse diameters from flaring of the ribs. The level of the diaphragm rises by about 4 cm early in pregnancy even before it is under pressure from the enlarging uterus. This would account for the decrease in residual volume since the lungs would be relatively compressed at forced expiration.

Table 1.1 Normal arterial blood gas values in pregnancy.

pH	7.40–7.45
$PaCO_2$	3.7–4.2 kPa
PaO_2	13.0–14.0 kPa
HCO_3^-	18–21 mmol/l

Physiology

During pregnancy minute ventilation increases by about 40% from 7.5 to 10.5 l/min and oxygen consumption increases by about 18% from 250 to 300 ml/min. Tidal volume increases gradually from the first trimester by up to 45% at term. Functional residual capacity is decreased by 20–30% at term due to reductions of 25% in expiratory reserve volume and 15% in residual volume.

Blood gases

$PaCO_2$ decreases to 3.7–4.2 kPa by the end of the first trimester and remains at this level until term. Metabolic compensation for the respiratory alkalosis reduces the serum bicarbonate concentration to about 18–21 mmol/l, the base excess by 2–3 mmol/l and the total buffer base by about 5 mmol/l. PaO_2 in upright pregnant women is in the region of 14.0 kPa, higher than that in non-pregnant women. This is due to lower $PaCO_2$ levels, a reduced arterio-venous oxygen difference and a reduction in physiological shunt. Pregnant women maintain a normal arterial pH of 7.4 to 7.45 (Table 1.1).

Renal system

Kidney size increases by about 1 cm in length. There is marked dilatation of renal calyces, pelvis and ureters. Increase in glomerular filtration rate (GFR) by about 50% reaches maximum at the end of first trimester and is maintained at this augmented level until at least the 36th gestational week. 24-hour creatinine clearance increases by 25% at 4 weeks after the last menstrual period and by 45% at 9 weeks. During the third trimester a consistent and significant decrease towards non-pregnant values occurs preceding delivery.

Gastrointestinal system

Gums may swell and bleed easily. Incidence of caries is increased. Barrier pressure (lower oesophageal sphincter (LOS) pressure minus gastric pressure) is reduced significantly during pregnancy compared with the non-pregnant state, due to increased intragastric pressure and reduced LOS pressure. LOS pressure appears to return to normal by 48 hours post delivery.

Endocrine system

Glucose metabolism

Pregnancy is associated with an insulin-resistant condition, similar to that of type II diabetes. Early in pregnancy, increasing oestrogen and progesterone levels, which lead to pancreatic β-cell hypertrophy and insulin excretion, alter maternal carbohydrate metabolism. Secretion of other hormones such as human placental lactogen, prolactin, cortisol, oestrogen and progesterone induce insulin resistance. These hormones are found to be in significantly greater levels in pregnant women.

Thyroid

There is increased synthesis of thyroxine binding globulin (TBG) by the liver in pregnancy. This increase leads to a compensatory rise in serum concentrations of total T4 and T3. There is, however, no change in the amount of free circulating thyroid hormones. There is iodine deficiency as a result of loss through increased glomerular filtration and decreased renal tubular absorption. Active transport of iodine to the fetoplacental unit and fetal thyroid activity also deplete the maternal iodide pool further from the second trimester.

Pituitary

There is significant enlargement of the pituitary gland during pregnancy. The growth is as a result of increase in the number of prolactin-secreting cells, with the proportion of lactotrophs increasing from 1% to 40%. This results in elevated prolactin levels to up to 10–20 times those of normal, non-pregnant values. These return to normal by 2 weeks postpartum, unless the woman breastfeeds. Gonadotrophin levels are suppressed by the high concentrations of oestrogen and progesterone, and are undetectable during pregnancy. Levels of basal growth hormone and antidiuretic hormone remain unchanged during pregnancy.

Adrenal

Plasma CBG (corticosteroid binding globulin) concentrations increase during pregnancy. Levels of both free and bound cortisol also increase and levels of serum and urinary free cortisol increase three-fold by term.

Adrenocorticotropic hormone (ACTH), which influences steroid secretion from adrenal cortex, remains within the normal range for non-pregnant women.

Skin

During pregnancy the skin undergoes a number of changes, mainly thought to be due to hormonal changes.

Pigmentation – Hyperpigmentation occurs in up to 90% of women during pregnancy. This begins in the first trimester and is prominently noticed in areas of normal hyperpigmentation such as nipples, areola, perineum and vulva. Both oestrogens and progesterone, which have melanogenic stimulant properties, are thought to be responsible for this hyperpigmentation.

Linea nigra – This appears as an area of pigmentation extending from symphysis pubis to xiphisternum. Although the pigmentation fades after delivery it rarely returns to pre-pregnancy levels.

Melasma – Develops in up to 70% of women, mainly in the second half of pregnancy. It appears as patches of light-brown facial pigmentation usually over the forehead, cheeks, upper lip, nose and chin.

Spider naevi – These present as a central red spot and reddish extensions which radiate outwards like a spider's web and occur on the face, the trunk and arms. Most appear in early pregnancy and regress following delivery, although in up to 25% of women they may persist. Recurrences are known to occur at the same site in subsequent pregnancies.

Striae gravidarum – They appear perpendicular to skin tension lines as pink linear wrinkles. They fade

Table 1.2 Pregnancy specific ranges for serum biochemistry.

Biochemistry	Pregnancy specific ranges
Full blood count	
Hb	10.5–14.0 g/dl
White blood cell count	5–11.0 g/dl
Platelets	$100–450 \times 10^9$/l
Liver function	
Alkaline phosphatase	< 500 IU/l
Alanine transaminase	< 30 IU/l
Aspartate transaminase	< 35 IU/l
Albumin	28–37 g/l
Bilirubin	3–14 micromol/l
Renal function	
Urea	2.8–3.8 mmol/l
Creatinine	50–80 micromol/l
Uric acid	0.14–0.2/0.35 micromol/l
Na	135–145 mmol/l
K	3.5–4.5 mmol/l
Protein excretion	< 0.3/24 hours
Thyroid function	
Free T4	11–22 pmol/l
Free T3	43–45 pmol/l
TSH	0–4 mu/l

and become white and atrophic, although never disappear completely.

Palmar erythema – Palmar erythema is reddening of the palms at the thenar and hypothenar eminences. This is thought to be due to high levels of oestrogen in pregnancy and is seen in up to 70% of women by the third trimester and fade within 1 week of delivery.

Key changes in pregnancy

Normal anatomical, physiological and biochemical changes and their key implications during pregnancy are given in Tables 1.2, 1.3 and 1.4.

Optimising clinical practice

Liver and gall bladder

Changes in bile acid composition can influence the likelihood of the occurrence of cholelithiasis. An increase in the bile acid pool, a decreased proportion of chenodeoxycholic acid, and an increased proportion of cholic acid are findings that cause increased lithogenicity of bile in pregnancy. Decreases in gall bladder emptying can also promote biliary stasis and thus predispose pregnant women to biliary disease.

Endocrine system

Thyroid – Physiological changes (see above) result in increased uptake of iodine from blood three-fold by the thyroid gland. In women with dietary insufficiency of iodine, the thyroid gland hypertrophies in order to trap a sufficient amount of iodine, which can result in enlargement and the appearance of goitre. Biochemical assessment of thyroid function in pregnancy should include assays of free T4 and in some cases, free T3. Management decisions should be principally based on these levels. Immunoradiometric assays of TSH are useful but should not be used in isolation because of the variable effects of gestation. As there is more conversion of T4 to T3, low levels of T4 are not necessarily indicative of hypothyroidism.

Haemorrhage

Due to the increase in circulating blood volume, compared with a non-pregnant woman, a pregnant woman could lose up to 1200–1500 ml of blood (35% of blood volume) before showing signs of shock. There could be a significant delay in the development of symptoms and signs of hypovolaemia in a pregnant woman. Therefore, efforts should be made to estimate postpartum blood loss and prompt treatment instituted to avoid the consequences of massive postpartum haemorrhage.

Asthma

Decreasing or stopping inhaled anti-asthmatic therapy during pregnancy is a frequent cause of potentially dangerous deterioration in disease control. Poorly controlled severe asthma presents more of a risk to the pregnancy than the medication used to prevent or treat it.

Epilepsy

The additional demand for folate during pregnancy leads to a rapid fall in red cell folate and to a high incidence of megaloblastic anaemia in those women taking anticonvulsant drugs for control of epilepsy. Folate supplements should be given to all epileptic women taking anticonvulsants in pregnancy as well as before conception.

Constipation

Sluggish bowel movement during pregnancy can lead to severe or chronic abdominal pain. The

Table 1.3 Anatomical and physiological changes during pregnancy.

Parameters		< 12 weeks	13–28 weeks	29 weeks
Haematological parameters	Plasma volume	↑10–15%	Further rise (gradual)	↑50%
	Red cell volume	Falls	Reaches 'non-pregnant' levels	↑30%
	Total blood volume	↑10%	↑30%	↑45%
	Platelet count	→/↓	→/↓	↓0–5%
	Haemoglobin	↓	↓	↓15%
	WBC/ ESR	→/↑	→/↑	↑
	Factors V, VII, VIII, IX, XII, fibrinogen, vWF	→/↑	→/↑	↑
	Prothrombin III, protein C, protein S, plasminogen activator inhibitor	→/↓	→/↓	↓
Cardiovascular physiology	Heart rate	↑15%	↑30%	↑30%
	Stroke volume	↑20%	↑30%	↑30%
	Cardiac output	↑30–40%	↑30–50%	Remains over 50%
	Systolic and diastolic blood pressure	↓	→/↓	Non-pregnant value
Respiratory changes	Tidal volume	↑	↑	↑45
	FRC			↓20–30%
	IRV			↑5%
	ERV			↓25%
	TLC			↓0–5%
Renal system	GFR	↑50%		Declines gradually
	Creatinine clearance	↑45%		Steady↓ towards non-pregnant values
	Glycosuria			↑
	Proteinuria			↑
Gastrointestinal	LOS pressure	↓	↓	↓
	Gastric acid secretion			↓
	Gastric emptying			↓
	Heartburn			↑

Abbreviations: WBC, white blood cell count; ESR, erythrocyte sedimentation rate; FRC, functional residual capacity; IRV, inspiratory reserve volume; ERV, expiratory reserve volume; TLC, total lung capacity; GFR, glomerular filtration rate; LOS, lower oesophageal sphincter.

presentation is widely varied. The most common is a dull, constant and sometimes colicky pain in the iliac fossae (the left more than the right). Care should be taken in prescribing laxatives as medications resulting in significant increase in bowel activity may induce preterm labour.

Appendicitis

Pregnant women may lack classic symptoms and signs of appendicitis due to the anatomical and physiological changes that take place during pregnancy. As a result of this, the diagnosis may be delayed, particularly in the third trimester. The location of pain may vary depending on the gestation at the time of presentation e.g. pain may be located in the right lumbar region in early gestation or even in the right hypochondrium in late gestation. This may be due to displacement of the caecum and therefore the appendix by the gravid uterus. In early pregnancy, the pain starts in the paraumbilical region and then settles in the right iliac fossa. Both delayed intervention with perforation and unnecessary intervention increase mortality and morbidity for both the fetus and the mother. The timing of intervention varies by trimester: 90% of patients in the first trimester usually undergo an operation within 24 hours of the onset of symptoms, whereas in the third trimester 64% of patients will have symptoms for more than 48 hours before

Table 1.4 Summary of key changes in pregnancy and their clinical implications.

	Physiological effects	Key clinical implications
Haematology	Hypercoagulable state Haemodilution of pregnancy	Predisposition for venous thromboembolism. Clots usually develop in the left leg or the left iliac venous system. The left side is most affected because the right iliac artery crosses the left iliac vein. The increased flow in the right iliac artery after birth compresses the left iliac vein leading to an increased risk for thrombosis (clotting) which is exacerbated if there is lack of ambulation following delivery The ↑ blood volume and the ↑ level of coagulation factors including fibrinogen and factors VII, VIII and X provide physiological protection against haemorrhage
Cardiovascular system	Gravid uterus pressing over inferior vena cava Increased heart rate and stroke volume and cardiac output Reduced peripheral resistance	Aorto-caval compression – supine hypotension. In supine position, the vena cava is completely occluded in 90% of women and the stroke volume may be only 30% that of a non-pregnant woman During cardiac arrest, in order to minimise the effects of the gravid uterus on venous return and cardiac output a maternal pelvic tilt to the left of greater than 15° is recommended. The tilt needs to be less than 30° for effective closed-chest compression to take place Women with heart disease and fixed cardiac output may not cope with the demands and may develop pulmonary oedema Fall in diastolic blood pressure
Respiratory system	Oestrogen-induced oedema, hyperaemia and hypersecretion Minute ventilation increases in pregnancy because of increased tidal volume. 20% decrease in the functional residual capacity due to the pressure from the gravid uterus on the diaphragm and the lungs. This is exacerbated by 20% increase in their resting oxygen demand	New-onset rhinitis, laryngeal oedema, hypertrophy of breasts → difficulty intubating pregnant women Dyspnoea is experienced by up to 50% of pregnant women by 20 weeks and by 75% by 30 weeks. Relative state of hyperventilation causes a fall in $PaCO_2$ which results in chronic respiratory alkalosis. Mothers become hypoxic more readily
Gastrointestinal system	Reduced lower oesophageal pressure, high intragastric pressure, delayed gastric emptying time Reduced colonic motility Course of IBD is not usually affected by pregnancy. Risk of flare is reduced if colitis is quiescent at the time of conception. Crohn's disease may experience postpartum flare	Reflux oesophagitis; heartburn; constipation; risk of aspiration during general anaesthetic. In patients at term undergoing elective caesarean section, 49% are at risk of acid aspiration. Approximately 50% of women in labour have gastric pH < 2.5 Constipation is commonly seen in pregnancy May prolong drug transit time. Prolonged contact time with the intestinal surface may result in a more complete absorption of drugs. If a drug is metabolised in the gut wall, less of the parent drug may reach the systemic circulation and therefore bioavailability will be reduced. Narcotic analgesics used in labour may further prolong gastric emptying and may result in accumulation of repeated medications leading to higher than desired levels Women with IBD should be encouraged to conceive during periods of disease remission. Caesarean section may be indicated in the presence of severe peri-anal Crohn's disease. Active peri-anal Crohn's may prevent healing of an episiotomy
Renal system	Retroverted gravid uterus pressing on the urethra-vesical junction Dextro-rotation of uterus, pressure from gravid uterus; dilatation of ureters	Acute retention of urine in early pregnancy Small ureteric stones may be passed easily. Increased risk of pyelonephritis and difficulty in interpretation of radiological studies of the urinary collecting system of pregnant women Treatment of asymptomatic bacteriuria reduces the incidence of pyelonephritis
Endocrine system	Increased secretion of anti-insulin hormones – HPL, glucagon and cortisol by placenta Physiological changes in pregnancy can significantly affect preexisting diabetes	Glucose tolerance decreases progressively with increasing gestation → increased insulin requirements in established diabetics and development of abnormal glucose tolerance in gestation diabetics, in whom there is insufficient insulin secretion to compensate for the insulin resistance Exacerbation of complications of diabetes such as nephropathy and retinopathy
Skin	Hyperpigmentation	Spider naevi, palmar erythema are normally seen in pregnancy

Abbreviations: IBD, inflammatory bowel disease; HPL, human placental lactogen.

undergoing an operation. This delay may increase perforation and abscess formation [1]. Perforation, the rate of which has been reported to be approximately 25–40% during pregnancy, increases the rates of spontaneous abortion, preterm labour, perinatal morbidity and mortality [2]. The non-obstetric differential diagnoses include ovarian cyst accidents, degenerating fibroid, acute cholecystitis, pyelonephritis, ureteric calculi and bowel obstruction. For appendicectomy the type of incision will depend on the gestation and the location of the appendix. In the first trimester, appendicectomy may be performed laparoscopically or through a classical McBurney's incision. However, a paramedian incision over the area of maximum tenderness may allow the best access and the option of extension should the need arise.

Glycosuria

As a result of increased GFR there is an increase in the amount of glucose delivered to the kidneys. Associated with this is a reduction in the renal threshold for glucose. During pregnancy about a third of women excrete more than 5.5 mmol of glucose in 24 hours (renal glycosuria) which is significantly higher than that excreted by non-pregnant women (up to 0.55 mmol/24 hours). Since most commonly available commercial glucose oxidase/peroxide paper strips have a sensitivity of approximately 5.5 mmol/l, they will identify glycosuria in between 5 and 50% of the pregnant population, depending on the timing and frequency of testing. The routine use of urinalysis for monitoring of glycaemic control during pregnancy is therefore unreliable.

Thyroid function tests

In general, thyroid-stimulating hormone (TSH) is useful in screening for thyroid disease. However, it can be misleading when used alone in individuals being monitored for known thyroid disease, women in the first trimester, those with hyperemesis gravidarum or in molar pregnancy. This is mainly due to HCG levels, which show thyrotropic (TSH-like) activity. In these situations free T3 or T4 should be obtained.

Skin changes

Certain changes occur in normal pregnancy that would otherwise suggest liver disease. Physical findings include spider angiomata and palmar erythema, probably due to elevated oestrogen levels.

Key pitfalls

- Interpretation of blood results may be difficult due to physiological haemodilution and changes in plasma proteins.
- Most standard liver function tests are normal in pregnancy; the fall in plasma albumin (dilutional effect) and rise in alkaline phosphatase do not reflect any liver disorder.
- Even in renal impairment, serum creatinine may be within 'normal range' due to haemodilution.

Key pearls

- Because of the anatomical and physiological changes that take place in pregnancy, it is important to interpret the investigations in the context of the changed values. Pregnancy specific reference ranges should be used in making clinical decisions.
- Women who have low levels of haemoglobin at the start of pregnancy should receive an iron supplement throughout pregnancy to compensate for the 'physiological anaemia' of pregnancy.
- Considerable problems are recognised in the accurate measurement of blood loss and a definition based on volume alone has some shortcomings. Both visual and measured loss can be highly inaccurate. Underestimation of blood loss may delay active steps being taken to prevent further bleeding.
- Pregnancy increases the risk of venous thromboembolism (VTE). Assessment of pregnant women for development of risk factors during the course of pregnancy and postpartum is crucial to take appropriate measures to prevent/minimise the risk of VTE. d-Dimer does not carry the same significance as it would in non-pregnant women.
- Symptoms and signs of various medical conditions may not follow the same clinical pattern as in non-pregnant women e.g. appendicitis [3, 4].
- Glucose – In pregnancy, the action of insulin is blunted; this unmasks latent diabetes and aggravates existing diabetes. The non-diabetic mother has slightly lower than normal blood glucose levels.
- Because of a fall in plasma albumin levels in pregnancy, drugs which are highly bound to

albumin may be found in reduced levels in the bound fraction, with a corresponding increase in the free drug concentration. It is important to consider these effects while prescribing certain drugs.

References

1. Andersen B, Nielsen TF. Appendicitis in pregnancy: diagnosis, management and complications. *Acta Obstet Gynecol Scand* 1999; 78: 758–762.

2. Yilmaz HG, Akgun Y, Bac B, Celik Y. Acute appendicitis in pregnancy – risk factors associated with principal outcomes: a case control study. *Int J Surg* 2007; 5: 192–197.

3. Chandraharan E, Arulkumaran S. Minor disorders in pregnancy. In Arulkumaran S (Ed.), *Essentials in Obstetrics*. New Delhi: Jaypee Brothers Medical Publishers, 2007.

4. Chandraharan E, Arulkumaran S. Acute abdomen and abdominal pain in pregnancy. *Obstet Gynaecol Reprod Med* 2008; 18: 205–212.

Chapter

2

Principles of resuscitation for maternal collapse

Renate Wendler

Key facts

- Definition: Maternal collapse is an acute life-threatening event where the mother becomes unconscious due to cardiorespiratory or neurological compromise at any stage in pregnancy or up to 6 weeks postpartum. The outcome for mother and fetus depends on effective resuscitation.
- Patients are most likely to survive if attended by providers skilled in basic and advanced life-support techniques. The mechanical and physiological changes of pregnancy can have an impact on a successful outcome and should be taken into account [1].
- In hospital, maternal collapse and sudden cardiac arrest are usually related to peripartum events [2]. Therefore staff on the delivery suite must be expertly trained in advanced life-support techniques and resuscitation equipment should be readily available.
- The incidence of maternal collapse and severe maternal morbidity is unknown. It is estimated that maternal cardiac arrest occurs in 1 in 30 000 deliveries. Despite a young age group, survival rates are poor.

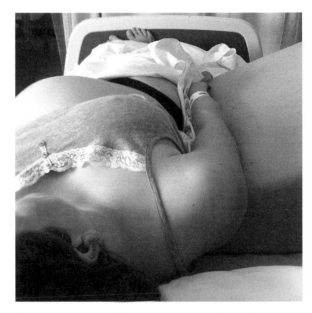

Figure 2.1 Patient in left lateral tilt position with Cardiff wedge.

performed with left lateral tilt of the pelvis greater than 15° to minimise aortocaval compression (see Figure 2.1). If the vena cava is partly occluded due to the pregnant uterus, cardiac output can be reduced by up to 40% [3]. This can in itself promote maternal collapse. During resuscitation, aortocaval compression further reduces cardiac output during chest compression [4].

Physiological changes in pregnancy affecting resuscitation

Aortocaval compression

Beyond 20 weeks' gestation (or in a noticeably pregnant patient) all resuscitation efforts must be

Changes in lung function/risk of hypoxia

Due to 20% reduced functional residual capacity of the lungs pregnant patients develop hypoxia much more rapidly [5]. Oxygen demand is increased in pregnancy making sufficient oxygen delivery difficult during resuscitation. This is further complicated by the increased weight of abdominal contents and breasts

Obstetric and Intrapartum Emergencies, ed. Edwin Chandraharan and Sabaratnam Arulkumaran. Published by Cambridge University Press. © Cambridge University Press 2012.

in late pregnancy, which can make effective rescue breaths difficult to perform.

Risk of aspiration

The risk of aspiration during resuscitation is increased due to a more relaxed lower oesophageal sphincter muscle and elevated gastric acid volume production [6]. Airway protection and effective ventilation via an endotracheal tube should be established as soon as possible. However, weight gain and laryngeal oedema can make intubation significantly more difficult and it should only be undertaken by experienced staff.

Perimortem caesarean section

The uteroplacental unit sequesters blood and hinders effective cardiopulmonary resuscitation (CPR). Case reports support the positive effect of evacuating the uterus on maternal outcome during CPR in later stages of pregnancy (beyond 20 weeks) [7]. Survival is inversely proportional to the time between maternal arrest and delivery. Current recommendations promote emergency caesarean delivery within 4 minutes of maternal collapse if no response to resuscitation efforts, to be completed within 5 minutes [8].

Key pointers – causes for maternal collapse

Whilst some underlying causes for maternal collapse are not preventable, it is important to note that maternal cardiac arrest occurs frequently due to deterioration of underlying critical illness. It is therefore important to introduce a maternal early-warning chart for the observation of all pregnant patients in a hospital setting, to detect critical illness at the earliest possible stage.

Haemorrhage

Worldwide, haemorrhage is still the leading cause of maternal mortality and it is the leading cause for maternal collapse on the delivery unit. Predisposing factors are multiple pregnancy, high parity, placenta praevia, uterine fibroids and multiple previous caesarean sections, prolonged labour, maternal clotting disorders and preeclampsia. It is important to memorise these risk factors as young pregnant women can lose a significant amount of blood without any

haemodynamic disturbance, therefore a high index of suspicion can be life saving. If haemodynamic changes become apparent, it can be estimated that the mother has already lost a third of her circulating blood volume.

Thromboembolism

A careful risk assessment for thrombotic complications should be performed in all pregnant patients. Multiple risk factors can make thromboprophylactic treatment necessary in pregnancy and postpartum [9]. Remember that deep vein thrombosis (DVT) of the pelvic venous system is often asymptomatic until pulmonary embolism develops.

Amniotic fluid embolism (AFE)

The incidence of AFE is estimated at 1.25–12.5 in 100 000 maternities. Whilst this is an unpreventable event, the speed of diagnosis determines the outcome. There is no diagnostic test to determine AFE; therefore the clinical picture should lead to a high index of suspicion. Clinical features include respiratory distress, followed by cardiovascular collapse with cardiogenic shock, frequently in combination with haemorrhage due to coagulopathy. AFE can also lead to fetal collapse of unknown origin that precedes maternal collapse. In all cases there is absence of any other significant medical condition or explanation for the rapid deterioration.

Maternal cardiac disease

Due to changes in lifestyle (later age of conception) and overall maternal health (obesity, diabetes and smoking, preexisting congenital heart disease), cardiac disease in pregnancy is increasingly common. In cases of known maternal cardiac disease a multidisciplinary approach is essential to predict complications and define antenatal and peripartum care. However, the majority of deaths secondary to cardiac disease occur with no previous cardiac history [10]. The risk of myocardial infarction is increased three- to four-fold in pregnancy (compared with a non-pregnant population) and is significantly greater in women beyond 36 years of age or black ethnicity. In addition, there is a greater risk of coronary artery or aortic dissection in pregnancy. It is important to remember that pregnant patients with cardiac disease frequently present with atypical symptoms.

Sepsis

Morbidity and mortality from pregnancy-related sepsis is common and has not significantly declined in recent years. Obstetric risk factors include prolonged rupture of membranes, cervical cerclage, retained placenta and operative trauma. Patient-related risk factors are obesity, anaemia, diabetes mellitus, sickle cell disease and group B streptococcus infection. Adequate antibiotic prophylaxis for patients at risk is crucial. Common clinical signs are temperature, tachycardia and anxiety. Special attention should be paid to changes in the respiratory rate as a first diagnostic sign as a physiological reaction to developing metabolic acidosis with sepsis.

Complications of labour analgesia

Even in a correctly sited epidural catheter a regular top-up can cause maternal collapse due to hypotension, therefore close blood pressure observation is required after every administration of local anaesthetic. More serious complications of epidural labour analgesia are high block (inadvertent spinal injection of an epidural top-up dose) and unintended intravascular injection of a large dose of local anaesthetic, both due to catheter misplacement. These are rare but serious complications that require advanced life support by a provider experienced in obstetric anaesthesia.

Drug toxicity

Drug overdose should be considered as a potential diagnosis in out-of-hospital cardiac arrest. In patients with preeclampsia and renal failure on magnesium infusion, careful monitoring should focus on signs of magnesium overdose, which are muscle weakness, loss of tendon reflexes, respiratory depression and bradycardia/cardiac arrest.

Eclampsia/ intracranial haemorrhage

Warning signs can be severe headache, flashing lights, hyperreflexia and confusion. Uncontrolled hypertension can lead to intracranial haemorrhage. Typical clinical signs are severe, 'never-experienced' headache preceding maternal collapse.

Anaphylaxis

The overall incidence of anaphylaxis is between 3 and 10/1000 patients, with a mortality of 1%. Typical signs are sudden skin changes (rash, flushing) and swelling (mucosal oedema), cardiovascular collapse and/or severe respiratory symptoms (upper airway obstruction, bronchospasm), leading to life-threatening hypoxia. Diagnosis is established with serial levels of mast cell tryptase.

Key diagnostic signs

Look out for reversible causes in cases of maternal collapse or maternal cardiac arrest. Very often risk factors exist and clinical signs precede maternal collapse. Recent enquiries into maternal deaths emphasised the importance of maternal early-warning scores in early recognition of clinical deterioration that can lead to collapse [11].

Reversible causes for maternal cardiac arrest – 4 Hs and 4 Ts

- *Hypovolaemia* – Common cause of maternal collapse and/or cardiac arrest. Very common due to bleeding, this can be obvious or concealed. There can also be a relative hypovolaemia due to sepsis with shock, neurogenic shock or high spinal block.
- *Hypoxia* – Pregnant patients can easily become hypoxic; therefore it is vital to pay attention to signs of respiratory failure (tachypnoea, respiratory pattern) to secure a competent airway early if necessary.
- *Hyperkalaemia/metabolic disorders* – These are not more likely in pregnancy. Check for electrolyte imbalances as soon as possible.
- *Hypothermia* – Mainly a problem if out-of-hospital collapse. It is important to establish the temperature of patients with out-of-hospital cardiac arrest. Resuscitation efforts can only be stopped once a patient is rewarmed!
- *Thromboembolism* – Very common in pregnancy. Thrombolysis in pregnancy is possible and should be performed in life-threatening cases.
- *Toxicity* – Mainly due to pregnancy-specific drugs. Local anaesthetic overdoses due to inadvertent

intravascular injection are related to an epidural top-up and show typical symptoms of dizziness, metallic taste, seizures and loss of consciousness. Cases of arrhythmia and cardiac arrest should be treated with intralipid infusion during resuscitation efforts [12]. Intralipid should be available in all maternity units. Watch out for magnesium toxicity in preeclamptic patients with impaired renal function. Calcium 1 g acts as an antidote.

- *Tamponade* – Cardiac tamponade in pregnancy occurs in cases of type A aortic dissection or trauma.
- *Tension pneumothorax* – Most likely following trauma, but also possible after central venous line insertion.

Key actions

Resuscitation efforts in pregnant patients should follow the standardised A, B, C approach. Modification to this algorithm should occur to take into account physiological changes in pregnancy that can hinder successful resuscitation.

First-line manoeuvres: 'S & T; A, B, C'

S & T

Shout for help and ensure **safe** environment. **Tilt** the patient left lateral if visibly pregnant or beyond 20 weeks' gestation. Use a wedge or ask another person to manually displace the uterus during resuscitation (see Figure 2.2).

A

Assess and open **airway**. Turn patient onto back (keep left lateral tilt or manually displace uterus). Check for airway obstruction. Use head tilt and chin lift.

B

Assess **breathing** for up to 10 seconds. Look for chest movements, listen for breath sounds and feel for air shifting. If breathing normally, turn onto left side and regularly reassess breathing, heart rate and blood pressure until help arrives. If not breathing normally start cardiopulmonary resuscitation (CPR).

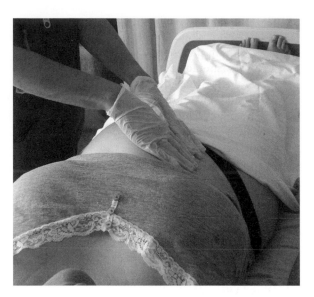

Figure 2.2 Manual uterus displacement to the left.

C

CPR – start immediately with 30 chest compressions, followed by two rescue breaths. Continue CPR with a ratio of 30 : 2 until signs of life or help arrives to provide advanced life support. Chest compressions should be performed slightly higher on the sternum than usual, as the maternal diaphragm is elevated in later stages of pregnancy. It is important to deliver efficient compressions with no interruption. In cases of CPR manual uterus displacement should be used if enough helpers are available, to maximise the effect of chest compressions, which can be less effective with a 15–30° tilt. Check that help is on the way.

Automated external defibrillator (AED)

Attach a defibrillator as soon as possible and assess the rhythm for no more than 10 seconds. If a shockable rhythm is detected, give 1 shock of 150–200 J biphasic and resume CPR immediately for a further 2 minutes. In cases where no shock is advisable continue CPR for further 2 minutes, followed by further assessment of the cardiac rhythm. There is a small risk for inducing fetal arrhythmias with defibrillation; however, external defibrillation is considered safe in all stages of pregnancy [13].

Advanced life support

With more help arriving, it is important to name a lead clinician for the management of the cardiac arrest. Documentation of all cases and contemporaneous note keeping should be allocated to a specific person. Underlying pathology and reversible causes for cardiac arrest should be treated accordingly.

As soon as advanced life support is available, the airway should be secured with an endotracheal tube. There is a higher incidence of failed intubation in pregnancy with significant maternal morbidity and mortality. Airway manoeuvres should therefore only be performed by an experienced operator and ideally capnography used to confirm correct tube placement. Intravenous access for drug administration should be obtained as early as possible above diaphragm level. Defibrillation and drug administration should follow standardised advanced life-support guidelines. As haemorrhage is the leading cause for maternal collapse and other underlying problems can lead to significant bleeding (AFE), blood products (red blood cells, fresh frozen plasma and platelets) should be made available at an early stage of the resuscitation.

Perimortem caesarean delivery

The gravid uterus acts as low-resistance high-volume unit that hinders venous return with reduced cardiac output. Delivery of fetus and placenta can reduce vena cava compression with improved venous return and increased effectiveness of CPR. In addition, chest compressions and ventilation will be easier and maternal oxygen demand is reduced. Survival of mother and fetus is inversely proportional to timing of delivery; however, perimortem caesarean delivery (PMCD) should be performed in the interest of maternal survival. If delivery is completed within 5 minutes of cardiac arrest, intact neurological outcome is most likely. Therefore, caesarean section should be performed after 4 minutes of maternal cardiac arrest in a patient beyond 20 weeks' gestation [8].

To perform PMCD the patient should not be transferred to an operating theatre, as this can waste valuable time. Bleeding is initially not expected, due to little or no circulation. Once haemodynamic stability is ensured, transfer to an appropriate environment should follow. In cases of successful resuscitation sedation and/or general anaesthetic for amnesia and pain relief should be instigated.

CPR must continue throughout the caesarean section and afterwards, as this can increase the chance of successful outcome for mother and fetus.

Key pitfalls

- Failure to anticipate and treat underlying critical illness in pregnancy and monitor accordingly on a maternal early-warning chart.
- Failure to recognise reversible causes for maternal cardiac arrest.
- Failure to adapt resuscitation techniques to maternal physiology.
- Failure to deliver adequate chest compression without interruption.
- Failure to apply left lateral tilt or manual uterus displacement.
- Failure to start perimortem caesarean delivery after 4 minutes of unsuccessful resuscitation.
- Failure to keep adequate records, including time keeping.

Key pearls

- All staff providing intrapartum care should undergo annual multidisciplinary skills and drills training on the management of maternal collapse and cardiac arrest.
- A dedicated protocol for the management of life-threatening maternal haemorrhage should be available on all maternity units.
- A cardiac arrest trolley and defibrillator, including wedge for left lateral tilt should be available on all maternity units and checked daily.
- Instrumentation for perimortem caesarean delivery should be available in all areas where maternal collapse may occur.
- All cases of maternal collapse and/or cardiac arrest should undergo review and debriefing for the staff involved. Good practice and substandard care should be highlighted to promote learning for all staff.

Management in low-resource settings

Key interventions to prevent maternal cardiac arrest should be immediate left lateral positioning or left lateral tilt to prevent vena cava compression syndrome. Compromised venous return and reduced cardiac output can precipitate cardiac arrest in critically ill pregnant patients. High-flow oxygen should be administered and venous access established, ideally above diaphragm level. Maternal hypotension (< 100 mmHg systolic or < 80% of baseline blood-pressure reading) should be treated with a fluid bolus of crystalloid or colloid infusion. Reversible causes of maternal collapse should be considered and treated as necessary.

At the onset of a cardiac arrest in a second- or third-trimester pregnant woman (if there is a visible pregnant uterus), basic life support should commence and if possible an automated external defibrillator (or other defibrillator) used as described above. Remember to restart CPR immediately after each shock for 2 minutes before checking for pulse. In addition a team for emergency caesarean section should be activated. The patient should not be moved into a theatre environment. A perimortem caesarean delivery can be performed with very little instrumentation (knife and forceps). Bleeding is usually not an issue due to poor peripheral circulation during cardiac arrest.

References

1. Belfort MA, Saade GA, Foley MR *et al*. *Critical Care Obstetrics*. Fifth edition. Oxford: Blackwell Publishing, 2010.

2. Dildy GA, Clark SL. Cardiac arrest during pregnancy. *Obstet Gynecol Clin North Am* 1995; 22: 303–314.

3. Chesnutt AN. Physiology of normal pregnancy. *Crit Care Clin* 2004; 20: 609–615.

4. Kerr MG. The mechanical effects of the gravid uterus in late pregnancy. *J Obstet Gynecol Br Commonw* 1965; 2: 513–529.

5. Prowse CM, Gaensler EA. Respiratory and acid-base changes during pregnancy. *Anesthesiology* 1965; 26: 381–392.

6. Mendelson CL. The aspiration of stomach contents onto the lungs during obstetric anaesthesia. *Am J Obstet Gynecol* 1946; 52: 191–205.

7. Katz V, Balderston K, DeFreest M. Perimortem cesarean delivery: were our assumptions correct? *Am J Obstet Gynecol* 2005; 192: 1916–1920.

8. Katz VL, Dotters DJ, Drogemueller W. Perimortem cesarean delivery. *Obstet Gynecol* 1986; 68: 571–576.

9. Royal College of Obstetricians and Gynaecologists. *Reducing the Risk of Thrombosis and Embolism during Pregnancy and the Puerperium*. Green-top guideline No. 37A. London: RCOG, 2009.

10. Malhotra S, Yentis SM. Reports on confidential enquiries into maternal deaths: management strategies based on trends in maternal cardiac deaths over 30 years. *Int J Obstet Anesth* 2006; 15: 223–226.

11. The Confidential Enquiry into Maternal and Child Health (CEMACH). *Saving Mothers' Lives: Reviewing Maternal Deaths to make Motherhood Safer – 2003–2005. The Seventh Report on Confidential Enquiries into Maternal Deaths in the United Kingdom*. London: CEMACH, 2007.

12. Weinberg GL, Palmer JW, Vade-Boncouer TR *et al*. Bupivacaine inhibits acylcarnitine exchange in cardiac mitochondria. *Anaesthesiology* 2000; 92: 5234–5238.

13. Vanden Hoek TL, Morrison LG, Shuster M *et al*. Cardiac arrest in special situations: 2010 American Heart Association guidelines for cardiopulmonary resuscitation and emergency cardiovascular care. *Circulation* 2010; 122: S821–S861.

Chapter

3

Deep vein thrombosis and pulmonary embolism

Tahir A. Mahmood and Adnan Hasan

Key facts

- Definition: Venous thromboembolism (VTE) is a condition in which a blood clot (thrombus) develops, commonly in the deep veins of the lower limbs, and this is called deep vein thrombosis (DVT). The majority of DVT in pregnancy are iliofemoral with a greater risk of both embolisation and recurrence. A thrombus may detach from its site of origin in the vein (embolus) and migrate through the blood stream to reach the lungs (pulmonary embolism (PE)). Venous thromboembolism has multiple contributory risk factors.

Classification:

- Distal or calf vein thrombosis.

   Acute DVT occurs in one of the three major paired veins, below the popliteal vein (posterior tibial, anterior tibial, peroneal) in the calf.

- Proximal venous thrombosis.

   Acute DVT in the popliteal vein or higher: superficial femoral or common femoral vein, iliac vein and vena cava.

- Upper extremity venous thrombosis.

   They are generally classified separately from classic DVT. They occur above the right atrium, most frequently in the subclavian, axillary or internal jugular veins.

- Incidence: 1–2/1000 pregnancies.

Key implications

Maternal

- Early identification of women at high risk of developing VTE during pregnancy, labour and postpartum.
- Pulmonary embolism has a case fatality rate of 1%.
- Recurrence of VTE during current pregnancy (1.15%) and in future pregnancies.
- Identification of women at increased risk of bleeding while on treatment with anticoagulants.
- Hospitalisation and access to high dependency unit (HDU) care secondary to low oxygen lung perfusion.
- Post-thrombotic syndrome including: leg pain, swelling, dermatitis, dependent cyanosis, ulcers and varicosities (risk 30–60%).

Complications related to long-term use of anticoagulants:

- Major postpartum haemorrhage (1.98%).
- Osteoporosis-related fractures (0.04%).
- Heparin-induced thrombocytopenia (HIT) which is substantially lower with low-molecular-weight heparin (LMWH).
- Allergic skin reaction (1.8%).

Radiological investigations/related complications:

- Increased life-time risk of breast cancer 13.6% (background risk of 1/200) with computerised tomography pulmonary angiography (CTPA).

Fetal

- V/Q scan carries an increased risk as compared to CTPA of childhood cancers to 1/280 000 (background risk of 1/1 000 000).

Obstetric and Intrapartum Emergencies, ed. Edwin Chandraharan and Sabaratnam Arulkumaran. Published by Cambridge University Press. © Cambridge University Press 2012.

- The radiation dose to the fetus from a chest X-ray performed during pregnancy is negligible.
- Hypothyroidism if iodinated contrast medium is used with CTPA.
- Fetal death: from the use of thrombolytic agents.

Medico-legal

- Clinical negligence claims due to delay in diagnosis and suboptimal treatment.
- Patient not appropriately counselled as regards long-term radiation risks to her and to the unborn baby.

Patient information

- Patients should be informed about all aspects of VTE including: seriousness of the disease process, risks related to each investigation and their implications. Counselling should include treatment benefits and risks. Every effort should be made to help women make informed choices about every aspect of their management where appropriate [1, 2].
- Patients who had a suspected DVT but negative US and on no treatment, should be advised that they should seek urgent advice and further assessment if they develop symptoms consistent with VTE such as: increased limb pains or swelling, sudden onset of breathlessness, chest or back pain, coughing or spitting up blood and any episode of collapse.
- Explain to the woman about the increased risk of VTE while using combined oral contraceptives/ hormone replacement treatment.

Key pointers

Magnitude of the problem

There is an approximately ten-fold increased risk during pregnancy compared with non-pregnant and 25-fold increased risk compared with non-pregnant/ non-puerperal during puerperium; and this risk is considerably increased among women with known thrombophilia. Pulmonary embolism has been the leading direct cause of maternal death in the UK (1.56/100 000 maternities) [3, 4].

Antenatal screening and thromboprophylaxis

The rationale for prophylaxis is based on its efficacy, the clinically silent nature of VTE, its prevalence in pregnant or puerperal patients and its potentially disabling or fatal consequences. Over 40% of antenatal VTE occur in the first trimester of pregnancy. The confidential enquiries into maternal deaths report in the UK found that two-thirds of antenatal fatal pulmonary embolism occurred in the first trimester [5]. Therefore every effort should be made to instigate antenatal thromboprophylaxis in the first trimester of pregnancy. Antenatal risk assessment should start at the time of first booking visit to the hospital. Women with multiple risk factors (three or more), those with a previous unprovoked VTE, previous recurrent VTE, and those with multiple thrombophilia defects should be offered thromboprophylaxis with LMWH antenatally [6].

Furthermore, women with a history of recurrent VTE who are on warfarin should be switched over to LMWH as soon as pregnancy is confirmed.

All known identifiable risk factors for VTE have been grouped together in Algorithm 1 so that women at booking visit can be classified at high, intermediate or low risk for VTE and managed accordingly. Each woman's risks need to be continually reviewed throughout pregnancy and during the intrapartum period. A note should also be made of conditions that can increase complications following thromboprophylaxis.

Key diagnostic signs

- Unilateral painful swelling and tenderness in one of the lower limbs (calf swelling > 3 cm as compared with other calf, measured 10 cm below tibial tuberosity).
- Chest pain, breathlessness, tachypnoea, tachycardia and haemoptysis.
- Low back or lower abdominal pain, low-grade fever.
- Haemodynamic instability (right ventricular strain or hypotension) and collapse.

Key assessment and actions

- Baseline investigation: full blood count (platelets), coagulation screen, liver and renal function tests.

Suggested algorithm (1) for risk identification and treatment of venous thromboembolism

Antenatal risk assessment for venous thromboembolism (VTE) – adjusted odds ratio (AOR) where available

High risk	Intermediate risk	Low risk
Single previous VTE (AOR: 24)	Single previous VTE with no family history or thrombophilia	Age > 35 years
• Thrombophilia or family history	Thrombophilia + but no VTE	Obesity (BMI > 30 kg/m^2) – 2- to 5-fold increase
• Unprovoked/oestrogen-related		Parity ≥ 3 (AOR: 3.4)
Previous recurrent VTE (> 1)	Medical comorbidities, e.g. heart or lung disease, systemic lupus erythematosus (ORA: 8.7), inflammatory conditions, nephrotic syndrome, sickle cell disease (2.5, 6.7), chronic HIV, intravenous drug user	Smoker (10–30/day): (AOR 1.4, 3.4)
		Gross varicose veins (AOR: 2.7), current systemic infection
		Heterozygous factor V
		Leiden and prothrombin G20210 A without prior Hx of VTE (risk < 1%)
	Surgical procedure, e.g. appendicectomy	Immobility, e.g. paraplegia, symphysis pubis dysfunction with immobility, long-distance travel, dehydration/hyperemesis
		Preeclampsia (AOR: 2.9, 3.1)
		Ovarian hyperstimulation syndrome (OHSS)
		Multiple pregnancy/Assisted reproductive treatment
Requires antenatal prophylaxis with LMWH	Consider antenatal prophylaxis with LMWH Seek expert team advice	Mobilisation and avoidance of dehydration: three or more risk factors, treat as intermediate

Additional intrapartum risk factors

Preeclampsia (AOR: 2.9, 3.1)
Dehydration/hyperemesis/OHSS (AOR: 2.5)
Multiple pregnancy or assisted reproduction (ART) (AOR: 4.3)
Caesarean section in labour (AOR: 2.7, 3.6)
Elective caesarean section (AOR: 2.1)
Mid-cavity or rotational forceps
Prolonged labour (> 24 hours)
PPH (> 1 litre or transfusion) (AOR: 4.1)

Transient risk factors

Postpartum infection (AOR: 4.1)
Immobility (AOR: 7.7)
Surgical procedure in pregnancy + haemorrhage or ≤ 6 weeks postpartum (AOR: 6.2, 12)
Obstetric haemorrhage (AOR: 9); transfusion (AOR: 7.6)

Antenatal and postnatal prophylactic dose of LMWH

Weight < 50 kg = 20 mg enoxaparin/2500 units dalteparin/3500 units tinzaparin daily
Weight 50–90 kg = 40 mg enoxaparin/5000 units dalteparin/4500 units tinzaparin daily
Weight 91–130 kg = 60 mg enoxaparin/7500 units dalteparin/7000 units tinzaparin daily
Weight 131–170 kg = 80 mg enoxaparin/10000 units dalteparin/9000 units tinzaparin daily
Weight > 170 kg = 0.6 mg/kg/day enoxaparin; 75 units/kg/day dalteparin/75 units/kg/day tinzaparin

Identification of women at increased bleeding risk when on anticoagulation treatment

Haemophilia or other known bleeding disorder (e.g. von Willebrand's disease or acquired coagulopathy)
Active antenatal or postpartum bleeding
Women considered at increased risk of major haemorrhage (e.g. placenta praevia)
Thrombocytopenia (platelet count < 75 × 10^9)
Acute stroke in previous 4 weeks (haemorrhagic or ischaemic)
Severe renal disease (glomerular filtration rate < 30 ml/minute/1.73 m^2)
Severe liver disease (prothrombin time above normal range or known varices)
Uncontrolled hypertension (blood pressure > 200 mmHg systolic or > 120 mmHg diastolic)

- Commence treatment with LMWH if no contraindication exists, until the diagnosis is excluded by objective testing.
- Baseline platelet count in order to monitor development of heparin-induced thrombocytopenia (HIT).
- Poor renal function is a risk factor for bleeding.
- Routine thrombophilia screening prior to start of treatment is not recommended.

- A positive d-dimer test is not necessarily consistent with VTE.

Confirmation of clinically suspected DVT

Compression duplex ultrasound is the preferred initial imaging test in pregnancy as this test has a high sensitivity (94–99%) and specificity (89–96%) when compared with contrast venography.

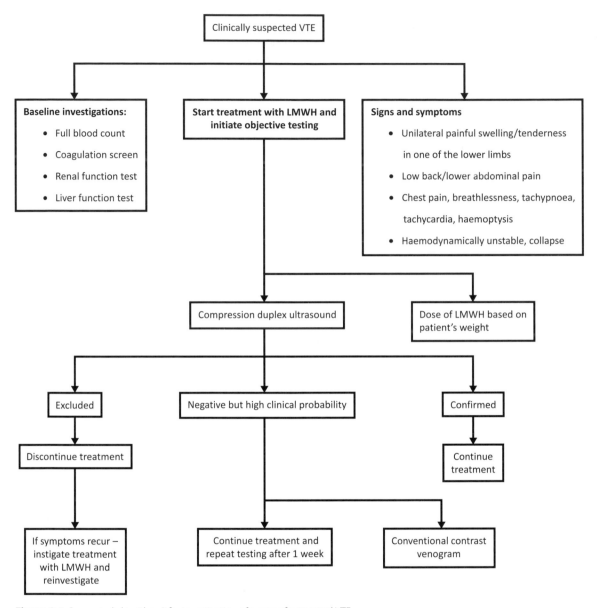

Figure 3.1 Suggested algorithm 2 for investigation of a case of suspected VTE.

If ultrasound is negative and there is a high level of clinical suspicion, treatment with anticoagulant should be continued (Figure 3.1). A repeat ultrasound examination or conventional venography should be carried out after 1 week.

If ultrasound is negative and there is a low level of clinical suspicion, anticoagulant treatment can be discontinued. However, women should be advised that if similar symptoms recur, they should report back to the hospital.

Treatment of acute-phase VTE

(1) In clinically suspected VTE (DVT or PTE), treatment with LMWH should be given until the

Table 3.1 Calculation of initial doses of drugs by early pregnancy weight to be used for acute phase venous thromboembolism (VTE).

	Early pregnancy weight (kg)			
Initial dose	< 50	50–69	70–89	90
Enoxaparin	40 mg bd	60 mg bd	80 mg bd	100 mg bd
Dalteparin	5000 IU bd	6000 IU bd	8000 IU bd	10 000 IU bd
Tinzaparin	175 units/kg once daily (all weights)			

bd, twice daily.

Table 3.2 Infusion rates according to activated partial thromboplastin time (APTT).

APTT ratio	Dose change	Additional action	Next APTT (hours)	(units/kg/ hour)
< 1.2	+ 4	Re-bolus	80 units/kg	6
1.2–1.5	+ 2	Re-bolus	40 units/kg	6
1.5–2.5		No change		24
2.5–3.0	– 2			6
> 3.0	– 3	Stop infusion	1 hour	6

diagnosis is excluded by objective testing, unless treatment is strongly contraindicated.

(2) For women with suspected DVT, the leg should be elevated and a graduated elastic compression stocking applied to reduce oedema and mobilisation should be encouraged.

(3) LMWH can be either given once daily or in two divided doses subcutaneously with dosage calculated according to the woman's most recent weight (Table 3.1).

(4) Once the woman's condition is stable, she can then be managed on an outpatient basis and followed up in a combined multidisciplinary clinic.

Confirmation of clinically suspected pulmonary embolism

- Chest X-ray should be performed (Figure 3.2). It is usually normal in > 50% of proven PTE but it may detect other lung pathology.
- If chest X-ray is normal, then bilateral compression duplex Doppler should be performed. If DVT is confirmed then treatment with LMWH is continued without further investigations.
- If the above two tests are negative and there is a persistent clinical suspicion of acute PTE, then a ventilation–perfusion (V/Q) lung scan (omitting the ventilation component) should be performed.
- If X-ray of chest is abnormal or if massive PTE is suspected, computerised tomography pulmonary angiography (CTPA) is the gold-standard investigation and has a high sensitivity (83–100%) and specificity (89–97%); CTPA/echocardiogram

should be arranged within 1 hour of admission when the woman is haemodynamically unstable. Assessment of right ventricular/left ventricular ratio as seen on CTPA is a useful indicator of severity of PE in the acute situation.

- For women where V/Q scan or CTPA and duplex Doppler are normal but the clinical suspicion of PTE is high, anticoagulant treatment should be continued until PTE is definitively excluded by repeating investigations a week later.

Routine measurement of peak anti-Xa activity for patients on LMWH for treatment of acute VTE in pregnancy or postpartum is not recommended except in women at extremes of body weight (less than 50 kg and 90 kg or more) or with other complicating factors (for example with renal impairment, GFR < 30%, or recurrent VTE).

Routine platelet count monitoring should not be carried out (unless unfractionated heparin has been given).

LMWH are considered to be associated with a lower risk of haemorrhagic complications and lower mortality than unfractionated heparin in the initial management of DVT. However there is equivalent efficacy of LMWH to unfractionated heparin in the initial treatment of PTE.

Treatment for massive PTE

- The woman should be admitted to the intensive care unit or high dependency unit.
- Intravenous unfractionated heparin is the preferred treatment in massive PTE with cardiovascular compromise (Table 3.2).
- Collapsed, shocked patients should be assessed by a team of experienced clinicians, including the on-call consultant obstetrician, to decide on an

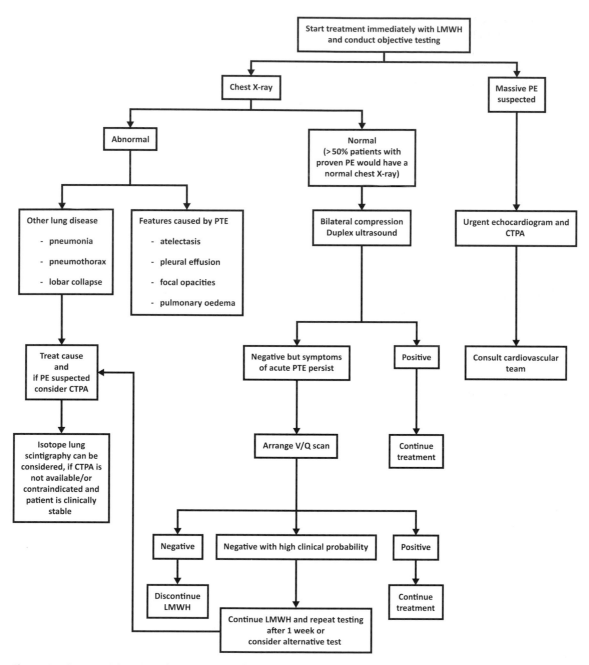

Figure 3.2 Suggested algorithm 3 for investigation of a case of suspected PTE.

individual basis whether a woman receives intravenous unfractionated heparin, thrombolytic therapy or thoracotomy and surgical embolectomy.

A recommended regimen for the administration of intravenous, unfractionated heparin:

- A loading dose of 80 units/kg, followed by a continuous intravenous infusion of 18 units/kg/hour can be started.
- If a woman has also received thrombolysis (Table 3.2), then the loading dose of heparin should be omitted and an infusion started at 18 units/kg/hour.

Activated partial thromboplastin time (APTT) should be measured 4–6 hours after the loading dose, and 6 hours after any dose change and then at least daily when in the therapeutic range. The therapeutic target APTT ratio is usually 1.5–2.5 times the average laboratory control value.

- The infusion rate should be adjusted according to the APTT using this weight-adjusted regimen, as shown in Table 3.2.

Women receiving therapeutic-dose unfractionated heparin should have their platelet count monitored at least every other day until day 14 or until the unfractionated heparin is stopped, whichever occurs first.

Use of inferior vena cava (IVC) shunt

Consideration should be given to the use of a temporary inferior vena cava filter in the perinatal period for women with iliac vein VTE, to reduce the risk of PTE or in women with proven DVT and who have continuing PTE despite adequate anticoagulation. However IVC filters are associated with an increase in the development of recurrent DVT.

Maintenance treatment of VTE

Treatment with therapeutic doses of subcutaneous LMWH should be employed during the remainder of the pregnancy.

Pregnant women who develop heparin-induced thrombocytopenia or have heparin allergy and require continuing anticoagulant therapy should be managed with heparinoid, danaparoid sodium or fondaparinux, under specialist advice.

Anticoagulant therapy during labour and delivery

The woman should stop treatment, once there are signs suggestive of onset of labour.

LMWH maintenance therapy should be discontinued 24 hours before planned delivery.

Regional anaesthetic or analgesic techniques should not be undertaken until at least 24 hours after the last dose of therapeutic LMWH.

A thromboprophylactic dose of LMWH should be given by 3 hours after a caesarean section (more than

4 hours after removal of the epidural catheter, if appropriate).

The epidural catheter should not be removed within 12 hours of the most recent injection.

Women delivered by caesarean section and on therapeutic doses of LMWH should have wound drains in the abdominal cavity and rectus sheath. The skin incision should be closed with staples or interrupted sutures to allow drainage of any haematoma.

Postnatal anticoagulation

- All women should be individually assessed on the delivery suite for postnatal thromboprophylaxis (Table 3.3).
- Women with multiple risk factors for VTE should be considered for postnatal prophylaxis.
- Women should be advised that neither heparin (unfractionated or LMWH) nor warfarin is contraindicated in breastfeeding.
- Postpartum warfarin should be avoided until at least the third day and for longer in women at increased risk of postpartum haemorrhage.

Postnatal clinic review

At postnatal review, women who develop VTE during pregnancy or the puerperium should be:

- Assessed for continuing risk factors.
- Counselled with regard to the use of contraception.
- Advised of their risk of developing recurrence of VTE in future pregnancies.
- Informed of other high-risk situations: long-distance travel, and concurrent illnesses.

Key pitfalls

- Delay in diagnosis as VTE is not considered at the initial assessment.
- Delay in initiating therapy or the use of inappropriate dose.
- Starting treatment in women at high risk of bleeding.
- Prolonged treatment without confirming the diagnosis.
- Vascular team not being involved in the management of massive PE where embolectomy could make a difference.

Table 3.3 Postnatal assessment and management.

Risk group	Patient group	Recommendation
High risk	Any previous VTE	At least 6 weeks postnatal prophylactic LMWH
	Anyone requiring antenatal LMWH	
Intermediate risk	Caesarean section in labour	At least 7 days postnatal prophylactic LMWH
	Asymptomatic thrombophilia (inherited or acquired) BMI > 40 kg/m^2	
	Prolonged hospital admission	
	Medical comorbidities, e.g. heart or lung disease, systemic lupus erythematosus, cancer, inflammatory conditions, nephrotic syndrome, sickle cell disease, intravenous drug user	Note: if persisting or > 3 risk factors, consider extending thromboprophylaxis with LMWH
Lower risk	Age > 35 years	
	Obesity (BMI > 30 kg/m^2)	
	Parity ≥ 3	
	Smoker	Two or more risk factors
	Elective caesarean section	
	Any surgical procedure in the puerperium	< two risk factors
	Gross varicose veins	
	Current systemic infection	
	Immobility, e.g. paraplegia, symphysis pubis dysfunction	
	Long distance travel	Mobilisation and avoidance of dehydration
	Preeclampsia	
	Mid-cavity rotational operative delivery	
	Prolonged labour (> 24 hours)	
	PPH > 1 litre or blood transfusion	

- Timing of inserting or removing regional anaesthesia catheter.

Key pearls

- All staff providing care to pregnant women should be aware of seriousness and presentations of VTE and initiate appropriate management as soon as possible.
- Protocols should be available in all sites of contact with pregnant women including A&E department and staff should have regular review of guidelines and protocols.
- Regular drills on managing collapsed obstetric patients.
- Clear protocols on how to contact radiology and other clinical staff.
- Women should be counselled and given information necessary to enable them to understand and share in informed choices with

regards to confirmatory tests and treatment options.
- The use of thrombolytic therapy during pregnancy should be reserved for women with severe pulmonary thromboembolism with haemodynamic compromise.
- If a woman is not suitable for thrombolytic treatment, a discussion with a cardio-thoracic surgeon with a view to urgent thoracotomy should be undertaken.

Management in low-resource settings

Venous thromboembolism is responsible for 2% of maternal deaths during pregnancy in developing countries. VTE may be under reported, undiagnosed and treatment is likely to be substandard.

This is particularly true in those settings where multiple risk factors are more common than in developed countries:

- Grandmultiparity.
- Age over 35.
- Prolonged labour.
- Dehydration.
- Higher incidence of comorbidities e.g. anaemia, sickle cell anaemia, thalassaemia, haemolytic anaemia and chronic HIV.
- Postpartum: higher incidence of postpartum haemorrhage (PPH), hypertension and dehydration.

Risk reduction

- Dissemination of information to increase women's and public awareness about VTE and its consequences.
- Developing local protocols and guidelines in delivery units and share with those who care for women throughout pregnancy, childbirth and in the postpartum period.
- Focus strategies to avoid dehydration during labour and proactively manage anaemia during antenatal periods.

References

1. Scottish Intercollegiate Guidelines Network (SIGN). *Prevention and Management of Venous Thromboembolism – A National Clinical Guideline.* NHS Quality Improvement Scotland, 2010.

2. Royal College of Obstetricians and Gynaecologists. *Thrombosis and Embolism during Pregnancy and the Puerperium, Reducing the Risk.* Green-top Guideline No. 37a. London: RCOG, 2009.

3. Royal College of Obstetricians and Gynaecologists. *The Acute Management of Thrombosis and Embolism during Pregnancy and the Puerperium.* Green-top Guideline No. 37b. London: RCOG, 2007.

4. Royal College of Obstetricians and Gynaecologists. *Standards for Maternity Care – Report of a Working Party.* London: RCOG, 2008.

5. Centre for Maternal and Child Enquiries (CMACE). *Saving Mothers' Lives: Reviewing Maternal Deaths to make Motherhood Safer – 2006–2008. The Eighth Report on Confidential Enquiries into Maternal Deaths in the United Kingdom. Br J Obstet Gynaecol* 2011; 118 (Suppl. 1): 1–208.

6. Mahmood T, Owen P, Arulkumaran S, Dhillon C (Eds.), *Models of Care in Maternity Services.* London: RCOG, 2010.

Chapter

4

Severe preeclampsia and eclampsia

Lucy Higgins and Alexander Heazell

Key facts

Definitions

- Preeclampsia: Pregnancy-induced hypertension ($\geq$ 140/90 mmHg) with significant proteinuria (see 'Key diagnostic signs'); developing after 20 weeks' gestation and resolving within 12 weeks of conclusion of pregnancy.
- Severe preeclampsia: pregnancy-induced hypertension $\geq$ 160/110 mmHg with significant proteinuria.
- Eclampsia: Occurrence of tonic–clonic seizures in a woman after 20 weeks' gestation (which may occur with preeclampsia) unless explicitly explained by alternative pathology.

Incidence

Estimates vary depending upon the population in which the condition is studied. Incidences of 1.5–7.7% have been reported in the developed world, and non-proteinuric pregnancy-induced hypertension is approximately twice as common (4.2–7.9%) [1]. The presence of risk factors increases the incidence 1.5–10-fold (see below).

Pathophysiology

The pathogenesis of preeclampsia is incompletely understood. Relatively shallow invasion and transformation of maternal spiral arteries leads to placental damage. The placenta releases inflammatory and vasoactive substances which act on maternal endothelium, activating platelets to release vasoconstrictory thromboxanes. This results in increased endothelial permeability and increased systemic vascular resistance accounting for the multisystem nature of preeclampsia. When the placenta is delivered the syndrome resolves.

Key implications

Table 4.1 shows the key effects of preeclampsia.

Table 4.1 Complications of preeclampsia: remember multisystem involvement

Organ/system	Implication /effect
Brain	Seizure Stroke
Lungs	Pulmonary oedema Pulmonary embolism
Cardiovascular system	Hypertension
Kidneys	Proteinuria Renal failure
Liver	Liver oedema Liver failure HELLP (**H**aemolysis, **EL**evated liver enzyme and **L**ow **P**latelets) syndrome Liver necrosis Hepatic rupture
Limbs	Brisk reflexes Clonus Peripheral oedema
Blood vessels	Deep vein thrombosis
Coagulation system	DIC (disseminated intravascular coagulation) Thrombocytopaenia
Feto-placental unit	Asymmetrical growth restriction Iatrogenic prematurity Placental abruption Intra-uterine death

Obstetric and Intrapartum Emergencies, ed. Edwin Chandraharan and Sabaratnam Arulkumaran. Published by Cambridge University Press. © Cambridge University Press 2012.

Maternal

Preeclampsia may affect multiple organ systems. Immediate effects:

- Peripheral vasoconstriction → hypertension → cerebrovascular haemorrhage, placental abruption.
- Oedema → peripheral, cerebral, hepatic (liver rupture/failure/necrosis), pulmonary (usually iatrogenic).
- Intravascular dehydration → renal failure (acute tubular necrosis).
- Venous thromboembolism (VTE).
- Deranged clotting/disseminated intravascular coagulation.
- HELLP syndrome (Haemolysis, Elevated Liver enzymes, Low Platelets).
- Eclampsia.

Medium-term effects:

- Protracted antihypertensive requirement.
- Prolonged hospital admission.
- Interventional delivery (induction of labour, caesarean section).
- Thrombophilic state.

Long-term effects:

- Recurrence of gestational hypertension or preeclampsia in future pregnancies.
- Increased incidence of hypertension, renal disease and death (due to cardiovascular events) [2].

Fetal/developmental

Immediate effects:

- Fetal growth restriction (FGR).
- Fetal death in utero.

Short-term effects:

- Prematurity → respiratory distress, necrotising enterocolitis.
- Neonatal death.

Long-term effects:

- Cerebral palsy (antepartum hypoxia).
- (Early onset) hypertension, diabetes and ischaemic heart disease in later life.

Table 4.2 Recognised risk factors for preeclampsia/eclampsia.

Patient	Partner	Pregnancy
Chronic hypertension	New partner	≥ 10 years since last pregnancy First pregnancy
Renal disease		Previous preeclampsia-affected pregnancy
Family history	Barrier contraception	Multiple pregnancy
Extremes of maternal age	Short sexual cohabitation	Molar pregnancy
Obesity	Donor insemination	Fetoplacental trisomy
(Pre-gestational) diabetes		
Antiphospholipid syndrome		
Systemic lupus erythematosus		
Other autoimmune disease		

Key pointers

A number of risk factors are recognised (Table 4.2), the most significant being preexisting renal disease (20-fold increase) or hypertension (five-fold increase).

Prediction

Early pregnancy

Currently no test can accurately predict who will develop preeclampsia early in pregnancy/preconceptually. A variety of clinical, biochemical and ultrasonic markers have been examined individually or in combination (including body mass index, early pregnancy blood pressure, alpha-fetoprotein, human chorionic gonadotrophin, oestriol, inhibin A, pregnancy-associated plasma protein-A, uric acid, placental growth factor and soluble vasculoendothelial growth factor 1). None is adequately specific or sensitive for widespread clinical use [3–7].

Later pregnancy

One in five women who demonstrate high resistance flow with (bilateral) notching of uterine artery Doppler waveforms at 20–22 weeks' gestation develop preeclampsia [8]. The sensitivity of this investigation increases with increasing gestation, however the test is time consuming, requires specific training and has large inter/intraobserver variability. It also has insufficient sensitivity for widespread clinical use.

At diagnosis of preeclampsia

The level of proteinuria (after diagnosis) is not effective in predicting who will develop severe disease [9].

Prevention

Preventing preeclampsia:

Various interventions have been tested; the majority unsuccessfully. The following are proven to reduce the risk of developing preeclampsia.

- Low-dose aspirin (75 mg); risk of preeclampsia reduced by 17% overall, 25% in high-risk women, 40% reduction in progression from non-proteinuric gestational hypertension to preeclampsia [10].
- Calcium; supplementation ≥ 1 g/day reduces the risk of preeclampsia by 55% overall, 88% in those at high risk [11].
- Tight blood pressure control for women who have preexisting hypertension; this is the subject of ongoing research [12].

Preventing eclampsia:

- Magnesium sulphate given prophylactically reduces the risk of eclampsia by 59% in women with severe preeclampsia [13].

Key diagnostic signs

Severe preeclampsia [1]:

- Blood pressure $\geq 160/110$ mmHg (mean arterial pressure (MAP) >125 mmHg = diastolic blood pressure + 1/3(systolic−diastolic blood pressure)) on at least one occasion, or two consecutive blood-pressure readings $\geq 140/90$ mmHg at least 4 hours apart with additional feature(s).
- Severe headache with visual disturbance.
- Epigastric pain.
- Clonus.
- Papilloedema.
- Liver tenderness.
- Platelet count $< 100 \times 10^9$/l.
- Alanine aminotransferase > 50 iu/l.
- Creatinine >100 mmol/l.
- Proteinuria ≥ 300 mg/24 hour urine collection, or urinary protein/creatinine ratio (PCR) > 30 mg/mmol [14].

- Pending results, bedside semi-quantitative analysis on mid-stream or catheter specimen urine of $\geq 1+$ protein.

Eclampsia:

- Occurrence of tonic–clonic seizure in pregnant woman (preeclampsia may be mild or undiagnosed prior to seizure) unless undoubtably explained by alternative pathology.

Key actions

For treatment algorithm see Figure 4.1.

General

- High-dependency obstetric care setting with one-to-one experienced midwifery care.
- Wide-bore intravenous access.
- Urinary catheter with hourly measuring chamber.
- Multidisciplinary review by senior obstetric and anaesthetic staff 4-hourly; low threshold for involvement of consultant obstetrician and anaesthetist.
- Inform neonatologist if delivery is considered < 34 weeks' gestation.

Monitoring

- Hourly measurement/documentation of maternal observations (blood pressure, pulse, respiratory rate, oxygen saturation, temperature, urine output, neurological status).
- Blood pressure (including MAP) and pulse measured every 15 minutes until stabilised.
- Oxygen saturations should be monitored continuously; medical review if $< 95\%$ on air.
- Meticulous fluid balance is essential to avoid pulmonary oedema.
- Deep tendon reflexes and clonus: 4-hourly.

Consider use of invasive arterial blood-pressure monitoring if:

- Unstable blood pressure.
- Persistent severe hypertension (more than one agent to control blood pressure).
- Inaccurate indirect maternal blood pressure measurement.
- Discrepant automated/manual readings.
- Obesity.
- Haemorrhage > 1000 ml/delivery complications.

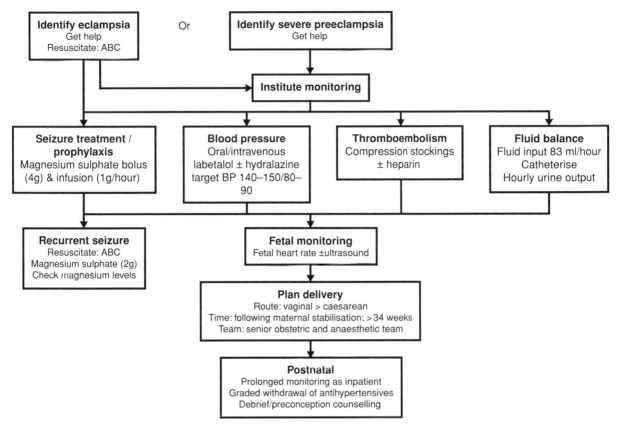

Figure 4.1 Management of severe pre-eclampsia / eclampsia.

- Hypoxia requiring arterial blood gas monitoring.
- Difficult venepuncture.

Request the following urgent investigations: full blood count, renal and liver function tests, urate, blood group and save serum.

- Clotting studies if platelet count $< 100 \times 10^9/l$.

Frequency of re-testing depends upon results, clinical situation and therapy.

Fetal well-being

- Once initial maternal management instituted, fetal heart rate monitoring should be commenced if gestation ≥ 24 weeks (intermittent fetal heart auscultation for viability < 24 weeks).
- Ensure the maternal condition is stable before acting upon fetal compromise.
- Following stabilisation, ultrasound assessment of fetal growth, liquor and umbilical artery Doppler to identify FGR/plan delivery.

Blood pressure

- Blood pressure trend can be measured using automated blood-pressure reading machines but should be verified with manual blood-pressure measurement (Korotkoff phase 5 to indicate diastolic blood pressure) as very few automated blood-pressure analysers are validated for use in pregnancy. Very high readings are particularly important to check manually as automated analysers tend to underestimate blood pressure.
- Control blood pressure to $< 160/105$ mmHg (MAP < 125 mmHg) gradually to reduce immediate risk of cerebral haemorrhage. A suggested protocol for initial management is:

(1) Oral labetalol 200 mg, repeated after 30 minutes if required.
(2) If oral medication fails to control hypertension then give intravenous labetalol 50 mg over 5 minutes, repeated after 10 minutes if required (maximum 4 doses).

27

(3) Intravenous labetalol infusion 20 mg/hour, doubling the infusion rate every 30 minutes if required (maximum 160 mg/hour).

(4) If labetalol is ineffective, intravenous hydralazine bolus 5 mg over 5 minutes, repeated every 20 minutes if required (maximum 4 doses).

(5) Intravenous hydralazine infusion 1 mg/hour, increasing every 30 minutes if required (maximum 5 mg/hour).

(6) Intravenous hydralazine bolus should be 2.5–5 mg over 5 minutes.

- Maintain blood pressure within the range 140–150/80–90 mmHg or booking blood pressure (whichever is higher) to ensure adequate utero-placental perfusion; rapid or prolonged hypotension may precipitate fetal compromise.

Seizure prophylaxis

- Magnesium sulphate should be commenced at diagnosis of severe preeclampsia/eclampsia; continuing until 24 hours following delivery/last seizure/commencement of magnesium sulphate therapy, whichever is the later.
- Administer magnesium sulphate according to the Collaborative Eclampsia Trial protocol [15]: 4 g magnesium sulphate over 5–10 minutes, followed by an infusion of 1 g/hour. Seizures treated with further 2 g magnesium sulphate bolus dose and increase infusion rate to 1.5 g/hour.
- Monitor renal function (not magnesium levels) 6-hourly during magnesium therapy. In the absence of oliguria (< 80 ml per 4-hour period), magnesium toxicity is rare. In oliguria consider cessation of magnesium sulphate until urine output improves.
- Signs of magnesium toxicity include respiratory rate < 12 per minute whilst awake and absence of deep tendon reflexes; check respiratory rate hourly and reflexes 4-hourly as a minimum.
- Treat magnesium toxicity with 10 ml of 10% calcium gluconate intravenously over 10 minutes and cessation of magnesium sulphate infusion. Involve senior obstetricians and anaesthetists.

Thromboprophylaxis

- Graded compression stockings should be applied provided no contraindications exist.

- Consider use of pneumatic compression devices e.g. 'Flotron boots', particularly in those with additional VTE risk factors or contraindication to compression stockings.
- Prophylactic heparin should be commenced as soon as possible (see below) and recommenced as soon as possible following delivery.
- Dose calculated according to pre/early pregnancy weight.
- Potential for imminent (< 12–24 hours) delivery should be assessed prior to every administration (withhold if necessary).
- Heparin should not be administered < 6 hours from insertion/removal of spinal/epidural anaesthesia.
- Epidural catheter not to be removed within 12 hours of heparin administration.
- Prophylactic heparin should be continued for a minimum of the duration of hospital stay.

Fluid management

- Limit input to 83 ml/hour (2 litres/24 hours) including therapeutic infusions (e.g. magnesium/antihypertensives); administer fluids orally where possible (if intravenous, via infusion pump/syringe).
- Large volume fluid losses should be replaced but not exceeded.
- Antenatal oliguria is not an indication for alteration of fluid input. If concerned involve senior obstetric/anaesthetic/renal physicians and expedite delivery.

Delivery

- The definitive treatment of preeclampsia/eclampsia is delivery, however this is inappropriate until the maternal condition is stable, even with fetal compromise.

Timing of delivery [1]

- > 37 weeks' gestation; after maternal stabilisation, regardless of severity of preeclampsia [16].
- 34–37 weeks' gestation; delivery is rarely associated with adverse maternal or fetal outcomes (consider betamethasone for fetal lung maturity; evidence lacking) therefore delivery should be considered. A randomised

controlled trial is currently addressing this issue [17].

- < 34 weeks; delivery indicated only if severe maternal/fetal compromise.

Individualised clinical/biochemical parameters for delivery < 34 weeks should be documented by the senior obstetrician.

If delivery is anticipated within 2 weeks, corticosteroids (e.g. 2 doses of betamethasone 12 mg intramuscularly 24 hours apart) should be administered to reduce the risk of surfactant deficiency lung disease.

- Severe, deteriorating disease in mothers of fetuses of pre-viable weight/gestational age is an indication to offer termination of pregnancy on maternal health grounds.

Place of delivery

- Due to potential sudden changes in maternal condition in utero transfer is generally inappropriate in severe preeclampsia/eclampsia; ex utero transfer of the baby to a relevant facility is usually preferred.
- If transfer is planned, all maternal observations must be stable, blood pressure maintained < 160/105 mmHg without evidence of fetal compromise. The patient should be accompanied by a senior midwife and anaesthetist. Transfer notes and investigation results with the patient.

Mode of delivery

- No benefit exists to elective caesarean over vaginal delivery, provided no contraindication to vaginal delivery exists [1]. However, under 32 weeks' gestation, caesarean section is preferred due to the high risk of failed induction of labour.
- There is no evidence to support limiting the duration of the active second stage of labour [1].
- The full range of analgesia options should be made available to women with severe preeclampsia during delivery.
  - Regional anaesthesia is generally safe if platelets $\geq 80 \times 10^9$/l.
  - Routine fluid loading should not be given; hypotension should be managed with judicious aliquots of phenylephrine.
- If general anaesthetic is necessary, anticipate pressor effects of intubation in preeclampsia and allow adequate time for its management, usually with opiates, even in the context of severe fetal compromise.
- H_2 antagonists (e.g. ranitidine) should be administered prior to caesarean delivery.

Management of the third stage

- Active management, with intramuscular oxytocin (10 iu) rather than ergometrine-containing products, is optimal due to increased risk of postpartum haemorrhage.

Eclampsia

Eclampsia affects 1/2000 pregnancies in the UK. It may occur prior to diagnosis of preeclampsia. Unless there is objective evidence to the contrary, any tonic-clonic seizure in the third trimester of pregnancy should be regarded as eclampsia until proven otherwise.

- Call all emergency personnel; inform consultant obstetrician and consultant anaesthetist.
- Ensure safety (patient and team).
- Systematic assessment of the patient as per Advanced Life Support algorithm [18] paying particular attention to prevention of supine hypotension by use of a wedge or tilt.
- Administer magnesium sulphate bolus (4 g over 10 minutes) as described above.
- In persistent seizures refractory to magnesium sulphate, consider diazepam, thiopentone or phenytoin. Intubation, ventilation and muscle relaxation may be required if seizures do not respond to second-line drug therapy.
- Send blood for magnesium level if patient was receiving magnesium sulphate prophylaxis prior to seizure (aim 2–4 mmol/l).
- Once seizure has resolved, perform full neurological examination, examine for other causes (electrolyte imbalance, sepsis, drug/alcohol withdrawal) and treat accordingly.
- Neuroimaging (CT/MRI) may be used to exclude other causes of seizure including intracerebral bleed, particularly if focal neurological signs persist.
- If antenatal, consider delivery when maternal condition stable.
- Emergency documentation should be of a high standard.
- Debrief the patient, family and clinical team.

- Report as an adverse incident for risk management.
- In the case of further seizures in a patient receiving magnesium sulphate administer a further 2 g bolus.

Treatment of HELLP

- No specific therapy exists, spontaneous resolution should occur postnatally as with severe preeclampsia.
- Corticosteroids lead to quicker improvement of haematological parameters but no improvement in maternal outcomes has been demonstrated and therefore should not be administered for this purpose.

Postpartum management

- Continue fluid restriction for the duration of magnesium infusion or until diuresis occurs.

  - Postnatal oliguria, e.g. urine output < 0.5 mg/kg/hour for 4 hours, in the presence of normal renal function tests, is not generally considered an indication for intervention; acute tubular necrosis is a rarer event than iatrogenic pulmonary oedema. However, monitor persistent oliguria with 6-hourly renal function tests.
  - In the presence of a rising creatinine, intervention may be considered, guided by accurate fluid balance.

- Monitor in hospital with measurement of maternal observations at least 4-hourly following discontinuation of magnesium sulphate, until at least the fifth postnatal day as per NICE guidance [1].
- Anticipate postnatal antihypertensive requirements to prevent delayed discharge. Recommended agents include labetalol or nifedipine (modified-release form).
- If methyldopa was used antenatally this should be withdrawn (replaced if necessary) after delivery [1].
- Ensure thromboprophylaxis is maintained.
- Discharge from hospital if asymptomatic of preeclampsia with stable blood pressure $< 150/100$ mmHg, if facility exists for alternate-days blood-pressure assessment as a minimum.

- Follow up with the general practitioner within 2 weeks of discharge and with hospital consultant 6–8 weeks following delivery.
- Antihypertensives often require a graded withdrawal. Approximately 20% of patients require ongoing antihypertensive medication 6 months after delivery and 13% of women will have chronic hypertension [19].
- Consider antiphospholipid antibody/inherited thrombophilia screen particularly if early-onset preeclampsia (< 28 weeks) or FGR.
- Ensure proteinuria has subsided, if still present re-check in 3 months and/or consider referral to renal physicians according to local protocol [1].
- Debrief regarding antenatal and postnatal events.

Preconceptual counselling prior to future pregnancies

- Risk of gestational hypertension is 13–53% dependent on severity/gestation of onset and persistence of additional risk factors (see Table 4.1) [1].
- Risk of preeclampsia is 16% (25% if severe preeclampsia, HELLP or delivery < 34 weeks, 55% if delivery < 28 weeks)[1].
- Long-term cardiovascular health; assess risk of chronic hypertension and modifiable risk factors for cardiovascular disease.

Key pitfalls

- Failure to recognise women at high risk of preeclampsia at first antenatal contact and institute appropriate consultant-led antenatal care.
- Failure to consider the diagnosis of preeclampsia in women with abdominal pain, other classical symptoms or involvement of organ systems involved in preeclampsia, particularly if they present to other specialities (primary care, emergency department).
- Failure to involve senior personnel at an early stage.
- Over-zealous initial reduction in blood pressure leading to placental underperfusion and fetal compromise.
- Inappropriate fluid management leading to pulmonary oedema.
- Failure to anticipate postpartum haemorrhage.

- Failure to assess risk of VTE and institute appropriate thromboprophylaxis.

Key pearls

- A departmental protocol should be in place for the management of women with severe preeclampsia/eclampsia.
- All members of staff involved in care of women with severe preeclampsia/eclampsia should receive annual training.
- Regular 'skills drills' should be conducted on management of severe preeclampsia/eclampsia.
- Care of all women with severe preeclampsia/eclampsia should be documented in an auditable form; lessons should be learned from good and suboptimal management alike.
- Set, and document, individualised parameters for delivery < 34 weeks' gestation.
- Consider invasive monitoring to guide antihypertensive management.

Management in low-resource settings

Severe preeclampsia and eclampsia are leading causes of global maternal mortality; the burden of mortality is heavier in low-resource settings yet safe management of severe preeclampsia/eclampsia is possible. A number of guides to the management of severe preeclampsia/eclampsia have been produced by the World Health Organization [20]. The management described above represents the standard to which all units should aim; a number of barriers to providing that care are recognised. The gestation at which termination rather than induction of labour is performed is likely to vary depending on expertise and resources.

Monitoring and care provision

- Recording of maternal observations on a standard chart enables visualisation of trends in vital statistics, and is invaluable in situations where one-to-one care is not possible.
- Careful attention should be paid to fluid balance.
- Collect and measure urine/other outputs.
- Where facility exists for monitoring haematological parameters, blood tests as described above should be taken at baseline and after any significant change in maternal condition/treatment.
- Fetal viability should be confirmed by auscultation.

- Induction of labour should be undertaken as soon as safely possible in fetal death in utero in order to prevent further maternal deterioration.

Magnesium sulphate

- Magnesium sulphate can be administered intramuscularly 4-hourly [20].

Antihypertensives

- Choice of antihypertensive should be based upon availability, cost and physician preference; no good evidence exists to value any particular antihypertensive.

Thromboprophylaxis

- As a minimum, the patient should be encouraged to mobilise/move legs to discourage venous stasis.

Delivery

- Mode: Account should be taken of maternal condition, chances of neonatal survival and facilities for care in future pregnancies.
- Timing: Delivery/termination may be required for maternal health. The gestation at which termination is performed rather than induction of labour is likely to vary depending on expertise and resources.
- Setting: Where safely possible, transfer women with severe preeclampsia/eclampsia to hospital. Consider referral to tertiary units for care of the newborn if preterm delivery is required for maternal health.

References

1. National Institute for Health and Clinical Excellence. *Hypertension in Pregnancy: The Management of Hypertensive Disorders during Pregnancy. CG107.* London: National Institute for Health and Clinical Excellence, 2010.

2. Jim B, Sharma S, Kebede T, Acharya A. Hypertension in pregnancy: a comprehensive update. *Cardiol Rev* 2010; 18 (4): 178–189.

3. Giguere Y, Charland M, Bujold E *et al.* Combining biochemical and ultrasonographic markers in predicting pre-eclampsia: a systematic review. *Clin Chem* 2010; 56 (3): 361–375.

4. Thangaratinam S, Ismail KM, Sharp S *et al.* Accuracy of serum uric acid in predicting complications of pre-eclampsia: a systematic review. *Br J Obstet Gynaecol* 2006; 113: 369–378.

5. Cnossen J S, Vollebregt KC, de Vrieze N *et al.* Accuracy of mean arterial pressure and blood pressure measurements in predicting pre-eclampsia: systematic review and meta-analysis. *BMJ* 2008; 336: 1117.

6. Cnossen JS, Leeflang MM, de Haan EE *et al.* Accuracy of body mass index in predicting pre-eclampsia: bivariate meta-analysis. *Br J Obstet Gynaecol* 2007; 114 (12): 1477–1485.

7. Polliotti BM, Fry A, Gordon MD *et al.* Second-trimester maternal serum placental growth factor and vascular endothelial growth factor for predicting severe, early-onset pre-eclampsia. *Obstet Gynecol* 2003; 101 (6): 1266–1274.

8. Cnossen JS, Morris RK, ter Riet G *et al.* Use of uterine artery Doppler ultrasonography to predict pre-eclampsia and intrauterine growth restriction: a systematic review and bivariable meta-analysis. *Can Med Assoc J* 2008; 178 (6): 701–711.

9. Thangaratinam S, Coomarasamy A, O'Mahoney F *et al.* Estimation of proteinuria as a predictor of complications of pre-eclampsia: a systematic review. *BMC Med* 2009; 24 (7): 10.

10. Duley L, Henderson-Smart DJ, Meher S, King JF. Antiplatelet agents for preventing pre-eclampsia and its complications. *Cochrane Database Syst Rev* 2007; 2: CD004659.

11. Hofmeyr GJ, Lawrie TA, Atallah ÁN, Duley L. Calcium supplementation during pregnancy for preventing hypertensive disorders and related problems. *Cochrane Database Syst Rev* 2010; 8: CD001059.

12. Magee LA, Von Dadelsczen P, Chan S *et al.* The Control of Hypertension in Pregnancy Study pilot data. *Br J Obstet Gynaecol* 2007: 114 (6): 770, e13–20.

13. Duley L, Gülmezoglu AM, Henderson-Smart DJ, Chou D. Magnesium sulphate and other anticonvulsants for women with pre-eclampsia. *Cochrane Database Syst Rev* 2010; 11: CD000025.

14. Papanna R, Mann LK, Kouides RW *et al.* Protein/creatinine ratio in pre-eclampsia: a systematic review. *Obstetrics and Gynaecology* 2008; 112 (1): 135–144.

15. Which anticonvulsant for women with eclampsia? Evidence from the Collaborative Eclampsia Trial. *Lancet* 1995; 345 (8963): 1455–1463; erratum in *Lancet* 1995; **346**: 258.

16. Koopmans C, Bijlenga D, Grown H *et al.* Induction of labour versus expectant monitoring for gestational hypertension or mild pre-eclampsia after 36 weeks' gestation (HYPITAT): a multicentre open-label randomised controlled trial. *Lancet* 2009; 374 (9694): 979–988.

17. HYPITAT-II Trial. *Study Information.* http://www.studies-obsgyn.nl/hypitat2/ [Accessed 17/03/2011].

18. Resuscitation Council (UK). *Resuscitation Guidelines: Adult Advanced Life Support. 2010.* http://www.resus.org.uk/pages/alsalgo.pdf [Accessed 28/02/2011].

19. Tuffnell DJ, Shennan AH, Waugh JJS, Walker JJ. *The Management of Severe Pre-Eclampsia/Eclampsia.* Guideline No. 10(A). London: RCOG, 2006.

20. World Health Organization, UNIFPA, UNICEF, The World Bank. *Pregnancy, Childbirth, Postpartum and Newborn Care: A Guide for Essential Practice.* Geneva: WHO, 2006.

Chapter

5

Massive obstetric haemorrhage

Vivek Nama and Edwin Chandraharan

Key facts

Definition

Blood loss of over 2000 ml (or > 30% of blood volume) is defined as massive obstetric haemorrhage (MOH). There is a tendency to underestimate rather than overestimate the actual blood loss.

Types

Massive obstetric haemorrhage can occur either in the antepartum (placenta praevia, placental abruption and placenta accreta) or postpartum period (postpartum haemorrhage (PPH) due to uterine atonia, genital tract trauma, retained placenta and membranes or coagulopathy). Rare obstetric disorders such as amniotic fluid embolism (AFE) or acute inversion of uterus may also present with massive obstetric haemorrhage.

Incidence

Antepartum haemorrhage (APH) occurs in about 3–5% of all pregnancies and placenta praevia accounts for approximately a third of all cases of antepartum haemorrhage. Placental abruption accounts for a quarter of all cases of antepartum haemorrhage.

Postpartum haemorrhage occurs in 2–10% of deliveries but the incidence of major obstetric haemorrhage is estimated to be 3.7–5/1000 maternities.

It is estimated that every year about 600 000 to 800 000 women die during childbirth around the world. In the developing world, PPH occurs in about 1 in 1000 deliveries. The Eighth Report of the Confidential Enquiries into Maternal Deaths in the UK has listed PPH as the third most common direct cause of maternal mortality [1]. Massive blood loss leads to sudden and rapid cardiovascular decompensation and coagulopathy.

Three delays have been identified as the causes of maternal deaths due to massive obstetric haemorrhage: delay in seeking medical care, delay in reaching healthcare facilities and delay in receiving appropriate care in a healthcare institution. The latter is common to both developing and developed countries. The Confidential Enquiries report has emphasised that deaths caused by PPH are due to 'too little done too late'.

Management of massive obstetric haemorrhage should follow a logical sequence of steps. Figure 5.1 provides an algorithm for the management of massive obstetric haemorrhage [2]. The mnemonic 'HAEMOSTASIS' [1] spells out the suggested actions that may facilitate the management of atonic PPH in a logical and stepwise manner (Table 5.1). Involvement of a multidisciplinary team of anaesthetists, haematologists and intensivists is essential to improve outcome [3]. Special Massive Haemorrhage Protocols such as 'Code Blue' should be in place for the effective, multidisciplinary management of massive obstetric haemorrhage.

Key implications

Massive obstetric haemorrhage causes significant maternal morbidity and mortality as well as many 'near misses'. Antepartum haemorrhage due to placental abruption and intrapartum haemorrhage due to uterine rupture are associated with increased perinatal mortality.

Moreover, massive obstetric haemorrhage due to placenta praevia may result in fetal complications secondary to prematurity as well as severe maternal hypovolumia and hypotension.

Obstetric and Intrapartum Emergencies, ed. Edwin Chandraharan and Sabaratnam Arulkumaran. Published by Cambridge University Press. © Cambridge University Press 2012.

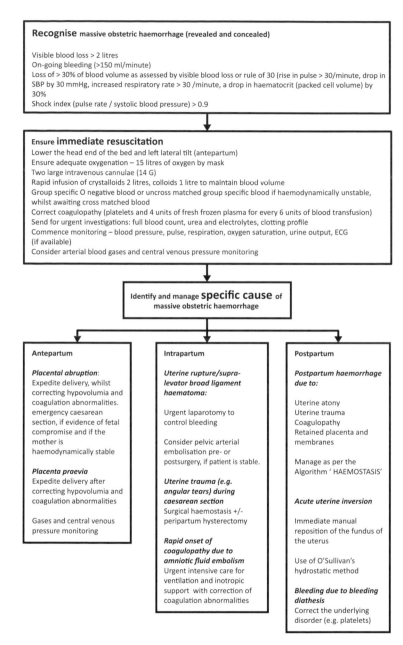

Recognise massive obstetric haemorrhage (revealed and concealed)

Visible blood loss > 2 litres
On-going bleeding (>150 ml/minute)
Loss of > 30% of blood volume as assessed by visible blood loss or rule of 30 (rise in pulse > 30/minute, drop in SBP by 30 mmHg, increased respiratory rate > 30 /minute, a drop in haematocrit (packed cell volume) by 30%
Shock index (pulse rate / systolic blood pressure) > 0.9

Ensure **immediate resuscitation**
Lower the head end of the bed and left lateral tilt (antepartum)
Ensure adequate oxygenation – 15 litres of oxygen by mask
Two large intravenous cannulae (14 G)
Rapid infusion of crystalloids 2 litres, colloids 1 litre to maintain blood volume
Group specific O negative blood or uncross matched group specific blood if haemodynamically unstable, whilst awaiting cross matched blood
Correct coagulopathy (platelets and 4 units of fresh frozen plasma for every 6 units of blood transfusion)
Send for urgent investigations: full blood count, urea and electrolytes, clotting profile
Commence monitoring – blood pressure, pulse, respiration, oxygen saturation, urine output, ECG (if available)
Consider arterial blood gases and central venous pressure monitoring

Identify and manage **specific cause** of massive obstetric haemorrhage

Antepartum

Placental abruption:
Expedite delivery, whilst correcting hypovolumia and coagulation abnormalities. emergency caesarean section, if evidence of fetal compromise and if the mother is haemodynamically stable

Placenta praevia
Expedite delivery after correcting hypovolumia and coagulation abnormalities

Gases and central venous pressure monitoring

Intrapartum

Uterine rupture/supra-levator broad ligament haematoma:

Urgent laparotomy to control bleeding

Consider pelvic arterial embolisation pre- or postsurgery, if patient is stable.

Uterine trauma (e.g. angular tears) during caesarean section
Surgical haemostasis +/- peripartum hysterectomy

Rapid onset of coagulopathy due to amniotic fluid embolism
Urgent intensive care for ventilation and inotropic support with correction of coagulation abnormalities

Postpartum

Postpartum haemorrhage due to:

Uterine atony
Uterine trauma
Coagulopathy
Retained placenta and membranes

Manage as per the Algorithm ' HAEMOSTASIS'

Acute uterine inversion

Immediate manual reposition of the fundus of the uterus

Use of O'Sullivan's hydrostatic method

Bleeding due to bleeding diathesis
Correct the underlying disorder (e.g. platelets)

Figure 5.1 Management algorithm for massive obstetric haemorrhage.

Immediate implications:

- Hypovolumia, hypoxaemia and cardiac arrest.
- Blood transfusion and effects of multiple blood transfusions including transfusion reactions, risk of infections and transfusion associated acute lung injury (TRALI).
- Acute renal failure.
- Pulmonary oedema.
- Coagulopathy.

- Risk of peripartum hysterectomy.
- Intensive care treatment.

Long-term implications:

- Psychological sequelae – delayed bonding with baby, post-traumatic stress disorder.
- Sheehan's syndrome (pituitary necrosis and failure due to massive obstetric haemorrhage leading to panhypopituitarism).

Table 5.1 Management algorithm 'HAEMOSTASIS' for postpartum haemorrhage.

H	Ask for **H**elp and **h**ands on uterus(uterine massage)
A	**A**ssess (**A**BC) and resuscitate (crystalloids 2 l, colloids 1 l, oxygen by mask (15 l/min))
E	**E**stablish aetiology (atonic, traumatic, coagulopathy or trauma), **e**nsure availability of blood and administer **e**cbolics (drugs that contract the uterus – oxytocin, ergometrine or syntometrine intramuscularly)
M	**M**assage uterus
O	**O**xytocin infusion/prostaglandins – IV/IM/per rectal (second-line medications to contract the uterus)
S	**S**hift to theatre – aortic pressure or anti-shock garment/bimanual compression as appropriate
T	**T**amponade balloon/uterine packing – after exclusion of **t**issue and **t**rauma
A	**A**pply compression sutures – B–Lynch/ modified
S	**S**ystematic pelvic devascularisation – uterine/ovarian/quadruple/internal iliac
I	**I**nterventional radiology and, if appropriate uterine artery embolisation
S	**S**ubtotal/total abdominal hysterectomy

- Impaired future fertility.
- Long-term anaemia.

Key aetiological factors

Antepartum

- Placenta praevia.
- Placental abruption.
- Rupture of an undiagnosed secondary abdominal pregnancy.
- Uterine rupture.

Intrapartum

- Amniotic fluid embolism (AFE) with coagulopathy.
- Uterine rupture secondary to previous uterine scar or grand multiparity, especially with injudicious use of oxytocin.
- Surgical complications (extension of uterine angular tear during caesarean section).

Postpartum

Uterine: Atonic uterus, ruptured uterus, uterine inversion. Broad ligament tears with resultant haematoma.

Placental: Placenta praevia, placental abruption, retained placenta.
Vaginal: Laceration and tears, haematoma.
Coagulopathy: Preexisting coagulopathy, treatment with anticoagulants, obstetric causes – HELLP, amniotic fluid embolism, chorioamnionitis.

Key pointers to massive obstetric haemorrhage

- Visible blood loss > 2 litres.
- Ongoing bleeding (> 150 ml/minute).
- Loss of > 30% of blood volume as assessed by visible blood loss (estimated blood loss or EBL expressed as the percentage of estimated blood volume = EBL/100 ml/kg).
- 'Rule of 30' (Rise in pulse > 30/min, drop in systolic blood pressure by 30 mmHg, increased respiratory rate > 30/minute, a drop in haematocrit (packed cell volume) by 30%) which is suggestive of at least 30% loss of blood volume.
- Shock index (pulse rate/systolic blood pressure) > 0.9. Normal shock index is between 0.5–0.7 as the pulse rate is less than systolic blood pressure.
- Tense, tender abdomen with evidence of intrauterine death (massive placental abruption).

Key actions: massive obstetric haemorrhage prior to delivery

Placental abruption

Placental abruption refers to the premature separation of a normally situated placenta. Maternal risks include haemorrhage secondary to accumulation of blood in the retro-placental space after separation of placenta as well as, in severe cases, bleeding into the uterine cavity as well as within the myometrial fibres. Activation of the extrinsic pathway of coagulation results in disseminated intravascular coagulation. Fetal risks include hypoxic cerebral injury as well as intrauterine death.

Predisposing factors

- Preeclampsia.
- Placental ischaemia secondary to vasculopathy (e.g. systemic lupus erythematosus (SLE), chronic renal disease).
- Multiparity.

- Abdominal trauma (road traffic accidents, domestic violence).
- Substance use (e.g. cocaine).

Clinical presentation

Vaginal bleeding that is associated with abdominal pain or discomfort ('revealed' bleeding). Sometimes, blood can accumulate behind the separated placenta and hence, no bleeding may be noted (concealed haemorrhage). Rarely, it may be 'mixed' (a combination of the above).

On examination, the patient may be pale and may be in constant pain. Abdominal examination may confirm a very tense, tender 'woody hard' uterus (especially in a concealed haemorrhage).

In severe cases of placental abruption, the fetal heart rate may be absent and the patient may show signs of coagulopathy. Observed blood loss may be out of proportion to the clinical condition and this may point to a 'mixed' haemorrhage.

Management

Immediate management involves active resuscitation to ensure a patent airway, breathing and maintaining circulation with intravenous fluids, blood and blood products as well as correction of coagulopathy. The role of 'left lateral tilt' and administration of high flow oxygen (15 l/minute) at the outset cannot be overemphasised. A multidisciplinary input involving haematologists and anaesthetists is essential. Delivery should be planned once the patient is haemodynamically deemed stable. Emergency caesarean section may be considered for fetal reasons (i.e. evidence of fetal compromise). If intrauterine death is diagnosed, delivery should be expedited by performing artificial rupture of membranes (ARM) and commencement of oxytocin infusion.

Postpartum haemorrhage should be anticipated due to coagulopathy as well as Couvelaire uterus (presence of blood within the myometrial fibres results in their disruption, leading to uterine apoplexy).

Placenta praevia

Placenta praevia refers to the extension of the placenta wholly or partially to the lower uterine segment. Massive obstetric haemorrhage ensues as the progressive uptake of the lower segment with advancing gestation leads to separation of the placenta, resulting from bleeding from the placental attachment. Such bleeding

is therefore maternal with no direct effect on the fetus. Iatrogenic preterm delivery in the 'maternal interest' as well as effects of prolonged maternal hypotension may result in detrimental effects on the fetus. Paucity of muscle fibres and hence the inability of the lower segment to contract and retract after birth increases the risk of atonic postpartum haemorrhage.

Clinical features

'Painless, causeless and recurrent' vaginal bleeding is typical of placenta praevia. 'Non-engaged' presenting part or abnormal lie or presentation with a soft non-tender uterus may help clinch the diagnosis. Uterine tenderness may be rarely present as placenta praevia may be associated with co-existing abruption in 10% of cases. Ultrasound examination will help confirm the diagnosis and a digital vaginal examination should be avoided in all cases of massive antepartum haemorrhage prior to excluding the diagnosis of placenta praevia.

Management

Initial management involves active resuscitation (please refer to placental abruption). However, vaginal birth is not possible in major degree placenta praevia. Hence, emergency caesarean section should be performed by an experienced operator, once the woman is stabilised. Postpartum haemorrhage should be anticipated and managed effectively (the lower uterine segment has fewer muscle fibres and hence is not effective in controlling bleeding from the placental site).

Massive obstetric haemorrhage: postpartum

As massive atonic postpartum haemorrhage is a major cause of maternal morbidity worldwide, we have discussed the management algorithm 'HAEMOSTASIS' in detail.

H – Ask for Help and Hands on the abdomen (uterine massage)

The first step should be to alert all members of the team (including the haematologist and the hospital porter) in case of an emergency through the hospital switchboard (e.g. 'Code Blue' protocol). A multidisciplinary approach would optimise the monitoring and management of fluid, electrolytes and coagulation parameters apart from providing input when necessary. Uterine massage should be commenced early, as 80% of postpartum haemorrhages occur secondary to uterine atony.

A – Assess (vital parameters, blood loss) and resuscitate

The woman should be positioned flat and resuscitation should begin with administration of high-flow oxygen (10–15 l/min) via a face mask regardless of her oxygen saturation. Body temperature should be maintained. Two large-bore cannulae (preferably 14 gauge) should be inserted in either arm and Hartmann's or normal saline infusion should be commenced. Up to 2 litres of crystalloids may be infused rapidly over 1–2 hours for initial stabilisation. Colloids like gelatin (Haemacel) or hydroxyethyl starch (1–2 litres) may also be needed to achieve haemodynamic stability. Pulse, blood pressure and respiration should be recorded every 15 minutes. Additional monitoring includes pulse oximetry and indwelling urinary catheter for hourly urine output. A central venous pressure (CVP) and an arterial line should be considered in cases of severe PPH.

E – Establish aetiology; ensure availability of blood, ecbolics (bolus of oxytocin, syntometrine, ergometrine)

The cause of massive postpartum haemorrhage (4Ts: tone, tissue, trauma and thrombin) should be identified. The uterus should be examined for contraction and retraction; it may also be worthwhile to check for 'free fluid' in the abdomen, if the history suggests trauma (previous caesarean section, difficult instrumental delivery) or if the patient's condition is worse than what would be expected based on the estimated blood loss. It is important to exclude any trauma to the genital tract and to ensure completeness of the placenta and membranes.

Ecbolics

Once atonic uterus has been identified as the cause of PPH, measures should be taken to ensure uterine contraction and retraction. Syntocinon (5 units) should be administered intramuscularly and if bleeding persists, syntometrine (combination of oxytocin 5 U and ergometrine 0.5 mg) or ergometrine (0.5 mg) should be administered (with caution in severe preeclampsia).

Ensure availability of blood and blood products

Replacement of the circulating blood volume with crystalloids and colloids should be followed by restoration of the oxygen-carrying capacity of the blood and correction of any derangements in coagulation. The aim of blood and fluids should be to replenish the previous loss in the first hour followed by maintenance fluids to replace continuing loss and maintain normal vital parameters. If coagulopathy is suspected, the haematologist should be involved and fresh frozen plasma (FFP), cryoprecipitate and platelets administered as required.

In massive obstetric blood loss, rapid infusion of FFP may be required to replace clotting factors other than platelets. It is recommended that with every 6 units of blood transfusion, 1 litre of FFP should be administered. It is important to maintain the platelet count above 50 000 by infusing platelet concentrates when indicated. Cryoprecipitate may also be needed if the patient develops disseminated intravascular coagulation (DIC) and her fibrinogen drops to less than 1 g/dl (10 g/l).

Massage the uterus

Uterine massage helps stimulate uterine contraction and retraction and should be commenced very early. It may act synergistically with the uterotonic drugs.

Compression of aorta may be used to gain temporary control of bleeding by applying the fist directly in the midline, just above the umbilicus and the uterus with the heel of the hand pressing down on the aorta. In a low-resource setting, anti-shock garments may also be used if available, during transfer to operating theatre or to another referral centre.

Oxytocin infusion/prostaglandins

Syntocinon 40 units can be added to 500 ml of normal saline and infused at a rate of 125 ml/hour [4]. It is important to avoid fluid overload, as fatal pulmonary and cerebral oedema with convulsions may occur secondary to dilutional hyponatraemia. An indwelling transurethral catheter is a requisite in these cases. In addition to monitoring urine output, it also helps to keep the bladder empty and promote uterine contractions.

Prostaglandins such as Hemabate (15-methyl prostaglandin 2 alpha) 250 µg can be administered intramuscularly, once every 15 minutes for a maximum of eight doses (2 mg). Intramyometrial injection of Hemabate has been tried, but serious complications, including severe hypotension and cardiac arrest, have been reported. Rectal misoprostol (600–1000 µg) may be tried, especially if oxytocin infusion was not used earlier. This is a valuable option in developing countries due to its low cost and relatively easier storage.

Tranexamic acid (starting dose of 1–4 g followed by 1 g 8-hourly) may be considered for PPH if administration of uterotonics has failed to stop the bleeding, or it is thought that the bleeding may be partly due to trauma.

S – Shift to theatre

If the patient continues to bleed despite initial management (i.e. 'HAEMO') it is best to transfer her to the theatre (for 'STASIS'). Theatre provides an environment suitable for continuous monitoring and resuscitation and facilitates an examination to exclude any retained placental tissue or membranes. A bimanual compression can be carried out at this stage to 'squeeze' the uterus between the abdominal and vaginal hands.

T – Tamponade balloon

Uterine tamponade with a balloon is easy to perform and takes only a few minutes. It arrests the bleeding and may prevent coagulopathy due to massive blood loss and the need for further surgical procedures. Although a Sengstaken–Blakemore oesophageal catheter (SBOC) is most commonly used, the Rusch urological hydrostatic balloon and the 'Bakri SOS' balloon may also be used. Usually a volume of about 300 to 400 ml may be required to exert the desired counter-pressure to stop bleeding from the uterine sinuses. If the tamponade arrests the bleeding (i.e. positive), the chances of the patient requiring any further surgical intervention are remote. Such a 'tamponade test' has a positive predictive value of 87% for the successful management of PPH [5].

Apply compression sutures

Failure of the tamponade test to arrest haemorrhage warrants an immediate laparotomy. Amount of blood loss, continuing bleeding, haemodynamic status and the patient's parity should be considered prior to attempting conservative surgical measures. This will help avoid 'too little being done too late'. It is prudent to discuss with the anaesthetist regarding the ability to withstand continued bleeding, whilst conservative surgical measures are attempted. This is vital in developing countries, where the patient might have lost a significant amount of blood by the time she reaches the referral centre. In such situations, radical measures such as total or subtotal hysterectomy to save the patient's life should be considered at the first instance.

Conservative surgical measures include compression sutures which include classical B-Lynch or vertical or horizontal brace sutures using a delayed absorbable suture material [6].

Systematic pelvic devascularisation

If the compression sutures fail, ligation of blood vessels supplying the uterus should be tried. These include ligation of both uterine arteries, followed by tubal branches of both ovarian arteries proximal to the ovarian ligament (called the 'quadruple ligation'). Uterine artery ligation is straightforward once the uterovesical fold of peritoneum is incised and the bladder is reflected down. A window is made in the broad ligament just lateral to the uterine vessels and the needle is passed through this opening. Medially, the needle is passed through the lower uterine myometrium, about 2 cm from the lateral margin, thus getting a good 'bite' and then the sutures are tied. The same procedure is repeated on the other side.

Internal iliac artery ligation is an option if bleeding persists. This requires an experienced surgeon who is familiar with the anatomy of the lateral pelvic wall. Bilateral internal iliac artery ligation has been found to reduce the pulse pressure by up to 85% in arteries distal to the ligation. This translates to an acute reduction in the blood flow by about 50% in the distal vessels.

The reported success rate of this procedure has been between 40% and 75% and it is invaluable for avoiding a hysterectomy. Potential complications include haematoma formation in the lateral pelvic wall, injury to the ureters, laceration of the iliac vein and accidental ligation of the external iliac artery. Ligation of the main trunk of the internal iliac artery may result in intermittent claudication of the gluteal muscles due to ischaemia. Examining the femoral pulse prior to completely ligating the internal iliac artery is vital.

Table 5.2 Symptoms and signs observed with massive obstetric haemorrhage.

	Class I	Class II	Class III	Class IV
Per cent blood loss	15	15–30	30–40	> 40
Amount of blood loss	1000	1500	2000	> **2500**
Respiration rate	14–20	20–30	30–40	> 40
Pulse	< 100	100–120	120–140	> 140
Systolic blood pressure	Normal	Normal	Decreased	Decreased
Diastolic blood pressure	Normal	Increased	Decreased	Decreased
Mental state	Anxious	Anxious and confused	Confused and agitated	Lethargic
Urine output /HR	> 30	20–30	5–15	Negligible

Interventional radiology

In women who are not acutely compromised or bleeding severely, interventional radiology can be considered. The success rates may be as high as 85–95% [7] and the entire procedure may take about 1 hour. Uterine artery embolisation helps to avoid radical procedures and preserve future fertility. Complications include vessel perforation, haematoma, infection and tissue necrosis.

Subtotal or total abdominal hysterectomy

If the bleeding is predominantly from the lower segment (as in PPH following a major degree placenta praevia), a total abdominal hysterectomy is warranted. A subtotal hysterectomy may be performed if the bleeding is mainly from the upper segment and the cause is 'unresponsive' uterine atony. Subtotal hysterectomy has lower morbidity and mortality rates and requires less time to perform. Due to the anatomical changes of pregnancy, it is important to exercise utmost care to prevent visceral trauma, especially of the bladder and ureters. It is also important to clamp the ovarian ligament medially to avoid non-intentional or inadvertent oophorectomy.

Postoperative care

Women with massive obstetric haemorrhage often need multi-organ support. Hence, transfer to an intensive care unit or high dependency unit should be considered for monitoring. Thromboprophylaxis should be considered once the coagulation parameters return to normal.

Complete the '3 Es' after every obstetric emergency

Examine – for heart rate, blood pressure, uterine contractility, vaginal bleeding and monitor urine output. Replenish lost fluid, blood and blood products adequately.

Explain the delivery events, possible reasons, complications and future plan of care to the patient (i.e. debrief).

Escalate – incident reporting form and to senior colleagues as well as to the team to identify learning points to continuously improve patient care.

Key pitfalls

- Failure to accurately estimate blood loss and involve senior and multidisciplinary input.
- 'Too little done too late' – 'too little' estimation of blood loss, 'too little' fluid replacement, 'too little' ecbolics, 'too little' replacement of blood and clotting factors, 'too late' referral or involvement of multidisciplinary team and 'too late' laparotomy and surgical haemostasis.

Key pearls

- Young fit women may maintain their blood pressure until significant blood loss occurs (Table 5.2).
- Systematic management of massive obstetric haemorrhage with the use of algorithms (Figure 5.1 and Table 5.1) with multidisciplinary input will help save lives.
- Use of 'Shock index' and 'Rule of 30' may help in estimating actual blood loss, when the vital signs are maintained despite significant blood loss.

References

1. Centre for Maternal and Child Enquiries (CMACE). *Saving Mothers' Lives: Reviewing Maternal Deaths to make Motherhood Safer – 2006–2008. The Eighth Report on Confidential Enquiries into Maternal Deaths in the United Kingdom. Br J Obstet Gynaecol* 2011; 118 (Suppl. 1): 1–208.

2. Chandraharan E, Arulkumaran S. Management algorithm for atonic postpartum haemorrhage. *J Paediatr Obstet Gynaecol* 2005; June: 106–112.

3. Chandraharan E, Arulkumaran S. Massive postpartum haemorrhage and management of coagulopathy. *Obstet Gynaecol Reprod Med* 2007; 17: 119–122.

4. Royal College of Obstetricians and Gynaecologists. *Prevention and Management of Postpartum Haemorrhage.* Green-top Guideline No. 52. London: RCOG, 2009.

5. Condous GS, Arulkumaran S, Symonds I *et al.* The tamponade test for massive postpartum haemorrhage. *Obstet Gynecol* 2003; 104: 767–772.

6. Chandraharan E, Arulkumaran S. Surgical aspects of postpartum haemorrhage. *Best Pract Res Clin Obstet Gynaecol* 2008; 22 (6): 1089–1102.

7. Ratnam LA, Gibson M, Sandhu C *et al.* Transcatheter pelvic arterial embolisation for control of obstetric and gynaecological haemorrhage. *J Obstet Gynaecol* 2008; 28 (6): 573–579.

Chapter

6

Sepsis and septic shock in pregnancy

Nicola Lack and Austin Ugwumadu

Introduction

The contribution of sepsis to maternal mortality in the UK has increased steadily over the last decade. In the 2000–2002 triennium sepsis accounted for 13 deaths, rising to 21 deaths in the 2003–2005 triennium and by the 2006–2008 triennium, sepsis has emerged as the leading cause of direct maternal deaths in the UK, accounting for a total of 29 deaths [1]. It is likely that there is a greater number of women who suffered significant sepsis related morbidity and survived. Therefore there is a particular need for vigilance on the part of healthcare professionals to detect the signs of sepsis during the antenatal, intrapartum or postpartum period.

Key facts

A proper understanding of sepsis begins with the definition of systemic inflammatory response syndrome (SIRS). SIRS is a complex, generalised but finely balanced and predictable network of non-specific inflammatory response of the body to a variety of severe insults such as massive haemorrhage, burns, trauma or pancreatitis. This non-specific inflammatory response includes temperature $> 38\,^{\circ}$C or $< 36\,^{\circ}$C, tachycardia > 90 bpm, tachypnoea > 20 or $PaCO_2 < 32$ mmHg, abnormal WCC (leukocytosis $> 12\,000$ or leukopenia < 4000) and acute phase reaction. Sepsis is defined when SIRS is due to a documented infection [2].

Other related definitions

- Bacteraemia: The presence of bacteria within the bloodstream.
- Severe sepsis: SIRS + organ dysfunction or hypotension.
- Septic shock: SIRS + systemic hypotension, which is unresponsive to adequate fluid resuscitation.
- Multiple organ dysfunction syndrome: SIRS associated with dysfunction in > 2 terminal phases of the spectrum.
- Septicaemia: The presence of bacteria and their toxins in the bloodstream leading to signs of infection – this term is no longer in use.

Incidence

Bacteraemia may be present in 0.1–0.4% of women after vaginal delivery and in 3–4% following caesarean section [3]. However the risk of progression to sepsis, septic shock and death is very small at < 1%. The common conditions encountered in pregnancy which may progress to sepsis and their frequencies are presented in Table 6.1 [4].

Key organisms involved

Beta-haemolytic Strep Lancefield group A (*Streptococcus pyogenes*) (GAS)

- A community-based organism.
- Asymptomatically carried in 5–30% of the population in throat or on skin.
- Droplet spread.
- More prevalent in December–April.
- Spread to pelvic organs by perineal contamination from the hands of colonised individuals.
- In the CMACE report 2006–2008, GAS was responsible for 50% of deaths from sepsis.

Other organisms

- *Escherichia coli.*
- *Streptococcus pneumoniae.*

Obstetric and Intrapartum Emergencies, ed. Edwin Chandraharan and Sabaratnam Arulkumaran. Published by Cambridge University Press. © Cambridge University Press 2012.

Table 6.1 Bacterial infections associated with septic shock found in the obstetric patient [4].

Bacterial infections	Incidence (%)
Chorioamnionitis	0.5–1.0
Postpartum endometritis Caesarean section Vaginal delivery	0.5–8.5 < 1.0
Pyelonephritis/UTI	1–4
Septic termination/miscarriage	1–2
Necrotising fasciitis (postoperative)	< 1
Toxic shock syndrome	< 1

- *Morganella morganii.*
- *Staphylococcus aureus.*
- *Clostridium septicum.*

Pathophysiology of sepsis

Host response to infection involves the activation of a mutually interactive array of cellular and humoral homeostatic systems including the activation of Th1 lymphocytes, which secrete proinflammatory cytokines. Cytokines stimulate the production of secondary mediators, which activate the coagulation and complement cascades. There is also activation of anti-inflammatory mediators to contain inflammation locally [5].

In severe sepsis the key pathology is endothelial dysfunction (endothelial apoptosis, increased expression of adhesion molecules and increased capillary permeability) and disordered coagulation homeostasis. There is a bias towards excess thrombosis and inadequate fibrinolysis. This results in widespread microvascular thrombosis and reduced tissue perfusion and oxygen availability leading to organ dysfunction and damage. Furthermore, there is reduced vasomotor tone because of disturbances of Ca^{2+} channel and electrolyte transport.

Key implications

- Maternal – ultimately multi-organ failure leading to death.

  · Haematological – Disseminated intravascular coagulation.
  · Cardiac – Myocardial dysfunction and failure.

Box 6.1 Clinical sequelae of infection.

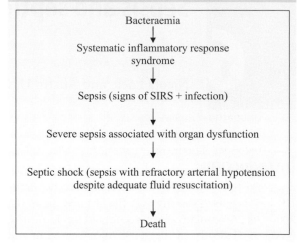

Bacteraemia

↓

Systematic inflammatory response syndrome

↓

Sepsis (signs of SIRS + infection)

↓

Severe sepsis associated with organ dysfunction

↓

Septic shock (sepsis with refractory arterial hypotension despite adequate fluid resuscitation)

↓

Death

  · Renal – Renal dysfunction leading to renal failure.
  · Liver – Hepatic encephalopathy.
  · Neurological – Encephalopathy and polyneuropathy.
  · Septic shock.
  · Death.

- Fetal.

  · Early pregnancy – miscarriage.
  · Late pregnancy – preterm labour.
  · Intra-uterine growth restriction.
  · Stillbirth.
  · Periventricular leukomalacia.
  · Intraventricular haemorrhages.
  · Cerebral palsy.
  · Neonatal death.

Key pointers
Possible origins of sepsis in the pregnant woman

- Chorioamnionitis – inflammation of the fetal membranes due to bacterial infection, more often associated with prolonged labour or PPROM (prolonged pre-labour rupture of membranes).
- Postpartum endometritis – infection of the endometrium, more common after emergency LSCS (lower segment caesarean section) or PROM (prolonged pre-labour rupture of membranes).

- Pyelonephritis.
- Wound infection.
- Other including peritonitis, pneumonia, cellulitis, pancreatitis.

Risk factors (particularly for women developing pelvic infection)

- Nulliparous women.
- Prolonged rupture of membranes.
- Prolonged labour with repeated vaginal examinations.
- Internal fetal monitoring.
- Bacterial vaginosis.
- The presence of beta-haemolytic Group B streptococcus.
- Meconium stained liquor.
- Preexisting disease (e.g. chronic anaemia, immunosuppression).

Key diagnostic signs

The development of sepsis in obstetric patients tends to be insidious followed by stepwise deterioration. In general, obstetric patients are young, fit and healthy women who compensate well, but deteriorate quickly. In order to treat sepsis effectively and prevent maternal deaths, it is important to pick up the signs as quickly as possible and initiate treatment in order to prevent the development of septic shock. It is also important to note that the signs and symptoms of sepsis can be non-specific.

Key actions

In 2003, the Society of Critical Care Medicine, the European Society of Intensive Care Medicine and the International Sepsis Forum jointly initiated a 'Surviving Sepsis Campaign'. The campaign focused on improving awareness and the management of sepsis with the aim of reducing the global mortality associated with sepsis. The two widely recognised care bundles and the key recommendations for the management of sepsis are discussed in greater detail below.

Patients with suspected or confirmed sepsis should be managed by a multidisciplinary team including obstetricians, anaesthetists, microbiologists and intensivists, with input from haematology and other specialities as and when required. The principles of treatment revolve around the basic elements of resuscitation (Airways, Breathing, Circulation), treatment of

Box 6.2 Signs and symptoms of sepsis.

Temperature	Raised temperature > 38 °C. Hypothermia < 36 °C – may indicate worseninginfection. Remember – patients may have a normal temperature, and this does not exclude sepsis. Swinging pyrexia – may indicate a persistent focus of infection and warrants investigation.
Tachycardia	HR > 90–100 bpm. NB – do not forget differential diagnosis including VTE, or an underlying cardiac problem – investigate fully.
Tachypnoea	RR > 20. Again, remember to exclude other pathologies including VTE, amniotic fluid embolism, pulmonary oedema, pneumonia.
Gastrointestinal signs	Diarrhoea. Vomiting. Abdominal pain.
Haematological signs	Leukocytosis. Leukopenia (often an indicator of worsening sepsis). DIC/ abnormal clotting.
Biochemistry	Rising inflammatory markers – CRP. Worsening renal function. Worsening liver function. Metabolic acidosis (rising lactate concentration).
Fetal	Fetal heart rate abnormality or intra-uterine death.

the underlying infection including surgical drainage or excision, and organ support until recovery [6].

Airways and breathing

Adult respiratory distress syndrome (ARDS) is a severe complication of sepsis and septic shock with a mortality of 36–52% [7]. These patients are likely to need mechanical ventilation in an intensive care setting. Careful monitoring of oxygen saturation and respiratory rate should be undertaken to alert the medical teams of the need for ventilatory support.

Circulation

Patients with sepsis may become hypotensive as a result of reduced peripheral vascular resistance and sequestration of fluid. Fluid resuscitation is the mainstay of treatment. This must be undertaken with caution to avoid fluid overload and potentially fatal pulmonary or cerebral oedema. Careful documentation of fluid balance should be undertaken including hourly urine output, and if necessary invasive monitoring with CVP lines should be considered. Patients who remain hypotensive despite adequate fluid resuscitation may require vasopressor therapy, with or without inotropic support.

Commence MEOWS chart

The use of Modified Early Obstetric Warning System (MEOWS) charts has been shown to minimise risk in the unwell obstetric patient (see Figure 6.1) [1]. In the obstetric setting, women may be cared for by any member of the multidisciplinary team and any number of different midwives and doctors during the course of their treatment. Therefore, continuity of care may be affected and there may be difficulty in recognising subtle trends and signs of deterioration in the patient's condition. MEOWS charts help to redress this problem and should be retained with the patient even if she moves between clinical areas.

Investigations in pregnant or recently confined women displaying signs or symptoms of infection:

- Haemoglobin.
- White blood cell (WBC) count (note that during pregnancy the WBC count may reach 15 000 and up to 20 000 during labour).
- Blood cultures if temperature $> 38\,°C$.
- Midstream sample of urine.
- Swabs including a vaginal swab.

Investigations in women who develop signs or symptoms of infection during labour or delivery:

- Swabs from placenta, baby and vagina.
- Placenta sent for histology and microbiology.

Investigations in the septic patient:

- Blood tests — Haematology – Full blood count, clotting.
  Biochemistry – U+Es, LFTs, LDH.
  Amylase.
  Arterial blood gases including lactate.

- Urine — Midstream urine/catheter specimen urine.
- Chest — Sputum sample (if appropriate).
- Swabs — Throat.
  Vagina.
  Wound.
  Other.
- Radiology — Pelvic ultrasound.
  Chest X-ray.
  Abdominal imaging – US or CT scan.
- Other — Lumbar puncture (if appropriate).
  Stool sample.

Antibiotics

Prophylactic antibiotic administration is recommended in a number of clinical scenarios to prevent infection in women considered to be at risk. These scenarios include caesarean section, prolonged prelabour rupture of membranes, prolonged rupture of membranes and anal sphincter injuries. The 'Surviving Sepsis' guidelines recommended the following approach to antibiotic therapy as well as appropriate antibiotic regimes [6]. These were endorsed in the CMACE report [1]:

- Obtain appropriate cultures before initiating appropriate antibiotic therapy.
- Avoid delay in commencing antibiotics. There is a direct relationship between each hour of delay in initiating effective antibiotics and increased mortality.
- Initial empirical antibiotic therapy should include:
  · One or more drugs that have activity against all likely pathogens.
  · Treatment that penetrates in adequate concentrations into the presumed source of sepsis.

Women with severe sepsis or septic shock warrant broadspectrum therapy until the causative organism and its antibiotic sensitivities have been defined.

- All women should receive a full loading dose of each antimicrobial, but as women with sepsis or septic shock often have impaired renal or hepatic function, measuring serum levels may be necessary, and advice about further doses should be sought from the critical-care team or a consultant physician.

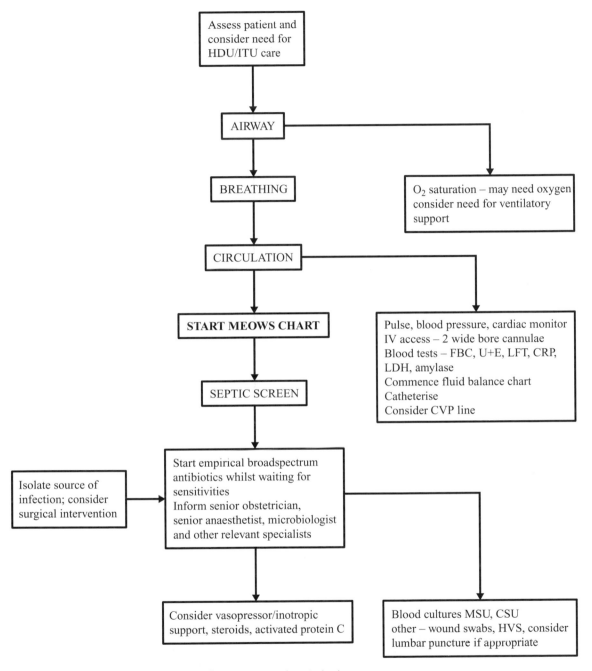

Figure 6.1 Algorithm for the management of severe sepsis and septic shock.

- The antimicrobial regimen should be reassessed daily to optimise activity, to prevent the development of resistance, to reduce toxicity and to reduce costs. If and when a specific organism is identified, antibiotic therapy can then be modified to the most appropriate regimen.

- Duration of therapy should be typically 7–10 days; longer courses may be appropriate in women who have a slow clinical response, undrainable focus of infection, or immunological deficiencies, including neutropenia. Blood cultures will be negative in > 50% of cases of severe sepsis or septic shock, even though these cases are very likely to be caused by bacteria or fungi, so that decisions to continue, narrow, reduce or stop antimicrobial therapy must be made on the basis of clinical judgement and clinical information.

- Choosing the most appropriate antibiotic regimen may be complex and advice should be sought from a consultant microbiologist as soon as possible. This should never delay urgent treatment, and some suggested choices of initial empirical intravenous antibiotic therapy in genital-tract sepsis are outlined below.

Where the organism is unknown and the woman is not critically ill:

- Co-amoxiclav 1.2 g 8-hourly plus metronidazole 500 mg 8-hourly.

or

- Cefuroxime 1.5 g 8-hourly plus metronidazole 500 mg 8-hourly.

or

- Cefotaxime 1–2 g 6- to 12-hourly plus metronidazole 500 mg 8-hourly.
- In cases of allergy to penicillin and cephalosporins, clarithromycin (500 mg twice daily) or clindamycin (600 mg to 1.2 g by intravenous infusion 3 or 4 times daily) plus gentamicin for Gram-negative cover are possible alternatives while waiting for microbiological advice.

In severe sepsis or septic shock (seek urgent microbiological advice):

- Piperacillin–tazobactam 4.5 g 8-hourly or ciprofloxacin 600 mg 12-hourly plus gentamicin (3–5 mg/kg daily in divided doses every 8 hours by slow intravenous injection).
- A carbapenem such as meropenem (500 mg to 1 g 8-hourly by intravenous injection over 5 minutes or by intravenous infusion) plus gentamicin may also be added.
- Metronidazole 500 mg 8-hourly may be considered to provide anaerobic cover.
- If Group A streptococcal infection is suspected, clindamycin (600 mg to 1.2 g by intravenous infusion 3 or 4 times daily) is more effective than penicillin as clindamycin inhibits exotoxin production.

- If there are risk factors for MRSA, add teicoplanin 10 mg/kg 12-hourly for three doses then 10 mg/kg daily or linezolid 600 mg twice daily.

Adjuvant interventions

There are other adjuvant interventions that may be required in the management of the septic patient, and these are outlined below.

Surgery

Infections within closed spaces, e.g. retained products of infection, or abscesses need to be drained or removed surgically.

Steroids

There is no place for the use of high-dose steroids in the management of sepsis.

However, there is good evidence that low-dose steroids ($<$ 300 mg/day hydrocortisone) may be beneficial in women who have been on vasopressors for more than 6 hours.

Activated protein C

Activated protein C is an exogenous anticoagulant with anti-inflammatory properties. The early stage of sepsis is a pro-coagulant state and the resultant microthrombi create a microvascular disease leading to end-organ damage. The Recombinant Human Activated Protein C Worldwide Evaluation in Severe Sepsis (PROWESS) trial showed that activated protein C improved outcome in patients with evidence of end-organ damage [8]. The current recommendations are that its use should be restricted to those patients with a high likelihood of death.

Key pitfalls

- Failure to recognise the early signs of infection and developing sepsis.
- Failure to use or respond to MEOWS charts (Modified Early Obstetric Warning System Charts).
- Delay in starting antibiotics.
- Delay in involving the multidisciplinary team.

Key pearls

- Scenarios/simulation training in the management of the septic patient.

- Isolate source of infection.
- Multidisciplinary team involvement at an early stage.
- Appropriate use of MEOWS charts.
- Early use of broadspectrum antibiotics.

References

1. Centre for Maternal and Child Enquiries (CMACE). *Saving Mothers' Lives: Reviewing Maternal Deaths to make Motherhood Safer – 2006–2008. The Eighth Report on Confidential Enquiries into Maternal Deaths in the United Kingdom. Br J Obstet Gynaecol* 2011; 118 (Suppl. 1): 1–208.

2. Bone RC, Balk RA, Cerra FB, *et al.* Definitions for sepsis and organ failure and guidelines for the use of innovative therapies in sepsis. The ACCP/SCCM Consensus Conference Committee, American College of Chest Physicians/Society of Critical Care Medicine. *Chest* 1992; 101 (6): 1644–1655.

3. Greer IA, Nelson-Piercy C, Walters B. *Maternal Medicine: Medical Problems in Pregnancy*. Edinburgh: Churchill Livingstone, 2007.

4. Leonardi MR, Gonik B. Septic shock. In: Dildy G III (Ed.), *Critical Care Obstetrics*, 4th edition. Malden, MA: Blackwell Science, 2004.

5. Howell C, Grady K, Cox C. (Ed.) *Managing Obstetric Emergencies and Trauma*, 2nd edition. London: RCOG, 2007.

6. Dellinger RP, Levy MM, Carlet JM *et al.* Surviving Sepsis Campaign: International guidelines for management of severe sepsis and septic shock. *Critical Care* 2008; 36: 296–327.

7. Neal Reynolds H, McCunn M, Borg U, Habashi N *et al.* Acute respiratory distress syndrome: estimated incidence and mortality rate in a 5 million-person population base. *Crit Care* 1998; 2(1): 29–34.

8. Vincent JL, Angus DC, Artigas A *et al.* Effects of drotrecogin alfa (activated) on organ dysfunction in the PROWESS trial. *Critical Care Medicine* 2003; 31(3): 834–840.

Amniotic fluid embolus

Derek Tuffnell and Hlupekile Chipeta

Key facts

Definition

Amniotic fluid embolus (AFE) is a rare obstetric condition that is characterised by one or more of the following features, in the absence of any other clear cause:

- Acute fetal compromise.
- Cardiac arrhythmias or arrest.
- Coagulopathy.
- Convulsion.
- Hypotension.
- Maternal haemorrhage.
- Premonitory symptoms, e.g. restlessness, numbness, agitation, tingling.
- Shortness of breath.
- Excluding women with maternal haemorrhage as the first presenting feature in whom there was no evidence of early coagulopathy or cardiorespiratory compromise [1].

Histological amniotic fluid embolus is the presence of fetal squames or hair in maternal lungs at postmortem [1].

International variations exist in the definition of AFE which may account for differences in incidence.

Amniotic fluid embolus is sometimes considered in two phases. The first phase is characterised by an almost anaphylactoid reaction with hypotension, dyspnoea with or without cardiac arrest. The second phase is marked by haemorrhage and coagulopathy.

Incidence

- No change in incidence over the last 4 years. Approximately 2.0 per 100 000 deliveries (95% CI 1.5–2.5) in the UK [1], 3.3 per 100 000 in Australia [2] and 6.0 per 100 000 singleton deliveries in Canada [3].

Mortality

Amniotic fluid embolus is the seventh commonest cause of all maternal deaths [4]. At 0.57 per 100 000 maternities (95% CI 0.33–0.98) it has reduced from the second to the fourth leading cause of direct maternal deaths in the UK. Maternal case fatality rates are between 16.5 and 61% in the UK, Australia and the USA [1, 4]. There is a fall in case mortality rates which is probably due to high-level supportive care and diagnosis of milder cases [5].

Key implications

- Maternal: Pulmonary oedema, acute respiratory distress syndrome, disseminated intravascular coagulopathy (DIC), pulmonary embolus, haemorrhage, right then left cardiac failure, cerebrovascular events, cardiorespiratory arrest, death.
- Fetal: Fetal distress, hypoxic ischaemic encephalopathy (HIE), learning difficulties, cerebral palsy, intrauterine and neonatal death.

Key pointers

The following risk factors have been identified:

- Maternal age greater than 35 years, odds ratio (OR) 9.85 (95% CI, 3.57–27.2).

Obstetric and Intrapartum Emergencies, ed. Edwin Chandraharan and Sabaratnam Arulkumaran. Published by Cambridge University Press. © Cambridge University Press 2012.

- Induction of labour, OR 3.86 (95% CI, 2.04–7.31).
- Multiple pregnancy, OR 10.9 (95% CI, 2.81–42.7).
- Caesarean delivery, OR 8.84 (95% CI, 3.70-21.1).

Other factors that were previously considered risk factors are now no longer considered causal [6]:

- Ethnicity – Black and other ethnic minorities.
- Assisted vaginal delivery.
- Placenta praevia.
- Placental abruption.
- Eclampsia.
- Fetal distress.
- Hyperstimulation.

Black or other minority ethnicity is associated with an increased case fatality rate.

Key symptoms and signs
- Maternal:

  · Symptoms: dyspnoea, loss of consciousness, cough, wheeze, headache, chest pain.
  · Signs: cyanosis, hypoxia, hypotension, transient hypertension, cardiac arrhythmia, cardiopulmonary arrest, seizure, signs of pulmonary oedema.

- Fetal:

  · Fetal distress, neonate with severe HIE.

Key actions
- Suspect a diagnosis of AFE in any woman during labour, after delivery or following surgical evacuation of the womb with the following features [7]: maternal haemorrhage, hypotension, shortness of breath and new-onset respiratory symptoms, coagulopathy, premonitory symptoms such as restlessness, agitation, numbness, tingling, acute fetal compromise, cardiac and/or arrhythmia, seizures.

A significant number of women present with maternal collapse. Therefore management will consider this presentation foremost.

First-line management – resuscitation
Call for help – early
Senior multidisciplinary involvement is important for a positive prognosis. The team should include obstetricians, anaesthetists, intensivists, haematologists and neonatologists.

Airway
Women are at risk of a compromised airway due to depressed level of consciousness.

- Maintain patency.
- Give high-flow oxygen at a rate of 15 l/minute through a face mask with reserve bag.
- Attach a pulse oximeter.
- Consider intubation if still pregnant, respiratory distress or cardiopulmonary collapse.
- Place into left lateral tilt.

Breathing
Women are at risk of compromised breathing due to pulmonary oedema.

- Assess breathing (including respiratory rate) and ventilate if there is evidence of respiratory distress.
- Positive end expiratory pressures may be necessary to maintain adequate oxygen saturations.

Circulation
Women are at risk of cardiac arrhythmias, cardiac arrest, massive haemorrhage and pulmonary embolus due to sudden fluid shifts and disseminated intravascular coagulation (DIC).

- Assess circulation and blood pressure.
- Start CPR and deliver fetus if cardiac arrest.
- Monitor blood pressure.
- Perform ECG.
- Insert two large-bore intravenous cannulae.
- Consider central monitoring especially if pulmonary oedema, haemodynamic instability or peripheral shutdown.
- Send venous blood samples urgently for FBC, clotting and cross match.
- Perform an arterial blood gas analysis.
- Get a chest X-ray.

Correct hypotension and coagulopathy

- Replace intravascular volume with clear fluids and blood.
- Liaise *early* with haematologist to treat DIC with fresh frozen plasma, cryoprecipitate, platelets or red blood cells.
- Liaise with intensivists and anaesthetists to maintain blood pressure with inotropic support.

Deliver fetus

The main aim of early delivery is to facilitate and improve outcome of maternal resuscitation.

The fetus remains at significant risk of morbidity and demise even with prompt delivery. Outcome statistics of fetuses and neonates are unlikely to be accurate due to the small numbers in UK case series but suggest a ~50% survival if born to a dead woman with ~77% surviving if born to a live woman. Either way, infants are at significant risk of long-term neurological deficits [8].

Following delivery, beware of uterine haemorrhage due to DIC.

- Consider medical treatments for atony including oxytocics, ergometrine, carboprost and misoprostol.
- Consider mechanical measures including bimanual compression, intrauterine tamponading balloons and brace techniques.
- Consider interventional radiology and uterine artery embolisation.
- Consider surgical options including internal iliac artery ligation and hysterectomy.
- Consider discussion with haematologist for factor VIIa as well as cryotherapy, FFP and platelets.

Second-line management – diagnosis and supportive care

Ascertain the diagnosis

With mortality from AFE falling, diagnosis is increasingly clinical. The long list of differential diagnoses reflects the breadth of symptoms and signs women present with. These must be excluded before a diagnosis is made but treatment of the acutely ill woman must *not* be delayed in the quest to find a diagnosis.

Box 7.1 outlines a list of differential diagnoses.

Box 7.1 Differential diagnosis of women with suspected amniotic fluid embolism [5].

Postpartum haemorrhage
Placental abruption
Uterine rupture
Preeclampsia/HELLP syndrome
Septic shock
Thrombotic embolus
Air embolus
Acute myocardial infarction
Peri-partum cardiomyopathy
Local anaesthetic toxicity
Anaphylaxis
Transfusion reaction
Aspiration of gastric contents

Various investigations should be performed in an effort to investigate the above differential diagnoses. Blood tests to perform include clotting, liver and renal function tests, arterial blood gases. An ECG (with or without an echocardiogram) may be helpful in showing myocardial problems. A ventilation/perfusion (V/Q) scan may reveal a perfusion defect. A computerised tomography pulmonary angiography (CTPA) scan would diagnose intrapulmonary abnormalities.

Zinc coproporphyrin and tryptase levels are not used routinely in the diagnosis of AFE.

Transfer to intensive care unit

The mainstay of management of AFE remains supportive. Rigorous, early supportive therapy saves mothers' lives.

The purpose of ICU is to monitor observations, maintain haemodynamic instability and reduce iatrogenic and disease complications. Options of treatment include diuretics, inotropes and steroids. Plasma exchange, haemofiltration and extracorporeal membrane oxygenation have been used in treatment.

Disclosure and documentation

At a local level, clear, chronological and contemporaneous documentation is essential preferably on a high-dependency chart. Incident reporting is important e.g. for transfer to the ICU, major postpartum haemorrhage, unexpectedly low cord pH and neonatal admission to NICU.

At a national level, UKOSS and the National Near-miss Surveillance Programme (UKNeS) are currently conducting an AFE study looking into incidence, risk factors, management and maternal and infant outcomes. Voluntary notification of cases to the database over a period of 3 years should collect data on an estimated 30 cases.

Key pitfalls

- Failure to suspect AFE in a collapsed or unwell peripartum woman.
- Failure to seek early input from intensivists, anaesthetists and haematologists.
- Failure to ensure ABC.
- Failure to consider early delivery of the fetus principally for maternal resuscitation.
- Failure to correct coagulopathy, stop haemorrhage and control fluid balance.
- Failure to keep adequate records.
- Failure to report to national registers.

Key pearls

- All staff providing intrapartum care should attend annual skills and drills training on the management of maternal collapse.
- Regular fire drills involving maternal collapse on the labour ward can ensure that a robust system is in place for the acute management of AFE.
- All staff should be encouraged to report any maternal collapse through incident forms.

References

1. Knight M, Tuffnell D, Brocklehurst P, Spark P, Kurinczuk JJ, on behalf of the UK Obstetric Surveillance System. Incidence and risk factors for amniotic fluid embolism. *Obstet Gynecol* 2010; 115: 910–917.

2. Roberts C, Algert C, Knight M, Morris J. Amniotic fluid embolism in an Australian population-based cohort. *Br J Obstet Gynaecol* 2010; 117: 1417–1421.

3. Kramer MS, Rouleau J, Baskett TF, Joseph KS; Maternal Health Study Group of the Canadian Perinatal Surveillance System. Amniotic-fluid embolism and medical induction of labour: a retrospective, population-based cohort study. *Lancet* 2006; 368: 1444–1448.

4. Centre for Maternal and Child Enquiries (CMACE). *Saving Mothers' Lives: Reviewing Maternal Deaths to make Motherhood Safer – 2006–2008. The Eighth Report on Confidential Enquiries into Maternal Deaths in the United Kingdom. Br J Obstet Gynaecol* 2011; 118 (Suppl. 1): 1–208.

5. Howell C, Grady K, Cox C. *Managing Obstetric Emergencies and Trauma – the MOET Course Manual.* 2nd edition. London: RCOG, 2007.

6. Conde-Agudelo A, Romero R. Amniotic fluid embolism: an evidence-based review. *Am J Obstet Gynecol* 2009; 201 (5): 445.e1–13. Erratum in *Am J Obstet Gynecol* 2010; 202 (1): 92.

7. Tuffnell D, Knight M, Plaat F. Amniotic fluid embolism – an update. *Anaesthesia* 2011; 66 (1): 3–6.

8. Tuffnell DJ. United Kingdom amniotic fluid embolism register. *Br J Obstet Gynaecol* 2005; 112: 1625–1629.

Uterine rupture

M. F. M. Rameez and Malik Goonewardene

Key facts

Types

Complete uterine rupture:

- A full thickness separation of the uterine muscle and the overlying visceral peritoneum, associated with the extrusion of fetus, placenta or both into the abdominal cavity.

Incomplete uterine rupture:

- Disruption of the uterine muscle but visceral peritoneum intact. Commonly due to dehiscence of a lower segment caesarean section (CS) scar.

Incidence

- Varies from 1 in 80–500 deliveries in low-resource settings [1, 2] to 1 in 3000–5000 deliveries in well-resourced settings [3]. The incidence is rising in well-resourced setting as a result of rising CS rates [4, 5].

Key implications

- Adverse consequences occur mainly with a complete uterine rupture.
- Maternal
  - Haemorrhage leading to hypovalaemic shock and collapse, with a risk of maternal death.
  - Bladder injury
  - Compromisation of future fertility due to hysterectomy or repair of
  - rupture and tubal sterilisation being carried out

- Adverse psychological effects especially in traumatic ruptures and in cases resulting in perinatal death.

- Fetal
  - Hypoxia or anoxia, acidosis and a high risk of death in utero
  - High risk of admission to neonatal intensive care unit and neonatal death.

- Partial rupture
  - Usually not life-threatening to the mother or fetus. However a lateral extension of an incomplete uterine rupture can lead to extensive haemorrhage into the broad ligament and be potentially life-threatening to both mother and fetus.

- Medico-legal
  - Clinical negligence claims are possible especially in uterine rupture following induction and/or augmentation of labour, operative vaginal delivery and trial of vaginal birth after previous CS (VBAC)
  - Involvement of judicial medical team essential in all cases of maternal death or traumatic uterine rupture.

Key pointers

- Uterine scar
  - Upper-segment caesarean section scar has a higher risk of uterine rupture compared with LSCS scar [6].

- Risk of uterine scar dehiscence in lower-segment vertical incisions is comparable with that of lower-segment transverse incisions [7, 8].
- Prior single-layer closure carries more than double the risk of uterine rupture compared with double-layer closure [9].
- Although sonographic assessment of lower uterine segment and measurement of its thickness is a strong predictor for its strength and integrity, standardised measurement techniques and ideal cut-off values are yet to be established [10].
- Risk of rupture following hysterotomy is similar to risk of an USCS scar [11].
- Risk of rupture following myomectomy is significantly increased if the endometrial cavity has been opened during the procedure. Laparoscopic myomectomy, if performed by an expert, does not carry an increased risk of subsequent uterine rupture compared with myomectomy via laparotomy [12, 13].
- Uterine perforation also could lead to a uterine rupture.

- Induction and/or augmentation of labour with prostaglandins or oxytocin

  - Especially when used during vaginal birth after caesarean (VBACS) or in the presence of a previous uterine scar or cephalopelvic disproportion [14].

- Obstructed labour, especially in low-resource settings.
- Grande multiparity [15].
- Obstetric manipulation

  - Internal podalic version and breech extraction for the delivery of the second twin.
  - Forceps delivery carried out in an unsuitable patient by an inexperienced obstetrician.
  - Rotational forceps delivery.

Key diagnostic signs

- Depends on the site, extent and timing of the uterine rupture.
- Broad spectrum of symptoms and signs:

  - A scar dehiscence could be asymptomatic while a complete rupture could lead to hypovalaemic shock, collapse, fetal demise and even maternal death.

- Impending or early uterine rupture: A knowledge of symptoms and signs and a high index of suspicion is needed:

  - Constant lower abdominal pain.
  - Tenderness over the LSCS scar is non-specific. However, an increasing point tenderness is significant.
  - Vaginal bleeding associated with fetal distress and/or previous uterine scar.
  - Haematuria and bladder tenderness especially with a previous lower segment scar.
  - Maternal tachycardia.
  - Fetal tachycardia, variable and late decelerations, and bradycardia.

- Classical intrapartum rupture:

  - Severe abdominal pain.
  - Cessation of uterine contractions.
  - Abdominal swelling and alteration in the shape of abdomen (fetal parts palpable easily/two swellings).
  - Symptoms and signs of severe haemorrhage and collapse.
  - Persistent fetal bradycardia or absent fetal heart sounds.

Key actions [16–19]

Assessment and resuscitation

- Assess vital signs.
- Initial supportive treatment.
- Management of haemorrhagic shock and resuscitation of a collapsed woman.

Definitive surgery

- Incision

  - Pfannenstiel incision: rupture of lower segment caesarean scar.
  - Lower midline incision: fundal rupture is suspected or rapid entry is needed or if it is a traumatic rupture.

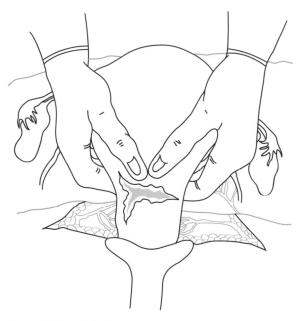

Figure 8.1 Exteriorisation of the uterus.

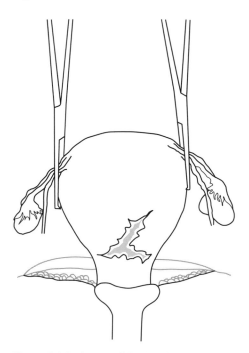

Figure 8.2 Reduction of bleeding from ovarian arterial supply.

- Delivery of the fetus and placenta
  - Through the partial or complete rupture.
  - Occasionally the fetus (sometimes together with placenta) may be completely extruded into the abdominal cavity.

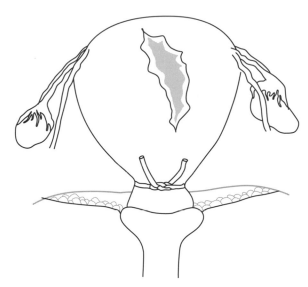

Figure 8.3 Reduction of bleeding from uterine arterial supply.

- Exteriorise the uterus (Figure 8.1)
  - Manually pulling the uterus out of the pelvis will reduce bleeding and also give a better view of the posterior aspect of the uterus and the broad ligament, and also help to identify the ruptured site/s and lacerations.

- Arrest bleeding
  - Apply Green Armytage forceps to the bleeding edges.
  - Apply two large straight clamps across the round ligament and fallopian tube along the uterine body to reduce bleeding from the ovarian arterial supply (Figure 8.2) if a total/subtotal hysterectomy is considered necessary.

- In a case of a simple laceration of the fundal region or upper segment of the uterus, a Foley catheter or a piece of intravenous tubing can be passed around the lower uterine segment and tightened to occlude the uterine arteries (Figure 8.3). Pull the uterus up and transilluminate the broad ligament to find a vascular space opposite the lower uterine segment to pass the tubes.

- In cases of heavy bleeding an assistant should manually compress the aorta until other measures are adopted to arrest bleeding.

- Clear the field

- Use suction and mopping to clean away the blood and properly visualise and assess the laceration/s.
- Decide on the surgery
  - In a case of simple lacerations or scar rupture (lower segment/classical) a simple repair of the laceration is appropriate. A continuous suture with No. 1 Vicryl in double layers will be appropriate in most cases. However, interrupted sutures may become necessary depending on the surgical complexity of the rupture. Always look for lateral extension of the laceration, as it could lead to a haematoma or haemorrhage into the broad ligament if undetected.
  - In cases of dehiscence of LSCS scars, it is advisable to trim the edges and suture the more viable parts. Consider tubal ligation in all cases of repair. Tubal ligation can be omitted in simple and uninfected ruptures if the woman has a strong desire to retain fertility. However, this should ideally be discussed with the woman before surgery if circumstances permit. If the uterine rupture warrants hysterectomy (extensive laceration), a subtotal hysterectomy is advisable where the cervix and paracolpos are not involved and there is no sepsis. This procedure can be performed rapidly and the risk of trauma to the bladder and ureters is minimal. However if the cervix and paracolpos are involved or if there is sepsis a total hysterectomy should be performed.
  - In all cases of lower segment rupture carefully check the bladder integrity as it is liable to get damaged because of its adherence to the lower segment. A marking medium could be used (methylene blue or sterile milk) in suspicious cases. Sterile milk is preferable to methylene blue as it could be re-used after repairing the laceration. A bladder laceration should be sutured in two layers in continuous running sutures using 3/0 Vicryl or its equivalent.
- Insert a drain if necessary.
- Give peri-operative antibiotics.
- Thromboprophylaxis should be considered in all cases.
- A proper documentation of the event which led to the uterine rupture as well as a description of the rupture along with the type of surgery undertaken is very important.
- The whole sequence of events should be discussed with the patient by an experienced obstetrician or the doctor who did the definitive surgery.
- In cases where the uterus is preserved and tubal ligation was not done, it is very important to give contraceptives for a minimum of 2 years. Any subsequent pregnancies should be monitored closely and an elective caesarean section should be considered soon after 34 weeks of gestation.

Key pitfalls

- Not suspecting scar rupture if there is vaginal bleeding in a woman undergoing trial of VBACS.
- Using oxytocin or prostaglandin injudiciously, especially in cases of scarred uterus or multiparous women.
- Ignoring gross haematuria even if it is after a successful vaginal delivery.
- Missing a lateral extension of the rupture into the broad ligament or an extension of the rupture into the cervix or vagina.
- Failing to identify bladder damage during the repair of a uterine rupture.
- Failing to appreciate that a uterine rupture could co-exist with or be mistaken for a placental abruption in a scarred uterus.
- Leaving unattended a woman complaining of persistent and increasing scar pain or tenderness.

Key pearls

- Anticipation of uterine rupture and early diagnosis is the key to good perinatal and maternal outcomes.
- Recognition of cephalopelvic disproportion or malposition is essential prior to augmentation of labour in all women, especially with secondary inertia or prolongation of the second stage of labour.
- Continuous electronic fetal heart monitoring is indicated for woman undergoing VBACS or trial of labour with a scarred uterus.

Management in low-resource settings

The causes for uterine rupture are different in low resource settings [20–22] and are more commonly due to neglected obstructed labour, unmonitored labour in a scarred uterus, high parity and injudicious use of oxytocin.

Primary precautions to prevent uterine rupture are most important. Increased motivation and encouraging early prenatal care will enable the detection of risk factors which could be managed appropriately. For women with high-risk factors for uterine rupture, contraceptive counselling and provision of long-term contraception is needed. All women with a risk of possible uterine rupture during labour should be referred well in advance to a tertiary care hospital with facilities for comprehensive emergency obstetric care such as blood transfusion services, operating theatres and good neonatal care. To complement early detection of risk factors and referral by improved prenatal care, the development of good transport and referral services and easy access for tertiary care are also needed.

Training of all maternity care-givers in the anticipation and early detection of symptoms and signs of impending rupture as well as diagnosis of a uterine rupture, and skills training on basic emergency life-saving skills in a case of suspected or diagnosed uterine rupture is needed. Training in the surgical management of a ruptured uterus is required in all tertiary care settings even in communities with limited resources.

Training and assessment

Simulation training for a situation such as management of uterine rupture in a routine skills and drills session is difficult.

However, this should be introduced in a feasible way to improve the clinical knowledge and skills as well as team working.

A suggested training scenario

A 31-year-old woman having an uncomplicated second pregnancy at 39 weeks' gestation after a previous caesarean section 3 years earlier for breech presentation, is undergoing a trial of VBAC.

The following equipment should be made available for the drill:

- A bed.
- An obstetric manikin with a detachable abdominal cover.
- Baby with cord.

- Pinard, handheld Doppler fetal heart monitor, cardiotocograph (CTG) machine.
- Intravenous cannulae without needles (22G + 16G).
- Normal saline and Ringer's lactate packs.
- Blood transfusion set.
- Foley catheter.
- Face mask and oxygen source.
- Case notes.
- Drug chart.
- Disposable syringes without needles.
- Gauze towels.
- Green Armytage forceps.
- Long and straight artery forceps.
- Tissue catch forceps.
- Needle holder.
- Suture materials.
- Scissors.

The trainer should ask the trainee: 'Demonstrate how you will manage her labour'.

The expected responses and actions would be:

- IV access with 16G cannula.
- Group and Save + Full Blood Count.
- Maintain partogram.
- Continuous close monitoring of fetus with best available facilities.
- Epidural anaesthesia/other appropriate pain relief (depending on setting).
- Ranitidine and metoclopramide 8-hourly.

'What are the warning signs for an impending scar rupture?'

The expected responses should be:

- Fetal heart rate (FHR) abnormalities:
  - Tachycardia.
  - Variable decelerations.
  - Prolonged decelerations or bradycardia.

- Severe/persistent lower abdominal pain.
- Vaginal bleeding.
- Haematuria.
- Receding presenting part on vaginal examination.

Scenario continues – the trainer states: 'After 8 hours of active labour there is a sudden onset of fetal bradycardia along with fresh vaginal bleeding [if CTG is available a trace with sudden bradycardia is shown]. What will you do?'

The expected responses and actions would be:

- Call for help.
- Quick assessment of pulse rate, BP and look for pallor.
- Abdominal examination to feel for the contractions, presenting part along with a vaginal examination to assess the cervical dilatation and station of the presenting part.
- Left lateral position.
- During this time other members of the team should have informed the operating theatre and the anaesthesiologist.
- Consultant obstetrician.
- Neonatologist and neonatal intensive care unit.
- Commenced oxygen by face mask 15 litres/minute.
- Transfer the patient to the operating theatre for 'Category 1 Delivery'.

On abdominal examination the fetal head is 2/5th palpable and on vaginal examination the cervix is 8 cm dilated.

The trainer asks: 'What actions you will take in the operating theatre?'

The expected responses and actions would be:

- Prepare for laparotomy.
- One team member explains the procedure to the patient and obtains verbal consent.
- Pfannenstiel incision.
- Delivery of the fetus and hand over to the neonatologist.
- Delivery of the placenta with the membranes.
- Exteriorise uterus after informing the anaesthetist.
- Achieve haemostasis by applying Green Armytage forceps.
- Clean the operative field by mopping and suction.
- Repair the laceration with No. 1 Vicryl continuous sutures, in double layers.
- Consider tubal ligation – depending on the severity of the laceration and patient's wishes for future fertility.
- By this time other members of the team should have:

    · Documented the events and treatment given in chronological order.
    · Commenced blood transfusion if the bleeding was severe or patient was haemodynamically unstable.

The training programme should consist of a brief account on key facts, key implications, key pointers and key diagnostic signs on uterine rupture. This should be followed by the case scenario and the drill.

At the end of the training session both the trainees and the trainer should give feedback on the performance. A repeat training programme should be planned to improve the skills of all members of the team.

Acknowledgement

Doctors Myuru Manawadu and D.V. Priyaranjana of the Department of Obstetrics and Gynaecology, University of Ruhuna contributed the figures.

References

1. Esike CO, Umeora OU, Eze JN, Igberase GO. Ruptured uterus: the unabating obstetric catastrophe in South Eastern Nigeria. *Arch Gynaecol Obst* 2011; 285 (5): 993–997.

2. Kara M, Toz E, Yilmaz E, Oge T, Avci I, Senturk S. Analysis of uterine rupture causes in Agri: a five-year experience. *Clin Exper Obstet Gynaecol* 2010; 37 (3): 221–223.

3. Gardeil F, Daly S, Turner MJ. Uterine rupture in pregnancy reviewed. *Eur J Obstet Gynaecol Reprod Biol* 1994; 56 (2): 107–110.

4. Guise JM, McDonagh MS, Osterweil P, Nygren P, Chan BK, Helfand M. A systematic review of the incidence and consequences of uterine rupture in women with previous caesarean section. *Br Med J* 2004; 329 (7456): 19–25.

5. Keiser KE, Baskett TF. A 10 year population based study of uterine rupture. *Obstet Gynaecol* 2002; 100: 749–753.

6. Green RA, Fitzpatrick C, Turner MJ. What are the maternal implications of a classical caesarean section? *J Obstet Gynaecol* 1998; 18 (4): 345–347.

7. Shipp TD, Zelop CM, Repke JT *et al*. Intrapartum uterine rupture and dehiscence in patients with prior lower uterine segment vertical and transverse incisions. *Obstet Gynaecol* 1999; 94 (5 pt 1): 735–740.

8. Naef RW, Ray MA, Chauhan SP *et al*. Trial of labour after caesarean delivery with a lower-segment, vertical uterine incision: is it safe? *Amer J Obstet Gynaecol* 1995; 172 (6): 1666–1673.

9. Bujold E, Goyet M, Marcoux S *et al*. The role of uterine closure in the risk of uterine rupture. *Obstet Gynaecol* 2010; 116 (1): 43–50.

10. Jastrow N, Chaillet N, Roberge S *et al.* Sonographic lower uterine segment thickness on risk of uterine scar defect: a systematic review. *J Obstet Gynaecol Can* 2010; 32 (4): 321–327.

11. Claw N, Crompton AC. The wounded uterus: pregnancy after hysterotomy. *Br Med J* 1973; 1: 21–23.

12. Seracchiodi R, Manuzzi L, Vianello F *et al.* Obstetric and delivery outcome of pregnancies achieved after laparoscopic myomectomy. *Fertil Steril* 2006; 86 (1): 159–165.

13. Sizzi O, Rosetti A, Malzoni M *et al.* Italian multicentre study on complications of laparoscopic myomectomy. *J Min Invas Gynaecol* 2007; 14 (4): 453–462.

14. Ravasia DJ, Wood SL, Pollard JK. Uterine rupture during induced trial of labour among women with previous caesarean delivery. *Am J Obstet Gynaecol* 2000; 103 (5): 1176–1179.

15. Golan A, Sandbank O, Rubin A. Rupture of the pregnant uterus. *Obstet Gynaecol* 1980; 56 (5): 549–554.

16. Plauche WC, Von Almen W, Muller R. Catastrophic uterine rupture. *Obstet Gynaecol* 1984; 64 (6): 792–797.

17. Schrinsky DC, Benson RC. Rupture of the pregnant uterus: a review. *Obstet Gynaecol Surv* 1978; 33 (4): 217–232.

18. Draycott T, Winter C, Crofts J, Barnfield S (Eds.) *PROMPT. Practical Obstetric Multiprofessional Training: Course Manual.* London: RCOG, 2008; pp. 3–10 and 69–85.

19. Rahman J, Al-Sibai MH, Rahman MS. Rupture of the uterus in labour. A review of 96 cases. *Acta Obstet Gynaecol Scand* 1985; 64 (4): 311–315.

20. Rizwan N, Abbasi RM, Uddin SF. Uterine rupture, frequency of cases and feto-maternal outcome. *J Pakistan Med Assoc* 2011; 64 (4): 322–324.

21. Osaikhuwuomwan JA, Ande AB. Reappraisal of ruptured uterus in an urban tertiary centre in the Niger-delta region of Nigeria. *J Matern Fetal Neonat Med* 2011; 24 (4): 559–563.

22. Ali AA, Adam I. Maternal and perinatal outcomes of uterine rupture in the Kossala Hospital, East Sudan: 2006–2009. *J Obstet Gynaecol* 2011; 31 (1): 48–49.

Chapter

9

Breech delivery

Osama Abu-Ghazza and Edwin Chandraharan

Definition

- The term 'breech' refers to the lower, rear part of the trunk of the body and is believed to be derived from the word 'britches', which is a cloth used to cover the loins and thighs.
- Breech presentation occurs when the buttocks and/or feet are in relation to the lower uterine segment, with the fetus in a longitudinal lie, and hence are the first to engage when labour commences.

Incidence

- The incidence of breech presentation decreases as the gestational age advances and by 36 weeks the majority of fetuses turn spontaneously to cephalic presentation, adopting the 'best fit' position that a normal gravid uterus provides.
- Incidence of breech presentation at 28 weeks' gestation is about 22%; it is 7% at 32 weeks and 1–3% of births at term [1, 2].

Types of breech

Three types of breech presentation have been described (Figure 9.1).

(a) Frank breech (50–70%): breech with extended legs (common in primigravidas).
(b) Complete breech (10–30%): breech with fully flexed legs (common in multiparous women).
(c) Footling breech (5–10%): with one or both thighs extended (rare, except in preterm labour).

(d) A fourth type, knee presentation (Figure 9.1d), is sometimes described but it is very rare.

Key implications

- Breech presentation at time of delivery is associated with increased perinatal mortality and morbidity. This higher perinatal mortality and morbidity with breech than cephalic presentation can be due to prematurity itself, congenital malformations and birth-related asphyxia or trauma [3, 4].
- Any factor that affects the uterine shape and tone, passenger (fetal size, maturity, structure and number) and passage (both bony pelvis and soft tissues) can predispose to breech presentation. Table 9.1 shows such predisposing factors for breech presentation. A high index of suspicion for possible breech presentation is recommended if any of these risk factors are identified during pregnancy.
- Antenatal and intrapartum identification of breech presentation may help improve perinatal outcome by optimising the individualised mode of delivery.
- Vaginal breech deliveries were the norm until 1959 when it was proposed that all breech presentations should be delivered by caesarean section to reduce perinatal morbidity and mortality; a more recent study favoured caesarean section over vaginal breech delivery for the same reasons [5, 6].
- Currently, in northern Europe and North America, caesarean section has become the accepted mode of delivery for breech presentation. However, a long-term follow-up of

Obstetric and Intrapartum Emergencies, ed. Edwin Chandraharan and Sabaratnam Arulkumaran. Published by Cambridge University Press. © Cambridge University Press 2012.

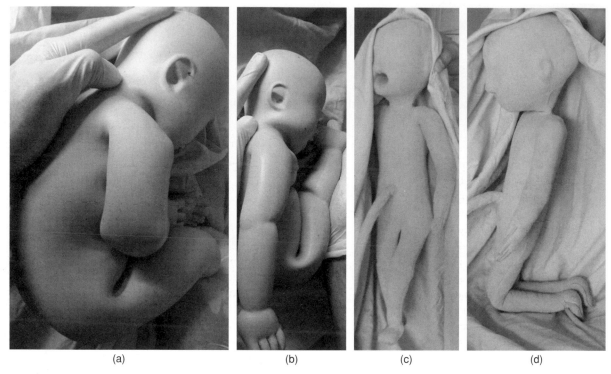

(a)   (b)   (c)   (d)

Figure 9.1 Types of breech. (a) Complete breech – flexion at hip and knee joints (elbows flexed too). (b) Extended breech – flexion at the hip but extension at the knee joint. (c) Footling breech – extension at both hip and knee joints. (d) Knee presentation.

Table 9.1 Predisposing factors for breech presentation.

Uterine
- Uterine malformation (e.g. bicornuate or septate uterus)
- Uterine fibroids
- Lax uterus (grand multiparity)
- Polyhydramnios (alters the pyriform shape of the uterus)
- Placenta praevia or cornual placental position

Fetal
- Prematurity
- Multiple pregnancy
- Previous breech presentation
- Fetal malformation (e.g. hydrocephalus, anencephaly)

Pelvis
- Fibroids in the lower uterine segment extending into the pelvis
- Pelvic masses (e.g. ovarian cysts, pelvic kidney)
- Abnormalities in the bony pelvis (congenital and acquired)

breech-presented babies suggested that whatever the mode of delivery, breech presentation is associated with increased risk of subsequent handicap [7]. There is a suggestion that failure to adopt the cephalic presentation may in itself be a marker for fetal neurological impairment and hence, the perinatal outcome may be uninfluenced by the mode of delivery.

Table 9.2 Options for management of breech presentation.

- External cephalic version (ECV)
- Spontaneous breech delivery
- Assisted vaginal breech delivery
- Total breech extraction
- Elective caesarean section

Management options of breech presentation

Management of breech presentation varies and depends on both clinical findings and a woman's choice. Table 9.2 illustrates the management options for a breech presentation. Management of breech presentation should be individualised by comparing the potential maternal and perinatal risks associated with different options, after considering the given clinical situation.

The Royal College of Obstetrician and Gynae-cologists in the UK currently recommends external cephalic version (ECV) to reduce the incidence of breech presentation at term, and consequently to reduce the risks associated with having a caesarean section [8]. The authors recommend ECV, provided there is no contraindication, to be performed from 36 weeks' gestation onwards. Antepartum ECV is outside the scope of this chapter as it is not part of managing an 'obstetric emergency'.

- **Spontaneous breech delivery.** Mother spontaneously delivers the baby without any traction or manipulation of the fetus. This usually occurs in severely preterm deliveries, often before viable gestations. Such an 'unassisted' breech delivery is not recommended at term.
- **Assisted vaginal breech delivery** is the recommended type of vaginal breech delivery. The accoucher usually conducts the delivery and initiates special manoeuvres to deliver the extended legs, arms and head as required.
- **Total breech extraction** refers to the procedure in which fetal feet are grasped, and the entire fetus is extracted. Total breech extraction is usually used at caesarean section for malpositioned babies and commonly for a non-cephalic second twin; it should not be used for a singleton fetus vaginal breech delivery because the cervix may not be adequately dilated to allow passage of the fetal head.

Key pointers to management: scientific evidence

- The Term Breech Trial recommended planned elective caesarean section for babies presenting by breech presentation at term [9]. This was because the perinatal morbidity and mortality were significantly higher in the vaginal delivery as compared with babies delivered by a planned caesarean section (5% vs 1.6%).

  - More recent observational prospective studies with an intent-to-treat analysis concluded that, in units where strict criteria are met before and during labour, planned vaginal breech delivery of a singleton at term remains a safe option that can be offered to women [10]. In this study, of the 2526 women with planned vaginal deliveries, 1796 delivered vaginally (71%). The rate of neonatal morbidity or death was considerably lower than the 5% in the Term Breech Trial (1.60%; 95% CI, 1.14–2.17) and not significantly different from the planned caesarean section group [10].

Table 9.3 Contraindications to assisted vaginal breech delivery.

- Any preexisting contraindications to vaginal birth (e.g. placenta praevia, compromised fetal condition, uterine malformations)
- Inadequate pelvis (on clinical examination or prior radiological evidence e.g. road traffic accident with pelvic fractures)
- Footling or kneeling breech presentation (Fig 9.1c, d)
- Large baby (usually defined as larger than 3800 g)
- Growth-restricted baby (usually defined as smaller than 2000 g)
- 'Star-gazing' appearance – Hyperextended fetal neck in labour (diagnosed with ultrasound or X-ray where ultrasound is not available)
- Unavailability of a clinician trained in vaginal breech delivery, *at the time of birth*
- Previous caesarean section (relative contraindication)

  - Caesarean section is associated with increased maternal morbidity in comparison to vaginal breech delivery [11]. In this regard, the methodology and findings of the Original Term Breech Trial have been questioned [12].
  - Two-years' follow-up of babies from the Term Breech Trial did not show any significant differences between assisted vaginal breech delivery and a planned caesarean section [13].
  - In view of the above evidence, women should be supported if they make an informed decision to attempt an assisted vaginal birth or arrive in advanced labour [14].
  - The findings of the Term Breech Trial, which was about elective delivery of term breeches, should not be blindly applied to preterm breech delivery, breech presentation in advanced labour and second of twins presenting by breech after the delivery of the first twin.

Key actions: how to conduct a vaginal breech delivery

Before allowing a vaginal breech delivery it is crucial to exclude the contraindications which are listed in Table 9.3.

A key role of the accoucher is to prevent fetal hypoxia and trauma that may arise from unrecognised cord prolapse, poor 'traumatic' handling of the fetus or due to difficulty or delay in delivering the after-coming head (Table 9.4).

Table 9.4 Potential complications of assisted vaginal breech delivery.

- Hypoxic ischaemic injury due to umbilical cord compression or cord prolapse
- Prolonged labour (ineffective cervical dilatation by the 'soft' breech)
- Intracranial haemorrhage
- Injury to 'intra-abdominal' abdominal organs
- Fracture of the bones (humerus, clavicle, femur and neck)
- Nerve injuries (cervical plexus, brachial plexus, spinal cord)
- Dislocation of the jaw (malconducted Mauriceau–Smellie–Veit manoeuvre by placing the fingers inside the mouth instead of on the malar eminences)

Principles and tips for assisted vaginal breech delivery

- In a hospital setting it is advisable to ensure a multidisciplinary approach when conducting an assisted vaginal breech delivery. This involves the presence of a skilled obstetrician, an anaesthetist, a paediatrician and a midwife.
- Before allowing vaginal breech delivery it is important to confirm the presenting part by performing a vaginal examination. Frank and complete breech are suitable for a trial of vaginal delivery provided cord prolapse or cord presentation is excluded on vaginal examination.
- The fetal sacrum is a landmark for breech presentation and is essential to identify the fetal position: whether the fetus is presenting sacro-anterior or posterior.
- It is preferable to leave fetal membranes if they are still intact as long as possible to act as a dilating wedge on the cervix to ensure maximum cervical dilatation before the fetal parts descend. At any stage if fetal membranes rupture, a vaginal examination is immediately recommended to rule out cord prolapse.
- Use of oxytocin during assisted vaginal breech delivery is controversial. In the authors' experience, oxytocin in the first stage of labour is safe for augmentation of labour to achieve optimum uterine contractions and to ensure recommended cervical dilation (0.5 cm–1 cm per hour) provided there is no evidence of fetal compromise. If oxytocin is used, it is essential to carefully monitor uterine contractions to ensure that there are no more than 3–4 contractions in 10 minutes, each lasting for 40–60 seconds. Continuous electronic fetal monitoring using a cardiotocograph (CTG) is also essential to timely recognise and appropriately intervene, if there is any evidence of fetal compromise.

- In second stage of labour, oxytocin should be used with caution and relative or absolute feto-pelvic disproportion should be excluded. A decision to use oxytocin in the second stage of labour, after excluding the above, should be made by a senior and experienced clinician, *directly supervising* the management of second stage of labour.
- An episiotomy may be performed as a prophylactic measure when the breech delivery is imminent, even in multiparous women. It has been advocated to prevent possibility of soft tissue dystocia.
- It is important to note that passage of thick meconium is a common finding as the breech (i.e. the rectum) is squeezed by the muscles of the maternal pelvic floor, as it descends through the birth canal. Such passage of meconium is usually not associated with meconium aspiration as the meconium passes out of the vagina and does not usually mix with the amniotic fluid.
- Once the buttocks of the fetus or feet are visible, it is crucial not to pull by the feet because this action may precipitate head entrapment in an incompletely dilated cervix or may precipitate nuchal arms by causing extension of the fetal arms. Instead it is a good practice to prevent a quick drop of feet or buttocks by putting the palm on the introitous and resisting the fetus for a couple of contractions; this may help in stretching the cervix and pelvic passages and prevent entrapment of the head.
- If the breech emerges out of the vagina with the sacrum facing posteriorly, the sacrum should be rotated 180° in order to maintain the sacro-anterior position. This is to ensure that the fetus will face down and will help to avoid deflexion of the fetal head that may lead to head entrapment.

Technique of assisted vaginal breech delivery

For simplicity, conduct of assisted vaginal breech delivery will be considered in three parts:

(a) Delivery of the legs and buttocks.
(b) Delivery of the trunk and shoulders.
(c) Delivery of the 'after-coming' head.

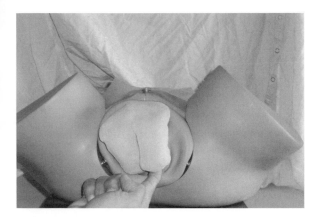

Figure 9.2 Pinard's manoeuvre: note the finger gently pressing on the popliteal fossa to enable flexion at the knee joint, followed by abduction and external rotation of the thigh to deliver the fetal lower limb.

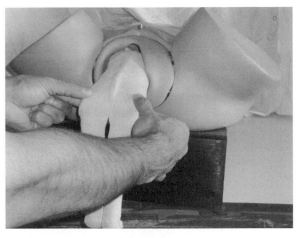

Figure 9.3 Holding the fetus at the hips and not on the abdomen to avoid injury to internal organs (hepatic or splenic rupture).

Delivery of the legs and buttocks

Spontaneous expulsion of both feet and buttocks with progressive uterine contractions and maternal effort is the norm, especially in flexed or complete breech. However, in cases of frank breech presentation, the 'Pinard manoeuvre' can be used to help delivering the fetal legs but only after the fetal umbilicus is at or just above the introitus. The Pinard manoeuvre involves application of pressure in the popliteal fossa of the knee joint which results in flexion of the knee. This is followed by abduction of the thighs with the lower leg swept medially out of the vagina (Figure 9.2).

Once the feet and buttocks are delivered, it is essential to ensure that the fetal sacrum is kept anterior. It is good practice to cover the fetal back with a warm towel to ensure that the cold air does not stimulate the 'first breath', whilst the head is still inside the vagina.

The umbilical cord should not be handled at this stage as this may stimulate spasm of umbilical vessels.

Delivery of the trunk and shoulders

It is best to allow uterine contractions to progressively expel the fetal trunk and shoulders. If necessary, the fetus should be held at the bony pelvis (i.e. at the hips) to ensure that the sacrum is maintained anteriorly whilst further descent occurs (Figure 9.3). This is to avoid inadvertent damage to internal organs by compression on the fetal abdomen by hands placed above the bony pelvis.

When the inferior angle of the scapula becomes visible (lower-most angle of the triangular 'shoulder

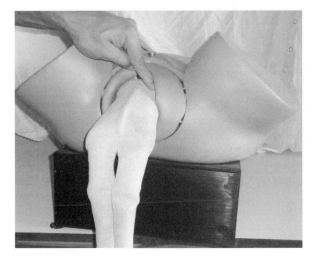

Figure 9.4 Identifying the 'inferior' angle of the scapula prior to delivering the shoulders

blade'), attempts should be made to deliver the shoulders (Figure 9.4). At this stage the position of the arms should be noted and if arms are flexed, they could be delivered one after the other by simply hooking down the elbows.

However, if extended or 'nuchal arms' are encountered, a Løvset's manoeuvre (Figure 9.5) may be used to deliver the extended or nuchal arms.

Løvset's manoeuvre involves rotation of the fetus 90° anticlockwise to deliver the anterior shoulder first by adduction and flexion of the shoulder followed by extension at the elbow; this helps to bring down the forearm and hand. Once the anterior arm is delivered,

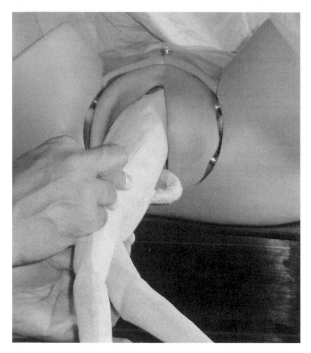

Figure 9.5 Løvset's manoeuvre: Initial rotation of the shoulders 90° anticlockwise to bring the anterior shoulder under the symphysis pubis.

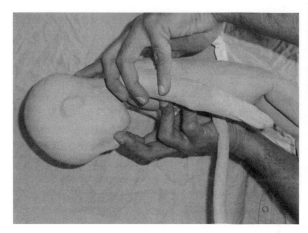

Figure 9.6 Mauriceau–Smellie–Veit manoeuvre: Flexion of the head by applying 'forward' pressure on the occiput and 'backward' pressure on malar eminences, whilst resting the fetal trunk on the accoucher's forearms.

the fetus should be gently rotated 180° clockwise. This movement would allow the posterior shoulder, which is below the sacral promontory, to become anterior below the symphysis pubis.

During Løvset's manoeuvre, the fetus should be held with thumbs on the sacrum and index fingers on the anterior superior iliac spines to avoid inadvertent injury to intraperitoneal organs during movements.

Delivery of the 'after-coming' head

This is the most crucial aspect of breech delivery that requires timely and purposeful assistance by the accoucher to avoid injury and trauma. The interval between delivery of umbilicus and delivery of mouth preferably should not exceed 10 minutes. Further delay in delivering the head is likely to lead to fetal hypoxia due to possible umbilical cord compression by the entrapped fetal head.

Appearance of the nape of the neck or the 'hairline' at the introitus indicates that the fetal head has now entered the lower pelvis and hence, assistance may be provided to deliver the head. The fetal head should be maintained in a flexed position during delivery to allow passage of the smallest diameter of the

head. Application of supra-pubic pressure by an assistant may aid this process.

Three methods may be employed to deliver the after-coming head:

(1) Mauriceau–Smellie–Veit manoeuvre.
(2) Burns–Marshall method.
(3) Forceps delivery.

The Mauriceau–Smellie–Veit manoeuvre is aimed at flexing the fetal head to reduce the presenting diameters to facilitate delivery in a controlled manner (Figure 9.6). This involves flexion of the head by applying 'forward' pressure on the occiput and 'backward' pressure on malar eminences, whilst resting the fetal trunk on the accoucher's forearms. The left hand supports the fetal neck, whereas accoucher's index and middle fingers of the right hand are placed on malar eminences on the fetal maxilla to help maintain flexion of the head.

The Burns–Marshall method involves allowing the breech to 'hang' by its weight until the nape of the neck (or the 'hair-line') is visible. This is followed by holding both feet and the fetus on to the maternal abdomen to deliver the fetal head. Care should be taken to avoid hyperextension of the fetal spine and also sudden 'popping out' of the fetal head that may cause intracranial bleeding.

Forceps may be used to facilitate delivery of the after-coming head as the primary mode of delivery if other methods are not successful or when traction of

During delivery of the head, it is essential to avoid extreme elevation of the body, which may result in hyperextension of the cervical spine and potential neurological injury.

Caesarean section for breech presentation

Principles of assisted vaginal breech delivery are applicable during caesarean section as well and the same manoeuvres could be employed. Sacrum should be maintained anteriorly.

Size of the skin and uterine incisions should be planned in accordance with the size of the fetus and any anticipated difficulties (transverse lie) during delivery.

It is good practice to use forceps to deliver the after-coming head. Hyper-extension of the fetal spine should be avoided and the assistant should be asked to exert downward pressure on the uterus to keep the fetal head flexed.

During emergency caesarean section, it is essential to avoid inadvertent fetal 'cut injuries' and the site of the uterine incision should be carefully selected, based on the peritoneal reflection of the utero-vesical fold to avoid inadvertent opening into the vagina.

Women in advanced labour should be re-examined in the operating theatre prior to commencing caesarean section to ensure that delivery is not imminent. If this is the case, women should be counselled and assisted vaginal delivery should be conducted to avoid maternal and fetal trauma.

During caesarean section, breech should be disengaged first, prior to delivery.

Total breech extraction

In modern obstetric practice, total breech extraction may be attempted during a caesarean section for transverse lie after an internal podalic version to convert transverse lie to a breech presentation. Alternatively, after the delivery of the first twin, total breech extraction may be carried out for the second twin presenting by transverse lie after successful internal podalic version or rarely, for fetal compromise of the second twin with a breech presentation.

The procedure involves holding a foot to bring both feet to the uterine incision (during caesarean section) or to the upper vagina (delivery of the second twin)

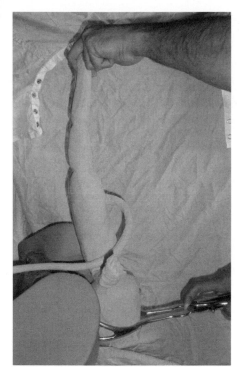

Figure 9.7 Use of forceps to deliver after-coming head.

the infant head is not required. Forceps are recommended in special clinical circumstances such as primiparous women or when the fetus is growth-restricted or premature as forceps may protect the fetal head and potentially avoid 'compression' of the fetal head by pelvic floor muscles followed by sudden 'decompression' as it emerges out of the introitus. Such sudden 'compression–decompression' may result in shearing of intracerebral veins resulting in intracranial haemorrhage.

Piper forceps and Elliot forceps are specially designed for this task but they are not universally available. Any forceps with a long shank (i.e. not Wrigley's) may be used. Forceps help to keep the fetal head flexed during delivery of the after-coming head. An assistant is required to hold the feet while the operator applies the blades of the forceps on the fetal head (Figure 9.7).

Piper forceps are specialised forceps used only for the after-coming head of a breech presentation. They are used to keep the fetal head flexed during extraction of the head. An assistant is needed to hold the infant while the operator gets on one knee to apply the forceps from below.

and then taking hold of both feet and gently applying traction to deliver both feet, legs, trunk and shoulders. The after-coming head should be delivered as described earlier.

Breech delivery in a low-resource setting

Breech delivery encompasses the old obstetric adage 'Masterly Inactivity and Timely Interference'. Most breech babies can be safely delivered without any obstetrical interventions even in low-resource settings. Hence a 'hands-off' policy is recommended in the early stages with intermittent auscultation of fetal heart rate to exclude fetal compromise.

During the second stage of labour, spontaneous expulsion of the feet, buttocks, trunk and shoulders should be encouraged with assistance if required (Pinard's manoeuvre, Løvset's manoeuvre). Suprapubic pressure may be useful in keeping the fetal head flexed during delivery of the after-coming head. If suitable forceps are not available, the Mauriceau–Smellie–Veit manoeuvre should be used.

Avoid unnecessary 'pulling' as it may result in nuchal arms and hyper-extension of the fetal head.

Key pitfalls

- Application of the findings of the Term Breech Trial to breech in advanced labour, preterm breech or second of twins presenting by breech.
- Undue panic and haste that cause additional problems such as hyperextension of fetal head or nuchal arms.
- Failure to conduct vaginal examination prior to an emergency caesarean section to exclude 'breech at the perineum'.
- Failure to avoid sudden compression–decompression injury by uncontrolled delivery of the fetal head.

Key pearls

- Recognise breech presentation early, determine suitability for assisted vaginal birth and counsel appropriately.
- Experienced clinician should be present at the time of birth.
- Avoid 'pulling' and undue assistance to avoid hyper-extension of the fetal head and nuchal arms.

- Regular skills and drills training in assisted vaginal breech delivery to improve knowledge and skills.
- Masterly inactivity and timely interference – 'Passive assistance up to the shoulders and active involvement for the after-coming head'.

Suggested algorithm for assisted vaginal breech delivery

B – *Breech to shoulder* – *Be calm*. Once contraindications for assisted vaginal breech delivery are excluded, **step back** and allow spontaneous expulsion (use Pinard's manoeuvre, if necessary) of the fetus up to the inferior angle of the scapula.

Be prepared – with neonatal team, anaesthetist and inform experienced clinician.

R – *Release* (flexed arms) or *Rotate* (Løvset's manoeuvre for nuchal or extended arms) when the inferior angle of the scapula is visible. *Reassure* the patient throughout birth.

E – *Exclude* cord compression or prolapse at all times – carefully monitor fetal heart rate.

E – *Episiotomy* and *epidural* (or suitable local analgesia) as required and *Experienced* clinician in attendance.

C – *Caution* against cervical spine injury and internal organ injury (sacrum should be kept anterior, baby should be held at the bony pelvis and there should be no hyperextension of the neck).

H – *Hair-line* (nape of the neck) at the introitus for the controlled delivery of the head (Mauriceau–Smellie–Veit manoeuvre, Burns–Marshall manoeuvre or forceps).

References

1. Hickok DE, Gordon DC, Milberg JA, Williams MA, Daling JR. The frequency of breech presentation by gestational age at birth: a large population-based study. *Am J Obstet Gynecol* 1992; 166 (3): 851–852.

2. Oats J, Abraham S. *Llewellyn-Jones Fundamentals of Obstetrics & Gynaecology*. 9th Edition. London: Mosby, 2010.

3. Pritchard JA, MacDonald PC. Dystocia caused by abnormalities in presentation, position, or development of the fetus. In Pritchard JA, MacDonald PC, Gant NF (Eds.), *Williams Obstetrics*. 17th Edition. Norwalk, CT: AppletonCentury Crofts, 1980, pp. 787–796.

4. Cheng M, Hannah M. Breech delivery at term: a critical review of the literature. *Obstet Gynecol* 1993; 82: 605–618.

5. Wright RC. Reduction of perinatal mortality and morbidity in breech delivery through routine use of cesarean section. *Obstet Gynecol* 1959; 14: 758–763.

6. Ghosh MK. Breech presentation: evolution of management. *J Reprod Med* 2005; 50: 108–116.

7. Danielian PJ, Wang J, Hall MH. Long-term outcome by method of delivery of fetuses in breech presentation at term: population based follow up. *Br Med J* 1996; 312: 1451–1453.

8. Royal College of Obstetricians and Gynaecologists. *External cephalic version and reducing the incidence of breech presentation*. Green-top Guideline No. 20a. London: RCOG, 2006.

9. Hannah ME, Hannah WJ, Hewson SA *et al*. Planned caesarean section versus planned vaginal birth for breech presentation at term: a randomised multicentre trial. *Lancet* 2000; 356 (9239): 1375–1383.

10. Goffinet F, Carayol M, Foidart JM *et al*. PREMODA Study Group. Is planned vaginal delivery for breech presentation at term still an option? Results of an observational prospective survey in France and Belgium. *Am J Obstet Gynecol* 2006; 194: 1002–1011.

11. Hofmeyr GJ, Hannah ME. Planned caesarean section for term breech delivery. *Cochrane Database Syst Rev* 2003; 2: Art. No. CD000166. doi: 10.1002/14651858. CD000166.

12. Glezerman M. Five years to the term breech trial: the rise and fall of a randomized controlled trial. *Am J Obstet Gynecol* 2006; 194: 20–25.

13. Whyte H, Hannah ME, Saigal S *et al*. for the Term Breech Trial Collaborative Group. Outcomes of children at 2 years after planned cesarean birth versus planned vaginal birth for breech presentation at term: the International Randomized Term Breech Trial. *Am J Obstet Gynecol* 2004; 191: 864–871.

14. Bewley S, Shennan A. Peer review and the Term Breech Trial. *Lancet* 2007; 369 (9565): 906.

Chapter

10

Umbilical cord prolapse

Malik Goonewardene

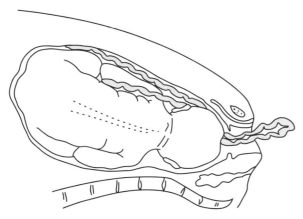

Figure 10.1 Overt cord prolapse.

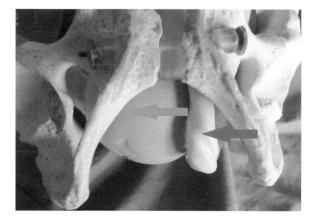

Figure 10.2 Occult cord prolapse. Arrow on right points to loop of umbilical cord protruding lying alongside the fetal head that may be easily missed on vaginal examination and hence, it is called 'occult' cord prolapse. Arrow on left (centre) shows fetal head (presenting part) lying alongside the umbilical cord.

Key facts [1, 2]

- Definition: Descent of the umbilical cord through the cervix, in the presence of ruptured membranes.
- Types: Overt – If the cord is below the presenting part and in the vagina or outside vulval introitus (Figure 10.1). Occult – If the cord is lying alongside the presenting part (Figure 10.2).
- Incidence: Varies from 0.1% – 0.6% (1–6 : 1000). Cord presentation occurs if the cord is below the presenting part but membranes are intact (Figure 10.3).

Key implications [1–5]

Cord prolapse is an obstetric emergency with a high risk of perinatal mortality (*c.* 10%).

Perinatal hypoxia, resulting from prolonged compression and mechanical occlusion of the prolapsed cord (e.g. by the fetal head which is presenting) or by vasospasm due to the relatively cooler temperatures in the vagina and especially outside the vulval introitus, is the leading cause of perinatal death.

Babies that survive may have cerebral palsy resulting from hypoxic ischaemic encephalopathy.

Cord prolapse occurring at home is associated with a higher risk of perinatal deaths.

Key pointers [1, 2, 6]

Presenting part of the fetus not fitting into the maternal pelvic inlet (e.g. small preterm baby or twin; especially the second twin, transverse lie, malpresentation such as footling or flexed breech, and polyhydramnios).

Obstetric and Intrapartum Emergencies, ed. Edwin Chandraharan and Sabaratnam Arulkumaran. Published by Cambridge University Press. © Cambridge University Press 2012.

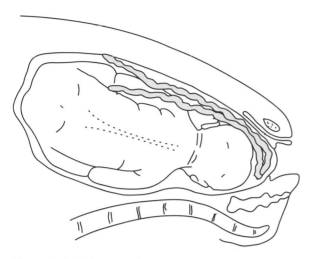

Figure 10.3 Cord presentation.

admission to hospital at 38 weeks' gestation. If this advice is declined, women should be advised immediate admission with any signs of labour or prelabour (prolonged) rupture of membranes (PROM) [2].

During labour the presence of the cord should be looked for, at each vaginal examination.

Amniotomy is contraindicated if the cord is palpable below or by the side of the presenting part during vaginal examination. Upward pressure and dislodging the head from the pelvis should be avoided during amniotomy, and amniotomy should be avoided if the presenting part of the fetus is high and mobile [2].

Women with unstable lies should be offered ripening of cervix and stabilising induction of labour after 39 weeks' gestation unless the cervix is favourable for induction by amniotomy and oxytocin infusion at that gestation. This involves external cephalic version (ECV) followed by an intravenous oxytocin infusion to stimulate uterine contractions that would stabilise the fetal head against the pelvic inlet, and then a careful controlled amniotomy after excluding a palpable cord. The same procedure could be adopted in cases of mild to moderate hydramnios. An assistant should steady the fetal head against the pelvic inlet during and after amniotomy. The amniotomy should be by minimal puncture and the fingers should be kept inside the vagina to carefully control the volume of liquor draining out. This will prevent the liquor gushing out, and the fetal head floating away from the inlet, predisposing to cord prolapse.

Grande multiparity, maternal pelvic abnormalities, relatively long cord or low placental implantations and male fetuses.

Obstetric interventions such as amniotomy, placement of internal monitoring devices, external cephalic version (ECV) and internal podalic version.

Intrapartum spontaneous rupture of membranes with advanced cervical dilation and high presenting part of fetus [6].

Key diagnostic signs

Prediction

Routine abdominal real-time colour Doppler ultrasound scan examination has not been shown to be effective in antenatal diagnosis of cord presentation and predicting the possibility of cord prolapse [7].

Selective transvaginal scanning in women with high-risk factors such as a transverse lie, malpresentation (e.g. footling or flexed breech) or high presenting part of fetus, may be useful [8].

Prevention

Women with a transverse or oblique lie or breech presentation should be offered an ECV at 37 weeks' gestation.

Women with persistent breech presentation or transverse, oblique or unstable lie should be offered

Diagnosis [2]

The possibility of cord prolapse should always be kept in mind in a woman with a risk factor for cord prolapse because signs of fetal distress may not occur immediately after cord prolapse.

Women with PROM should be offered a speculum examination irrespective of the period of gestation. A digital vaginal examination is best avoided if there is no cardiotocograph (CTG) abnormality or risk factors for cord prolapse.

A digital vaginal examination is indicated in the presence of PROM or preterm PROM (PPROM) with CTG abnormalities such as variable decelerations, prolonged decelerations and bradycardia and a suspicion of cord prolapse.

The cord may be visible outside the vulva or at the introitus or may be seen on speculum examination or felt on vaginal examination.

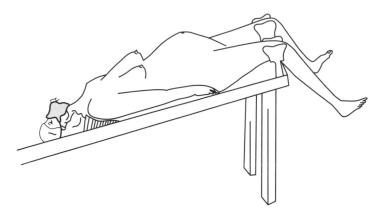

Figure 10.4 Head low position.

Key actions

Initial management

Additional help (obstetric colleagues, nurses and mid-wives) should be called for immediately, and the anaes-thesiologist and neonatologist (and the feto-maternal specialist if the gestational period is 24–28 weeks) informed.

The aim is to prevent or minimise fetal hypoxia, resulting from mechanical compression or vasospasm of the prolapsed cord, until the delivery is achieved.

Establish whether fetus is alive by palpating for cord pulsations, or using the fetal (Pinard's) stetho-scope or hand-held Doppler fetal heart detector or CTG and ultrasound scan (USS), depending on the facilities available. If USS facilities are available, visu-alisation of the fetal heartbeat is a possibility even if the fetal heart sounds cannot be detected [9]. If the fetus is dead, delivery is not urgent and the safest mode of delivery for the mother should be adopted. If the fetus is alive the measures described below should be adopted.

The mother should be placed in a head low (Tren-delenburg) position (Figure 10.4) or in the 'knee-chest' position (Figure 10.5).

The mother should be counselled regarding the problem and the plan of action, and verbal consent obtained for further management including caesarean section (CS) [1, 2].

If the cervix is not fully dilated and an assisted or operative vaginal delivery is not feasible within the next 15 minutes or so, the following steps are indicated [1, 2, 10–12].

The fetal presenting part should be manually dis-placed away from the pelvic inlet to prevent the cord

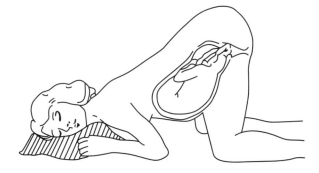

Figure 10.5 Knee–chest position.

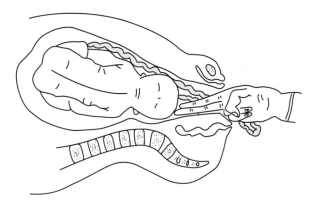

Figure 10.6 Displacement of presenting part away from pelvic inlet.

being compressed between the pelvic wall and the pre-senting part of the fetus. This could be achieved digi-tally through the vagina (especially if the cord prolapse occurs during vaginal examination or amniotomy) and maintained abdominally by an assistant thereafter (Figures 10.6 and 10.7).

The cord should be gently cradled in the hand and replaced within the vagina (Figure 10.8), and a gauze

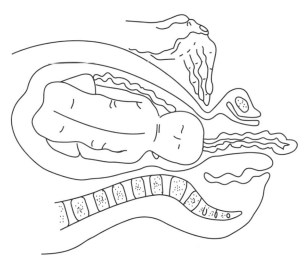

Figure 10.7 Maintaining displacement of presenting part away from pelvic inlet.

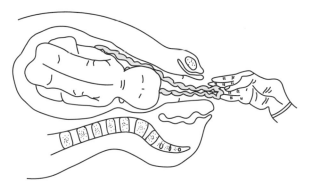

Figure 10.8 Replacement of cord within the vagina.

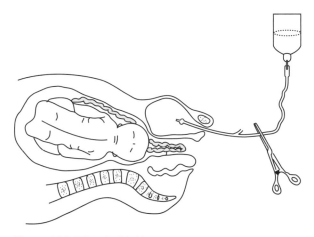

Figure 10.9 Filling the bladder.

towel, vaginal pack or tampon soaked in warm saline should be inserted into the vagina below the cord, if it tends to come out of the introitus.

Using a Foley catheter and an IV infusion set the bladder should be filled with 500–750 ml of normal saline, until it is visibly distended above the pubic symphysis, and then the catheter should be clamped (Figure 10.9). The full bladder will relieve the pressure on the cord by moving the presenting part away and may also inhibit uterine contractions.

An assistant should insert a 14 or 16 G intravenous cannula if it is not already in place, obtain blood for group and save and full blood count (FBC), and commence a Ringer's lactate or normal saline infusion.

If the woman is on an intravenous oxytocin infusion it should be stopped.

Oxygen should be given by face mask, 8 l/min.

Tocolytics (terbutaline 0.25 mg subcutaneously is preferable to salbutamol 0.5 mg intravenously slowly over 2 minutes) may be of value in cases with fetal bradycardia or pathological decelerations.

Measures to relieve compression of the cord should be continued during transfer of the woman to the operating theatre but they should not unduly delay the transfer.

If the cord prolapse occurs at home or in a well-resourced setting:

The woman should adopt the knee–chest position (Figure 10.5) until an ambulance arrives.

Medical assistants need to ensure that the presenting part is displaced away from the pelvic inlet, replace cord within the vagina and fill the bladder (Figures 10.6–9).

The woman should be in a head low, left lateral position with pillow under pelvis during transfer (Figure 10.10).

Definitive management [1, 2, 10–12]

Reconfirmation that the fetus is alive.

If suitable for an assisted breech delivery, breech extraction, vacuum or forceps delivery, it should be carried out urgently.

Emergency caesarean section would be indicated in most instances if the fetus is alive, as cord prolapse frequently occurs prior to full dilation of the cervix.

It has been suggested that a calm approach should be taken and intrauterine resuscitation with 100% oxygen, elevation of presenting part and maternal positioning with head low, left lateral position to enable spinal analgesia, is a suitable procedure and that the

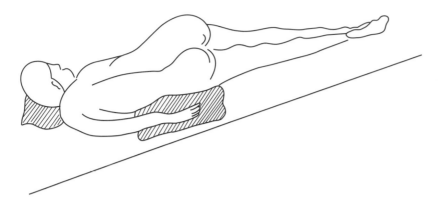

Figure 10.10 Head low left lateral position for transfer to hospital.

'emergency' situation could be converted to an 'urgent' situation [13]. This could be the case if there is no prolonged deceleration.

The bladder should be emptied by removing the clamp on the Foley catheter, prior to opening into the peritoneal cavity at CS.

Caesarean section within 30 minutes of diagnosis is recommended to improve perinatal outcome [2]. Although diagnosis to delivery intervals (DDI) of more than 60 min may be associated with adverse perinatal outcomes, it has been shown that the perinatal outcomes are poorly correlated with the cord pH of the neonates in women who are delivered within 30 minutes, even in well-resourced settings [2]. This suggests that in addition to decreasing the DDI, in utero resuscitation may be needed to reduce the effects of cord compression and improve the perinatal outcome.

Appropriate neonatal resuscitation and intensive care facilities should be ready prior to delivery.

Conservative management – in cases of extreme prematurity

May be considered with parental consent if the fetus is alive, has no gross fetal anomalies and PPROM with cord prolapse has occurred at the limits of gestational viability (c. 24–26 weeks) [1, 2].

Decision depends on neonatal facilities available in the centre.

An in-depth discussion involving the obstetrician, feto-maternal specialist, neonatologist, the woman and her partner is needed regarding chances of unexpected fetal demise, chances of survival if delivered now rather than later and the risks of long-term morbidity due to extreme prematurity.

The cord should be gently cradled in the hand and replaced in the vagina, and the woman placed in the Trendelenburg position, and managed as described under initial management above.

In-utero transfer to a centre with better neonatal facilities (the concern of cord spasm and fetal demise should be explained). If the fetus was > 26 weeks it may be best to consider delivery and an urgent ex-utero transfer.

A gauze towel or tampon soaked in warm saline should be inserted into the vagina if the cord tends to come out of the vulval introitus (especially during bowel motions with prolonged conservative management), to keep the cord warm and moist within the vagina and to prevent it going into spasm. The gauze/tampon needs to be removed just prior to delivery.

Antibiotics, tocolytics and corticosteroids can be administered as per PPROM management if it is decided to have prolonged conservative management [14].

The mother and fetus need very close monitoring and the conservative management terminated in cases of fetal demise.

In cases where a prolonged conservative approach is adopted because of extreme prematurity a CS will be needed if chorioamnionitis is suspected, fetal distress is detected, or spontaneous labour is established.

Post delivery

Parents, especially the mother, may be greatly affected psychologically.

Adequate debriefing and counselling of parents are needed.

Cord prolapse needs to be documented, reported and discussed at the next risk-management meeting.

Suggested management of cord prolapse in low-resource settings

In Nigerian women with cord prolapse, perinatal mortality rates of up to 68% have been reported, and up to 76% of the associated fetal deaths have been reported to occur prior to admission to hospital. Inadequate prenatal care was reported to be a high-risk factor for the occurrence of cord prolapse in these women [15]. The actions listed below are suggested for the management of cord prolapse in low-resource settings.

- Health education in the community and motivation of pregnant women to attend prenatal clinics.
- Education of all prenatal caregivers regarding the key risk factors for cord prolapse.
- Education of all maternity caregivers regarding the possible measures that could be taken to prevent cord prolapse.
- Education of women and any available caregivers in the community that women with PPROM, PROM or in labour should ideally lie flat, in left lateral position with a pillow under their hips (Figure 10.10) and be transported to hospital as soon as possible.
- On arrival in hospital, establishing the viability of the fetus and adapting the management algorithm in Figure 10.11 according to the resources available, and carrying out the most appropriate actions.
- Training all the staff involved in maternity care in the management of cord prolapse and conducting refresher training courses annually.

Key pitfalls

- Failure to anticipate cord prolapse in women with a high risk.
- Failure to carry out a speculum examination in PROM and PPROM.
- Carrying out amniotomy with a high head or when the fetal head is not fitting the pelvic inlet.
- Dislodging the head upwards during amniotomy.
- Failure to exclude cord presentation or occult cord prolapse during early intrapartum vaginal examination.
- Failure to relieve compressions and vasospasm of cord prior to emergency delivery.

- Failure to appreciate that fetal distress does not always occur immediately after cord prolapse.
- Failure to appreciate that the fetus may still be alive although the fetal heart sounds are not detectable.

Key pearls

- Cord prolapse is a life-threatening situation for the fetus.
- Immediately call for help and also request the anaesthesiologist and neonatologist to be informed.
- Immediate displacement of the fetal presenting part away from the pelvic inlet and gently replacing the cord within the vagina are essential primary steps in the management.
- Bladder filling maintains displacement of fetal presenting part away from the pelvic inlet and prevents cord compression.
- Emergency CS is frequently needed but assisted or operative vaginal delivery may be possible if the cervix is fully dilated.
- Post-delivery debriefing and counselling of parents and risk-management discussions are needed.
- Regular multiprofessional training programmes on the management of cord prolapse need to be conducted.

Training and assessment

Courses have been designed to enable simulation training of the multiprofessional obstetric team to manage obstetric emergencies including cord prolapse [10–12].

Training has been found to improve clinical knowledge and skills as well as team working and result in better overall management and reduces DDI [16].

A suggested training scenario

A primigravida at 38 weeks' gestation is admitted to the labour ward in advanced labour. The fetal head is 3/5th palpable abdominally, and the fetal heart rate is *c.* 128 bpm and regular. You proceed with a vaginal examination and find that the cervix is 6 cm dilated and the membranes are bulging. The membranes spontaneously rupture during your vaginal examination, and the cord prolapses out of the vagina.

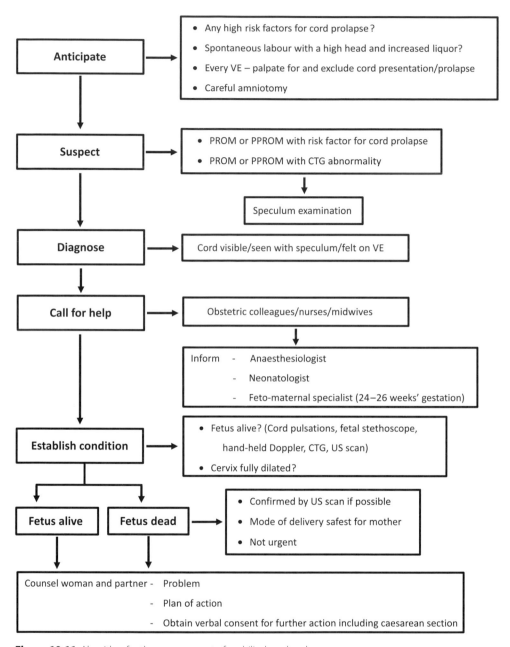

Figure 10.11 Algorithm for the management of umbilical cord prolapse.

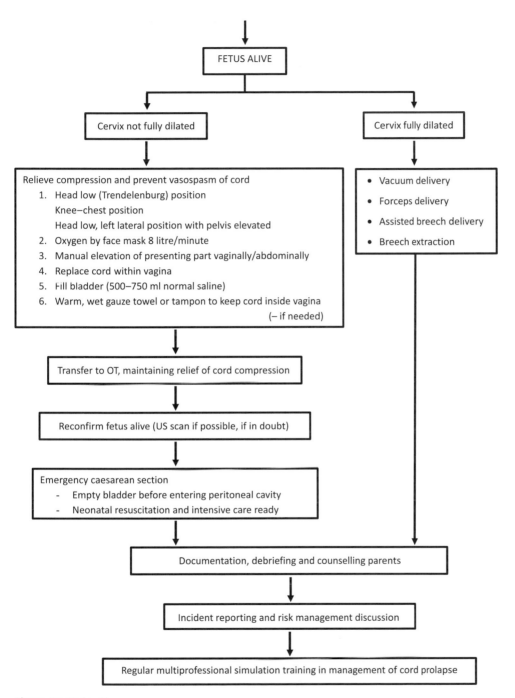

FETUS ALIVE

Cervix not fully dilated

Cervix fully dilated

Relieve compression and prevent vasospasm of cord
1. Head low (Trendelenburg) position
   Knee–chest position
   Head low, left lateral position with pelvis elevated
2. Oxygen by face mask 8 litre/minute
3. Manual elevation of presenting part vaginally/abdominally
4. Replace cord within vagina
5. Fill bladder (500–750 ml normal saline)
6. Warm, wet gauze towel or tampon to keep cord inside vagina
                                                    (– if needed)

- Vacuum delivery
- Forceps delivery
- Assisted breech delivery
- Breech extraction

Transfer to OT, maintaining relief of cord compression

Reconfirm fetus alive (US scan if possible, if in doubt)

Emergency caesarean section
- Empty bladder before entering peritoneal cavity
- Neonatal resuscitation and intensive care ready

Documentation, debriefing and counselling parents

Incident reporting and risk management discussion

Regular multiprofessional simulation training in management of cord prolapse

Figure 10.11 *(cont.)*

The following equipment will be available for the drill:

Delivery bed.

Obstetric manikin with perineum.

Baby with cord.

Fetal (Pinard's) stethoscope.

Hand-held Doppler fetal heart detector, CTG machine, US scanner (depends on centre).

Intravenous cannulae without needles.

Normal saline packs.

Blood transfusion set.

Foley catheter.

Face mask and oxygen source.

Cushion.

Case notes.

Drug chart.

Terbutaline and salbutamol vials.

Ranitidine and metoclopramide vials.

Disposable syringes without needles.

The trainer will ask the trainee 'What will you do?' The expected responses and actions would be:

Call for help.

Relieve compression and prevent vasospasm of cord.

Immediately elevate the fetal head digitally and disimpact it from the pelvic inlet.

While maintaining the above, instruct an assistant to adjust the delivery bed to a head-low position and place the mother in the Trendelenburg position or place the woman in the knee–chest position.

Instruct an assistant to abdominally ensure that the displacement of the fetal head is maintained.

Cradle the cord gently in the palm and replace it within the vagina.

Insert a Foley catheter and fill the bladder with 500–750 ml normal saline using an IV infusion set, until the bladder is palpable supra-pubically.

During this time other members of the team should:

Insert a 16 G intravenous cannula and obtain blood for group and save and FBC.

Inform the operating theatre and the anaesthesiologist.

Inform the neonatologist and the neonatal intensive care unit.

Commence oxygen by face mask 8 l/min.

Recheck the fetal condition: palpating for cord pulsations, fetal stethoscope, hand-held Doppler fetal heart detector, CTG and/or US depending on the facilities available and confirm that the fetus is alive.

Explain to the woman and her partner the problem, the state of the fetus and the proposed plan of action and obtain verbal consent for a caesarean section.

Terbutaline 0.25 mg subcutaneously or salbutamol 0.5 mg intravenously slowly over 2 min.

Ranitidine 50 mg and metoclopramide 10 mg intravenously.

Transfer to the operating theatre for emergency caesarean section maintaining the woman's head at a lower level than her pelvis.

Chronologically document accurately all the above steps.

The training programme should consist of a preliminary lecture based on the key facts, key implications, key pointers, key diagnostic signs, key actions, key pitfalls and key pearls. This should be followed by the case scenario and drill.

At the end of the drill the participants should be requested to identify what they did well and what they think they should improve on. The trainer should then give them feedback as to what they did well and what they could improve on. The drill should be repeated after these inputs until the trainer is satisfied that the team could efficiently manage a cord prolapse. The team too should be confident about their ability to manage a cord prolapse in real life.

An effective training programme will lead to the trainees performing the required clinical tasks in a coordinated manner, communicating with each other well and working as a team with a clear understanding of individual roles and responsibilities.

Frequent rehearsals will need to be conducted until the multiprofessional team acquires adequate skills. This should be followed by annual refresher training sessions [2].

Acknowledgement

Doctors Myuru Manawadu and D.V. Priyaranjana of the Department of Obstetrics and Gynaecology, University of Ruhuna contributed the figures.

References

1. Lin MG. Umbilical cord prolapse. *Obstet Gynaecol Surv* 2006; 61 (4): 269–277.

2. Royal College of Obstetricians and Gynaecologists. *Umbilical Cord Prolapse*. Green-top Guideline No. 50. London: RCOG, 2008.

3. Murphy DJ, MacKenzie IZ. The mortality and morbidity associated with umbilical cord prolapse. *Br J Obstet Gynaecol* 1995; 102: 826–830.

4. MacLennan A, for the International Cerebral Palsy Task Force. A template for defining a casual relation between acute intrapartum events and cerebral palsy: international consensus statement. *Br Med J* 1999; 319: 1054–1059.

5. Johnson KC, Daviss BA. Outcomes of planned home birth with certified professional midwives: large prospective study in North America. *Br Med J* 2005; 330: 1416–1422.

6. Dilbaz B, Ozturkoglu E, Dilbaz S *et al*. Risk factors and perinatal outcomes associated with umbilical cord prolapse. *Arch Gynaecol Obstet* 2006; 274: 104–107.

7. Ezra Y, Strasberg SR, Farine D. Does cord presentation on ultrasound predict cord prolapse? *Gynaecol Obstet Invest* 2003; 56: 6–9.

8. Kinugasa M, Sato T, Tamura M *et al*. Antepartum detection of cord presentation by transvaginal ultrasonography for term breech presentation: potential prediction and prevention of cord prolapse. *J Obstet Gynaecol Res* 2007; 33 (5): 612–618.

9. Driscoll JA, Sadan O, Van Geideren CJ, Holloway GA. Cord prolapse: can we save more babies? *Br J Obstet Gynaecol* 1987; 94: 594–595.

10. Draycott T, Winter C, Crofts J, Barnfield S (Eds.) *PROMPT. Practical Obstetric Multiprofessional Training: Course Manual*. London: RCOG, 2008, pp. 117–124.

11. Giswami K. Umbilical cord prolapse. In Howell C, Grady K, Cox C (Eds.) *Managing Obstetric Emergencies and Trauma – the MOET Course Manual*. Second Edition. London: RCOG, 2007, pp. 233–237.

12. van den Broek N (Ed.) *Life Saving Skills Manual – Essential Obstetric and Newborn Care*. London: RCOG, 2006.

13. McKeen D, Geeorge RB, Shukla R. We "can do it" does not mean we "should do it": obesity, umbilical cord prolapse, and spinal anesthesia in the knee-chest position. *Can J Anesthes* 2009; 56: 168–169.

14. Royal College of Obstetricians and Gynaecologists. *Preterm Prelabour Rupture of Membranes*. Green-top Guideline No. 44. London: RCOG, 2006.

15. Enakpene CA, Odukogbe AT, Morhason-Bello IO, Omigbodun AO, Arowojulu AO. The influence of health-seeking behavior on the incidence and perinatal outcome of umbilical cord prolapse in Nigeria. *Int J Womens' Health* 2010; 9 (2): 177–182.

16. Siassakos D, Hasafa Z, Sibanda T *et al*. Retrospective cohort study of diagnosis-delivery interval with umbilical cord prolapse: the effect of team training. *Br J Obstet Gynaecol* 2009; 116: 1089–1096.

Chapter

11

Fetal compromise: diagnosis and management

Edwin Chandraharan

Key facts

- Increasing strength, frequency and duration of uterine contractions during labour reduce oxygen supply to the utero-placental bed increasing the risk of intrapartum hypoxia.
- Intrapartum hypoxia and subsequent metabolic acidosis may lead to short-term complications, such as admission to a neonatal unit, hypoxic ischaemic encephalopathy (HIE) and neonatal death, or long-term implications such as cerebral palsy or learning difficulties.
- Intrapartum sentinel hypoxic events such as uterine scar dehiscence (or rupture), placental abruption or cord prolapse may cause acute hypoxic injury.
- Fetuses with chronic utero-placental insufficiency (intra-uterine growth restriction), congenital or acquired infection (chorioamnionitis), pre- or postmaturity may have less physiological reserve to deal with intrapartum hypoxic insults.
- The main aim of fetal monitoring is to timely identify and hence to salvage fetuses that are at risk of intrapartum hypoxic injury, whilst avoiding unnecessary operative intervention to fetuses that are normoxic or those who are mounting a good compensatory response.
- Intrapartum hypoxia accounts only for less than 10–30% of all cases of cerebral palsy and long-term neurological sequelae. The vast majority of fetuses are damaged antenatally.
- As a test of intrapartum hypoxia, a cardiotocograph (CTG) has a very high

false-positive rate (approximately 50–60%) and the positive predictive value of abnormal features of a CTG for intrapartum hypoxia is less than 30% [1, 2].
- Except in cases of acute hypoxia, management decisions should not be taken based on CTG patterns alone. Interventions should be based on understanding the wider clinical picture, fetal reserves and compensatory mechanisms and the results of additional tests of fetal well-being (fetal blood sampling, fetal ECG or fetal scalp lactate), if these are indicated [3].

Key implications

- Cardiotocography has been used for over 40 years to identify intrapartum hypoxia and when CTG was introduced into obstetric practice it was hoped that it would help reduce the cerebral palsy rate.
- Unfortunately, the incidence of cerebral palsy has remained fairly stable over the last 40 years, whereas there has been a significant increase in the incidence of operative delivery since the introduction of CTG [4].
- The 4th Confidential Enquiries into Stillbirths and Deaths in Infancy (CESDI) Report concluded that issues with interpretation and failure to act when a CTG abnormality was detected may have contributed to over half of all intrapartum-related deaths [5].
- Lack of knowledge to interpret CTG traces, failure to incorporate the clinical picture (meconium

Obstetric and Intrapartum Emergencies, ed. Edwin Chandraharan and Sabaratnam Arulkumaran. Published by Cambridge University Press. © Cambridge University Press 2012.

staining of amniotic fluid, intrapartum bleeding, maternal pyrexia, pre- and postmaturity), failures in communication and team working as well as delay in action contribute to intrapartum injury.

- CTG interpretation based on 'pattern recognition' leads to unnecessary interventions as well as lack of action as all the CTG patterns of fetal neurological injury are not currently known and the 'specific' CTG patterns do not correlate with poor neonatal outcomes.
- It is therefore essential to understand the pathophysiology of intrapartum fetal hypoxia to improve outcomes and to reduce unnecessary interventions. 'CTG patterns' are results of an investigation that has to be interpreted carefully with the understanding of the pathophysiology that causes that pattern. Actions should be based on this understanding and the clinical situation [6].

Key pointers

- Recognition of the fetus that is at an increased risk of intrapartum hypoxic insult.
- Prematurity and postmaturity, intra-uterine growth restriction, maternal disorders (severe preeclampsia, diabetes mellitus, immunological disorders such as systemic lupus erythematosus), maternal infections including pyrexia with or without clinical chorioamnionitis.
- Recognition of markers of sentinel hypoxic events during labour: fresh thick meconium, intrapartum bleeding, cord prolapse, prolonged deceleration, uterine hyperstimulation, sudden cessation of uterine contractions suggestive of uterine rupture.

Key diagnostic signs

Intrapartum hypoxia should be suspected when there are changes in the baseline heart rate (i.e. below 110 beats per minute (bpm) or above 160 bpm) and/or presence of decelerations (on auscultation for 1 min after a uterine contraction) on intermittent auscultation. Similarly, if any of the risk factors listed in Table 11.1 are present, continuous electronic fetal monitoring (EFM) using a CTG should be commenced.

Table 11.1 Indications for electronic fetal heart rate monitoring in labour.

Maternal problems

Any condition that increases the risk of utero-placental insufficiency, including:

Induced labour

Diabetes

Prolonged rupture of membranes ($>$ 24 hours)

Antepartum haemorrhage (placental abruption)

Previous caesarean section (scar dehiscence)

Preeclampsia (placental insufficiency)

Post-term pregnancy ($>$ 42 weeks)

Other maternal medical disease (systemic lupus erythematosus, renal disease)

Fetal problems

Any condition that reduces fetal blood flow or compromises fetal response to hypoxic insults:

Prematurity

Oligohydramnios (possible cord compression/utero-placental insufficiency)

Fetal growth restriction

Abnormal Doppler artery velocimetry

Multiple pregnancy

Meconium-stained liquor

Intrauterine infection

Intrapartum risk factors

Events that occur in labour and rapidly reduce fetal oxygenation:

Vaginal bleeding in labour (abruption, vasa praevia)

Oxytocin augmentation (hyperstimulation)

Epidural analgesia (maternal hypotension)

Maternal pyrexia (fetal inflammatory damage)

Fresh meconium-stained liquor (meconium aspiration syndrome)

Any deceleration or abnormal baseline on intermittent monitoring

Commencing CTG monitoring: getting the basics right – the machine and the trace

The patient's details and maternal pulse should also be recorded at the beginning of the trace.

Check the date and time are right, and it is very important to set the paper speed at the correct rate. In most countries, including the UK, the paper speed is set at 1 cm/min, while in the USA it is set at 3 cm/min.

If the paper speed is incorrectly set, the appearance of the CTG may change. For example, increase in the speed from 1 cm/min to 3 cm/min may create an erroneous impression that the variability has reduced. This may result in an incorrect classification and unnecessary intervention.

It is also important to record vaginal examinations, applications of scalp electrodes etc. on the CTG paper so as to optimise contemporaneous interpretation.

If there is any doubt that the machine is recording the maternal pulse (e.g. repeated accelerations with increased amplitude and duration with uterine contractions), check maternal pulse again.

Interpreting the CTG trace

Consider the following four features of a CTG trace prior to classification of CTG.

Baseline fetal heart rate (normal 110–160 bpm)

Baseline fetal heart rate (FHR) changes include baseline tachycardia (an increase in the baseline FHR above 160 bpm) and baseline bradycardia (baseline FHR below 110 bpm). The former may be physiological in a preterm fetus due to the immaturity of the parasympathetic system or secondary to maternal pyrexia, dehydration or rarely due to medication (e.g. betamimetics). Similarly, a post-term fetus may have a lower baseline heart rate (100–110 bpm) due to a mature parasympathetic system.

Baseline fetal heart-rate variability ('the bandwidth': 5–25 bpm)

The 'bandwidth' or the variation of the heart rate above and below the baseline on the CTG trace is called baseline fetal heart-rate variability. This reflects oxygenation of the central autonomic nervous system (CNS – the sympathetic and parasympathetic) that is responsible for the control of the fetal heart rate. The normal baseline variability of 5–25 bpm implies that cerebral hypoxia is unlikely. Reduced baseline variability of 0–5 bpm may represent a quiet sleep phase or may indicate depression of the central nervous system due to causes such as pharmacological agents (CNS depressants), fetal CNS infections, fetal strokes or hypoxia.

An increase in the baseline variability (more than 25 bpm) is termed a 'saltatory' pattern and should

be viewed with caution, if this persists for more than 30 minutes. This may reflect a rapidly developing intrapartum hypoxic insult if it is present with decelerations that may cause instability to the fetal autonomic nervous system. This is particularly important in the second stage of labour or in the presence of CTG features suggestive of a sub-acute hypoxic process.

Accelerations (transient increase in the baseline fetal heart rate)

A sudden transient increase in the fetal heart rate > 15 bpm from the baseline rate and lasting for > 15 seconds is termed 'acceleration'. A CTG trace with at least two such episodes in 20 minutes is called a reactive trace. Accelerations 'appear' to reflect the integrity of the somatic nervous system as they are almost always associated with fetal movements and are not present in the absence of fetal movements due to hypoxia, infection or cerebral haemorrhage. A paralysed fetus and an anencephalic fetus also show accelerations and this denotes that the accelerations are not due to the physical movement or due to the highest centres but could be due to some activity at a subcortical level.

Decelerations (any decrease in the heart rate below the baseline)

A sudden transient decrease of the fetal heart rate below the baseline heart rate (15 bpm and lasting for more than 15 seconds) is termed 'deceleration'. The decelerations are classified as early, late and variable in relation to the uterine contractions. It is important to appreciate that labour is a complex process with several pathophysiological processes occurring at any given time. Hence, it is possible to have decelerations that have characteristics that combine the two or three standard types of decelerations described below.

Early decelerations

These are 'mirror-image' decelerations and are due to head compression and the resultant stimulation of the parasympathetic nervous system. Hence, early decelerations are observed during the late first stage or second stage of labour. They commence with the onset of uterine contractions, reach the nadir with the peak of

Table 11.2 Feature classification of cardiotocograph (CTG) using NICE guidelines [7].

Feature	Baseline (beats per minute (bpm))	Variability (bpm)	Decelerations	Accelerations
Reassuring	110–160	≥ 5	None	Present
Non-reassuring	100–109 161–180	< 5 for 40–90 minutes	Typical variable decelerations with over 50% of contractions, occurring for over 90 minutes Single prolonged deceleration for up to 3 minutes	The absence of accelerations with otherwise normal trace is of uncertain significance
Abnormal	< 100 > 180 Sinusoidal pattern ≥ 10 minutes	< 5 for 90 minutes	Either atypical variable decelerations with over 50% of contractions or late decelerations, both for over 30 minutes Single prolonged deceleration for more than 3 minutes	

Table 11.3. Cardiotocograph (CTG) classification (NICE guidelines).

Category	Definition
Normal	A CTG where all four features fall into the 'reassuring' category
Suspicious	A CTG where one of the features falls into 'non-reassuring' category and the remainder of the features are 'reassuring'
Pathological	A CTG whose features fall into two or more 'non-reassuring' categories or one or more 'abnormal' categories

contractions and return to the baseline at the end of the contraction.

Late decelerations

Late decelerations are so termed because, in relation to uterine contractions, they occur 'late': both the onset of deceleration as well as the subsequent recovery to the baseline occur after the beginning and after the end of a uterine contraction, respectively. The nadir of these decelerations is seen after the peak of uterine contraction and they return to baseline at least 20 seconds after the contraction wanes off.

Presence of late decelerations indicates uteroplacental insufficiency, mediated through the fetal chemo-receptor mechanism secondary to fetal hypoxaemia, hypercarbia and acidosis. Based on the other features of the CTG trace and the clinical situation further tests of fetal well-being may be indicated to exclude fetal hypoxia, if it is intended to continue with labour.

Variable decelerations

Variable decelerations are due to umbilical cord compression and therefore, the commonest decelerations occurring during labour. They have a precipitous fall and recovery and are termed variable because they vary in shape, form and timing in relation to the uterine contractions. A 'typical' or 'uncomplicated' variable deceleration consists of a slight rise in the fetal heart rate (called 'shouldering') both before and after the deceleration and lasts for less than 60 seconds and usually within the confines of the onset and offset of the contraction.

Atypical or 'complicated' variable decelerations

Any variable decelerations that do not conform to the typical features as described above are termed 'atypical' or 'complicated' variable decelerations. These may last for more than 60 seconds and may lose their shouldering, have a slow recovery, have an 'overshoot' or be combined with a late deceleration. They may have 'U', 'V' or 'W' patterns or total loss of variability during a deceleration. Unlike 'typical' variable decelerations, 'atypical' variable decelerations are not due to umbilical cord compression alone. They may signify co-existing utero-placental insufficiency and hence the recovery to baseline in relation to the offset of the contraction may signify the importance of classifying this as an abnormal feature in the CTG interpretation.

Once the 'pattern analysis' is performed on a CTG trace using the four features described above, it is

Consider four features of CTG Trace (Baseline fetal heart rate, baseline variability, accelerations and decelerations)

Classify CTG according to NICE Guidelines (normal, suspicious or pathological)

Consider clinical picture: MOTHERS

M – Meconium staining of liquor (?fresh thick) / ?Maternal pulse
O – Oxytocin
T – Temperature (maternal pyrexia)
H – Hyperstimulation, haemorrhage (?abruption, vasa praevia)
E – Epidural
R – Rate of progress of labour, reserve of the fetus (pre- or postmaturity)
S – Scar (previous caesarean section or myomectomy)

Consider the type of hypoxia

Acute – sudden drop in baseline fetal heart rate below 80 beats per minute, persisting for more than 3 minutes (rate of fall in pH > 0.01/minute)

Sub-acute – Fetus spends < 60 seconds on the stable baseline and decelerates for more than 90 seconds (rate of fall in pH > 0.01 in every 2–3 minutes)

Gradually evolving hypoxia – occurrence of hypoxic or mechanical stress (decelerations) followed by loss of accelerations, a rise in baseline heart rate and possible loss of baseline variability

Long standing hypoxia – possible antenatal hypoxia characterised by a high baseline (150–180/min), loss of variability and presence of 'shallow' decelerations with uterine contractions

Pre-terminal CTG – a fetus that has exhausted all its compensatory mechanisms or in the final phases of a prolonged deceleration/terminal bradycardia

---

Consider *fetal compensation* to hypoxic or mechanical insult

Is the fetus maintaining a stable baseline heart rate? Stable heart rate reflects optimum functioning of CNS sympathetic and parasympathetic nervous system

Is the fetus using its adrenal glands to compensate? A fetus that is exposed to evolving hypoxic stress would release stress hormones (adrenaline and noradrenaline) to increase the heart rate and cause peripheral vasoconstriction to divert oxygenated blood to central organs

Is the baseline variability normal and with no saltatory pattern? CNS is well perfused

Figure 11.1 Algorithm for diagnosis of intrapartum hypoxia.

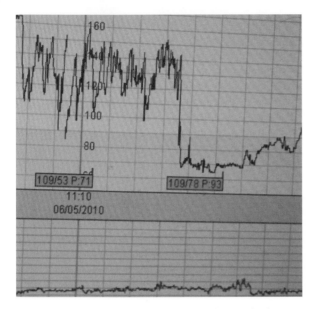

Figure 11.2 Cardiotocograph (CTG) pattern that may lead to acute hypoxia – prolonged deceleration – leading to build-up of hypoxia and metabolic acidosis.

important to classify each of the features into 'reassuring', 'non-reassuring' and 'abnormal' (Table 11.2).

Overall classification of the CTG

Once feature classification is completed, overall CTG classification should be performed as shown in Table 11.3.

Importance of further discussion about the significance of the observed CTG

The classification system recommended by the National Institute of Health and Clinical Excellence (NICE) is a useful tool to analyse the patterns observed on a CTG trace and to classify the CTG trace based on the features observed (Table 11.3). It is a good tool for communication among clinicians and helps avoid terminologies such as 'good', 'bad', 'suboptimal' or 'reassuring' CTG that cause confusion.

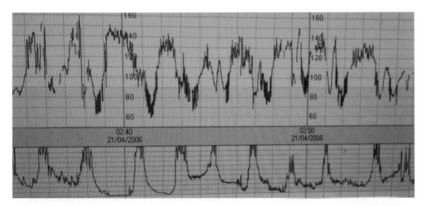

Figure 11.3 Cardiotocograph (CTG) pattern that may lead to sub-acute hypoxia. Note the fetus is spending less than 60 seconds at the baseline and more than 90 seconds below the baseline with the fetal heart rate decelerating to < 80 beats per minute.

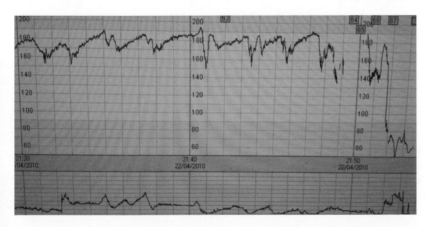

Figure 11.4 Cardiotocograph (CTG) pattern as a result of gradually evolving hypoxia. The type of decelerations suggests the mechanism causing the hypoxia; absence of accelerations and a rise in baseline heart rate (due to release of adrenaline) is followed by loss of baseline variability (reduction of the function of the autonomic nervous system due to hypoxia). If decelerations take a longer and longer time to recover it might suggest myocardial hypoxia.

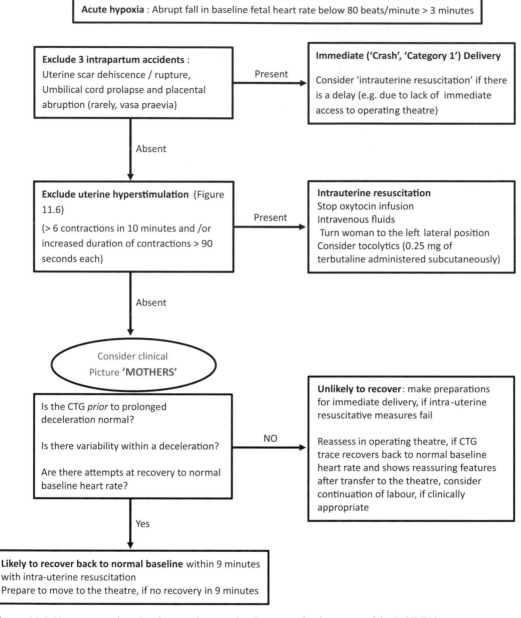

Acute hypoxia : Abrupt fall in baseline fetal heart rate below 80 beats/minute > 3 minutes

Exclude 3 intrapartum accidents :
Uterine scar dehiscence / rupture,
Umbilical cord prolapse and placental
abruption (rarely, vasa praevia)

→ Present →

Immediate ('Crash', 'Category 1') Delivery

Consider 'intrauterine resuscitation' if there
is a delay (e.g. due to lack of immediate
access to operating theatre)

Absent

Exclude uterine hyperstimulation (Figure
11.6)

(> 6 contractions in 10 minutes and /or
increased duration of contractions > 90
seconds each)

→ Present →

Intrauterine resuscitation
Stop oxytocin infusion
Intravenous fluids
Turn woman to the left lateral position
Consider tocolytics (0.25 mg of
terbutaline administered subcutaneously)

Absent

Consider clinical
Picture **'MOTHERS'**

Is the CTG *prior* to prolonged
deceleration normal?

Is there variability within a deceleration?

Are there attempts at recovery to normal
baseline heart rate?

→ NO →

Unlikely to recover: make preparations
for immediate delivery, if intra-uterine
resuscitative measures fail

Reassess in operating theatre, if CTG
trace recovers back to normal baseline
heart rate and shows reassuring features
after transfer to the theatre, consider
continuation of labour, if clinically
appropriate

Yes

Likely to recover back to normal baseline within 9 minutes
with intra-uterine resuscitation
Prepare to move to the theatre, if no recovery in 9 minutes

Figure 11.5 Management algorithm for acute hypoxia. See Figure 11.1 for description of the 'MOTHERS' mnemonic.

However, it must be understood that this classification is merely an 'interpretation' of a test (such as haemoglobin level (HB%)) and does not consider the wider clinical picture (as to the cause of low HB% e.g. iron deficiency or thalassaemia). Clinical decision on management needs to be based on the understanding of the inherent physiological reserves of the fetus, fetal compensatory response or the severity and rapidity of the hypoxic process. Only three types of decelerations due to head compression (early deceleration), umbilical cord compression (variable deceleration) or utero-placental insufficiency (late deceleration) are defined

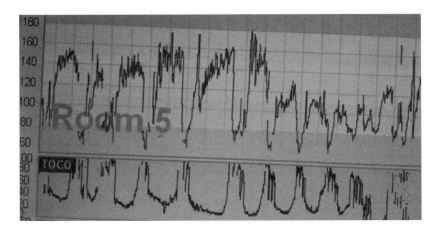

Figure 11.6 Uterine hyperstimulation with associated fetal heart rate changes on the cardiotocograph (CTG).

based on the basic pathophysiology. It is difficult and will become unwieldy to describe decelerations due to two or three mechanisms acting together such as head and umbilical cord being compressed together. This classification deals only with the description of the fetal heart rate. However the changes to the heart rate would be influenced by the frequency, amplitude and duration of uterine contractions. Uterine hyperstimulation ($>$ 5 contractions in 10 minutes) may contribute to fetal hypoxic injury [8]. Hence interpretation of the CTG test has to be related to parity, cervical dilation, rate of progress of labour, clinical risk factors and contraction frequency and duration. In the clinical setting some use a mnemonic DR C BRAVADO to encompass 'clinical monitoring':

DR – Define risk
C – Contractions
BR – Baseline Heart Rate
A – Accelerations
VA – Variability
D – Decelerations
O – Overall Assessment

Key pitfalls

- Lack of knowledge to interpret CTG traces, failure to incorporate clinical picture, delay in taking timely and appropriate action as well as failures in communication, team working and 'common-sense' approach lead to intrapartum hypoxic injury.

- Cardiotocograph is associated with increased false-positive rate (60%) and a low positive predictive value for intrapartum hypoxia ($<$ 30%). Hence, if it is used alone without understanding the pathophysiology of fetal hypoxia, the wider clinical picture, fetal response to hypoxic stress and without additional tests of fetal well-being, CTG may increase operative delivery rates without improving perinatal outcome.

Key pearls

- Clinicians should move from 'pattern-based' CTG interpretation to pathophysiology-based CTG interpretation.
- Consideration of the types of hypoxia (acute (Figure 11.1), sub-acute (Figure 11.2) and gradually evolving (Figure 11.3)) whilst interpreting CTG may help institute timely and appropriate action to improve perinatal outcome.
- Fetal response to hypoxic stress (Figure 11.4) is essential in planning management as a fetus responding to hypoxic or mechanical stress (decelerations) with a stable baseline heart rate and variability shows good compensation. A fetus that increases its baseline heart rate demonstrates release of adrenaline to compensate and additional tests of fetal well-being may be required, if the underlying cause of stress cannot be alleviated.

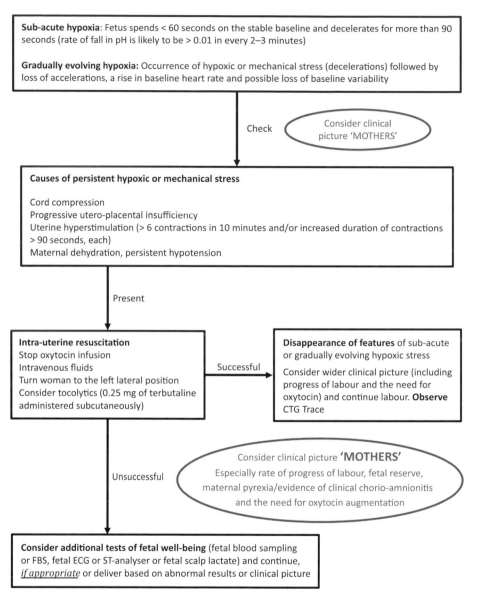

Sub-acute hypoxia: Fetus spends < 60 seconds on the stable baseline and decelerates for more than 90 seconds (rate of fall in pH is likely to be > 0.01 in every 2–3 minutes)

Gradually evolving hypoxia: Occurrence of hypoxic or mechanical stress (decelerations) followed by loss of accelerations, a rise in baseline heart rate and possible loss of baseline variability

Check

Consider clinical picture 'MOTHERS'

Causes of persistent hypoxic or mechanical stress

Cord compression
Progressive utero-placental insufficiency
Uterine hyperstimulation (> 6 contractions in 10 minutes and/or increased duration of contractions > 90 seconds, each)
Maternal dehydration, persistent hypotension

Present

Intra-uterine resuscitation
Stop oxytocin infusion
Intravenous fluids
Turn woman to the left lateral position
Consider tocolytics (0.25 mg of terbutaline administered subcutaneously)

Successful

Disappearance of features of sub-acute or gradually evolving hypoxic stress

Consider wider clinical picture (including progress of labour and the need for oxytocin) and continue labour. **Observe** CTG Trace

Consider clinical picture **'MOTHERS'**
Especially rate of progress of labour, fetal reserve, maternal pyrexia/evidence of clinical chorio-amnionitis and the need for oxytocin augmentation

Unsuccessful

Consider additional tests of fetal well-being (fetal blood sampling or FBS, fetal ECG or ST-analyser or fetal scalp lactate) and continue, _if appropriate_ or deliver based on abnormal results or clinical picture

Figure 11.7 Management algorithm for sub-acute or gradually evolving hypoxia. See Figure 11.1 for description of the 'MOTHERS' mnemonic.

References

1. Beard RW, Filshie GM, Knight CA, Roberts GM. The significance of the changes in the continuous fetal heart rate in the first stage of labour. *J Obstet Gynecol Br Commonw* 1971; 78: 865–881.

2. Curzan P, Bekir JS, McLintock DG, Patel M. Reliability of cardiotocography in predicting baby's condition at birth. *Br Med J (Clin Res Ed)* 1984; 289 (6455): 1345–1347.

3. Chandraharan E. Rational approach to electronic fetal monitoring in all resource settings. *Sri Lanka J Obstet Gynaecol* 2010; 32: 77–84.

4. Alfirevic Z, Devane D, Gyte GML. Continuous cardiotocography (CTG) as a form of electronic fetal monitoring (EFM) for fetal assessment during labour. *Cochrane Database Syst Rev* 2006; 3: Art. No. CD006066. doi: 10.1002/14651858. CD006066

5. Maternal and Child Health Research Consortium. *Confidential Enquiry into Stillbirths and Deaths in Infancy: 4th Annual Report, 1 January–31 December 1995.* London: Maternal and Child Health Research Consortium, 1997.

6. Chandraharan E, Arulkumaran S. Prevention of birth asphyxia: responding appropriately to cardiotocograph (CTG) traces. *Best Pract Res Clin Obstet Gynaecol* 2007; 21 (4): 609–624.

7. National Institute of Clinical Excellence. *Intrapartum care: Care of Healthy Women and their Babies during Labour.* NICE Clinical Guideline No. 55. London: NICE, 2007.

8. Ingemarsson I, Arulkumaran S, Ratnam SS. Single injection of terbutaline in term labour: effect of fetal pH in cases with prolonged bradycardia. *Am J Obstet Gynecol* 1985; 13: 859–865.

Chapter

12

Shoulder dystocia: diagnosis and management

Edwin Chandraharan and Sabaratnam Arulkumaran

Key facts

- Definition: Shoulder dystocia occurs when the baby's head has been born but a shoulder becomes stuck behind the mother's pelvic bone, resulting in a delivery that requires additional obstetric manoeuvres to release the shoulder after gentle downward traction has failed. This is a 'bone–bone problem' at the level of the pelvis inlet (Figure 12.1).
- Types: Anterior (impaction of anterior shoulder above symphysis pubis). Posterior (impaction of posterior shoulder above sacral promontory).
- Incidence: Approximately 0.5% (5/1000).

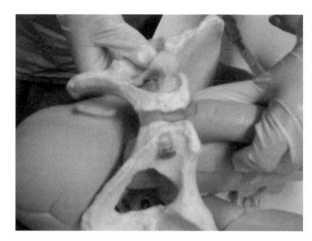

Figure 12.1 Demonstration of shoulder dystocia as a 'bony problem' at the pelvic inlet.

Key implications

- Maternal: Perineal trauma including third-degree perineal tears (3.8%), postpartum haemorrhage (11%) and psychological trauma secondary to traumatic birth experience.
- Fetal: Peripartum hypoxia resulting in stillbirths, neonatal admission for convulsions and multi-organ support, long-term neurological outcomes (learning difficulties, cerebral palsy), neonatal injuries such as fractures (clavicle, humerus), brachial plexus injuries (4–16%), Erb's palsy (10%).
- Medico-legal: clinical negligence claims due to delay in delivery, inappropriate or excessive traction to deliver the shoulders.

Key pointers

- Fetal macrosomia (~50%) and/or maternal diabetes mellitus/high maternal body mass index (BMI).
- Previous shoulder dystocia.
- Slow progress (first and second stages of labour).
- Instrumental vaginal birth.

Key diagnostic signs

- Failure of external rotation of the fetal head.
- 'Turtle sign' – retraction of the fetal head into the vagina from the perineum.

Key actions

Various mnemonics have been described to aid remembering the many manoeuvres that have been

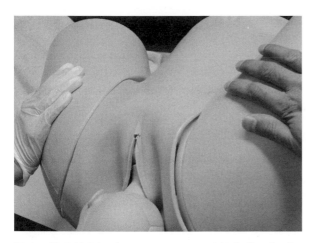

Figure 12.2 McRobert's manoeuvre: maternal thighs flexed at the hip, abducted and externally rotated by two birth attendants.

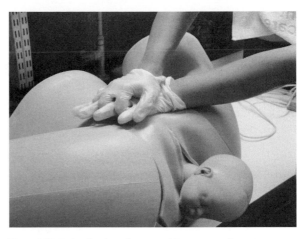

Figure 12.3 Application of supra-pubic pressure after identification of the fetal back.

described to manage shoulder dystocia. However, the choice of a manoeuvre should depend on the specific clinical situation (e.g. 'all fours' may be the manoeuvre of first choice in homebirths but not in a hospital setting in a woman having epidural analgesia), skill and experience of the accoucher (e.g. some clinicians may prefer delivery of the posterior arm to rotatory manoeuvres), patient characteristics (e.g. McRoberts manoeuvre may not be appropriate in a woman with a history of hip injury) and fetal condition (e.g. shoulder dystocia in a large macrosomic fetus who has sustained an intra-uterine death will not require alerting the neonatal team and cleidotomy may be considered early) [1, 2].

We have classified the manoeuvres into 'first line' (SPR) and 'second line'. The latter should be used when the first-line manoeuvres fail and are associated with increased maternal and fetal morbidity. Therefore, consultant obstetric presence is recommended during the performance of second-line manoeuvres.

Manoeuvres are described assuming that the fetal back is facing maternal left side. If the fetal back faces maternal right, it is recommended that clinicians use their opposite hand to facilitate these manoeuvres.

First-line manoeuvres (SPR)

S

Shout for help (experienced midwives and obstetricians, neonatologist, anaesthetist) as soon as shoulder dystocia is diagnosed and **Specify** emergency ('shoulder dystocia'). If shoulder dystocia has been anticipated based on risk factors, experienced midwives and obstetricians should be on 'stand-by', when active pushing commences and delivery is imminent.

Stop traction and advise the woman to stop pushing.

Scribe – assign someone to keep record of the time and to alert every minute.

P

Position the buttocks at the edge of the couch to enable manoeuvres that may later become necessary. **Position** the thighs – flexed at the hip over the maternal abdomen and externally rotated (McRobert's manoeuvre) by two attendants (Figure 12.2). This will achieve delivery of the shoulders in approximately 90% due to sliding of the sacral promontory upwards. Attempt 'roll over' or 'all fours' position, which may increase the diameter of the maternal pelvis due to 'sliding' of the sacral promontory upwards. This manoeuvre may be attempted first in settings where placing a woman in a McRobert's manoeuvre may not be immediately feasible (i.e. homebirths) and when the woman does not have epidural analgesia (i.e. no restriction of movements).

Pressure – (supra-pubic pressure) – first in a continuous motion for 30 seconds and later in a 'rocking motion' similar to cardiopulmonary resuscitation (CPR) after identifying the fetal back (Figure 12.3). A birth attendant should stand facing the fetal back and attempt to push the anterior shoulder away from the symphysis pubis. This will help the shoulders enter into the maternal pelvic inlet through the larger transverse diameter.

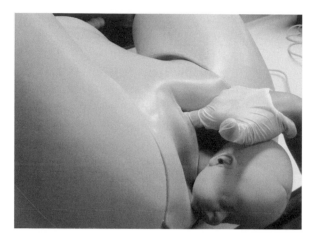

Figure 12.4 Two fingers inserted on to the posterior aspect of the anterior shoulder to displace the shoulder in the opposite direction – the Wood's screw manoeuvre.

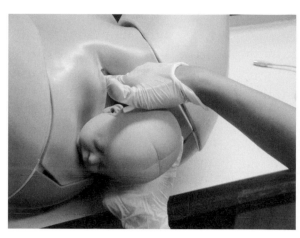

Figure 12.5 Two-handed technique to rotate the anterior shoulder.

Perineum – consider the need for episiotomy prior to rotational manoeuvres.

R

Rotate shoulders – aimed at moving the impacted anterior shoulder away from the symphysis pubis into the larger transverse diameter of the maternal pelvic inlet (Wood's screw or reverse Wood's screw manoeuvres). As shown in the illustrations, two fingers of the right hand are initially inserted into the vagina and placed on the posterior aspect of the anterior shoulder to 'push' the anterior shoulder into the transverse diameter (Figure 12.4). If this fails, the clinician should place two fingers of the left hand on the anterior aspect of the posterior shoulder. This enables the right hand to push the anterior shoulder into the transverse diameter whilst the fingers of the left hand assist this process by pushing the posterior shoulder in the opposite direction (Figure 12.5). If this manoeuvre fails, a 'reverse Wood's screw manoeuvre' could be tried, which involves the clinician now sliding the fingers of the right hand downwards onto the posterior aspect of the posterior shoulder and fingers of the left hand upwards onto the anterior aspect of the anterior shoulder (Figure 12.6). This will enable rotation of the shoulders onto the transverse diameter on the pelvic inlet in the opposite direction.

Release – the posterior arm. Clinician should insert the left hand and move it posteriorly (hollow of the sacrum) along the posterior fetal arm to reach the cubital fossa. The index finger should be used to flex

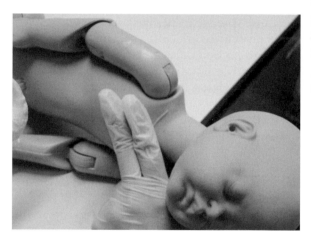

Figure 12.6 'Reverse' Wood's screw manoeuvre: the fingers are placed on the anterior aspect of the anterior shoulder to rotate the shoulder in the opposite direction.

the fetal forearm and sweep it across the fetal chest so as to release the posterior arm (Figure 12.7). This would create an additional space to facilitate the entry of the shoulders into the pelvic inlet by reducing the fetal diameter by 1–3 cm. It is recommended that the clinician should insert the hand directly posteriorly into the hollow of the sacrum (Figure 12.8) and that the fingers should be positioned in a manner similar to that adapted while putting on a bangle [3].

Repeat the above procedures until further senior help (i.e. consultant obstetrician) arrives or consider second-line procedures (below).

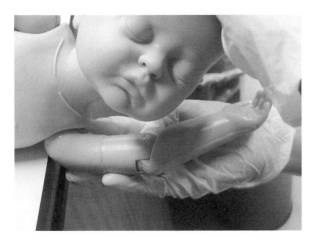

Figure 12.7 Release of the posterior arm.

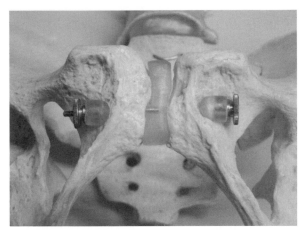

Figure 12.9 Symphysiotomy: site of incision in the midline over the joint.

Second-line procedures (SPR)

Shoulders – Cleidotomy or intentional fracture of the fetal clavicles. This may be considered earlier in intrauterine fetal death.

Pelvis – Partial or complete division of the maternal symphysis pubis (Figure 12.9). A metal catheter should be first inserted into the urethra to displace the urethra to one side as the incision is made on the cartilage of the pubic symphysis, to avoid inadvertent injury to the urethra. This procedure is recommended in low-resource settings where resources for immediate and safe emergency caesarean section are not readily available (see end of this chapter for further discussion).

Replacement of the fetal head and caesarean section. This is called the Zavanelli manoeuvre and should only be considered as the last resort if the above manoeuvres fail. Mechanism of labour should be initially reversed (i.e. 'de-restitution' and flexion) prior to caesarean section (Figure 12.10).

Complete the '3 Es' after every obstetric emergency

Examine – for maternal (genital tract trauma, postpartum haemorrhage) and fetal complications (hypoxic injury, neurological or skeletal injuries).

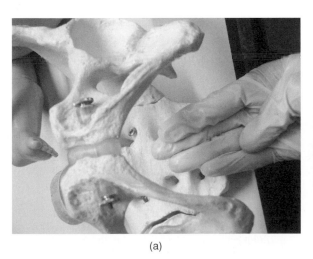

(a)

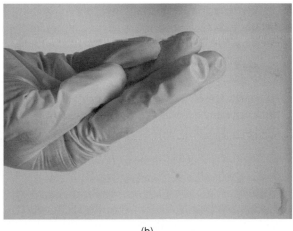

(b)

Figure 12.8 (a) Entering the hollow of the sacrum with the hands in a 'putting on a bangle' position. (b) Demonstration of the correct hand position.

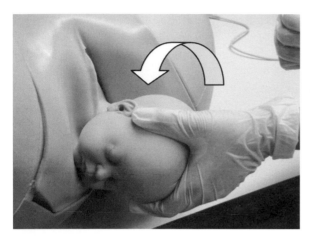

Figure 12.10 Zavanelli's manoeuvre: reversal of mechanism of labour.

Explain the delivery events, possible reasons, complications and future plan of care to the patient (i.e. debrief).

Escalate – incident reporting form and to senior colleagues as well as to the team to identify learning points to continuously improve patient care.

Key pitfalls

- Failure to anticipate shoulder dystocia/involve experienced clinicians.
- Failure to call for help/communicate clearly in an emergency.
- Failure to avoid excessive or inappropriate traction.
- Failure to anticipate postpartum haemorrhage.
- Failure to recognise and repair perineal trauma.
- Failure to keep adequate records, including time keeping, and documentation of cord gases.

Key pearls

- All staff providing intrapartum care should undergo annual skills and drills training on the management of shoulder dystocia.
- Regular fire drills on shoulder dystocia should be conducted in the labour ward.
- Lessons learned from adverse incidents due to shoulder dystocia should be disseminated to the entire team through the 'Maternity Dashboards' and Clinical Governance Seminars.

- All new staff should have hands-on training on shoulder dystocia as part of their induction.

Management in low-resource settings

Shoulder dystocia is an obstetric emergency that requires immediate and systematic management to improve maternal and perinatal outcome. The steps described in the section on first-line manoeuvres are applicable in all settings.

If facilities for safe and immediate emergency caesarean sections are not available, then clinicians should be trained on 'symphysiotomy' as the main second-line measure. A metal catheter, scalpel handle and blade and suitable local anaesthetic should be made available in birth settings.

Procedure of symphysiotomy

Instil 10 ml of 1% lignocaine on the skin overlying the symphysis pubis and insert a metal catheter into the urethra. Use the index and middle fingers of the left hand to displace the metal catheter (i.e. the urethra) laterally and make an incision on the skin overlying the symphysis pubis with a scalpel blade. Deepen the incision until the cartilage is divided to 'separate' the two innominate bones from their anterior midline attachment at the symphysis pubis (Figure 12.9). The end of the scalpel handle may be inserted vertically into the incision and then rotated to separate the pubic bones. Once the fetus is delivered, the patient should be 'strapped' to keep the innominate bones together at the pubic symphysis. Alternatively, if orthopaedic facilities are available, the pubic bones could be 'wired' together.

References

1. Chandraharan E, Arulkumaran S. Female pelvis and details of operative delivery; shoulder dystocia and episiotomy. In Arulkumaran S, Penna LK, Basker R (Eds.), *Management of Labour*. Orient Longman (India), 2005.

2. Royal College of Obstetricians and Gynaecologists. *Shoulder Dystocia*. Green-top Guideline No. 42. London: RCOG, 2005.

3. Draycott T, Winter C, Crofts J, Barnfield S (Eds.). *PROMPT. Practical Obstetric Multiprofessional Training: Course Manual*. London: RCOG, 2008.

Chapter

13

Twin delivery

Deepal S. Weerasekera

Key facts

- Zygosity in twins – 80% are dizygotic and 20% are monozygotic.
- Dizygotic twins arise from fertilisation of two ova and monozygotic twins arise from one ovum. Therefore all dizygotic twins have separate placentas and separate chorionic amniotic sacs.
- Monozygotic twins can divide into two at different stages resulting in three types:

  (1) Dichorionic diamniotic (DCDA) – twins have separate placentas and chorionic and amniotic sacs – approximately 30% of monozygotic twins are DCDA and they are of the same sex.

  (2) Monochorionic diamniotic (MCDA) – Each twin develops in its own amniotic cavity but the placenta and chorion are shared. Approximately 70% of monozygotic twins are MCDA.

  (3) Monochorionic monoamniotic (MCMA) – the placenta and chorionic and amniotic cavities are shared. Less than 1% of monozygotic twins are MCMA.

- Incidence – Currently around 15 per 1000 maternities. The incidence has increased by 50% in developed countries over the past two decades. Monozygous twin rate more constant at 4 per 1000 maternities and dizygous twin rate is more variable depending on the population and prevalence of assisted reproductive practices. In late pregnancy both fetuses are:

  · vertex in 31–47%
  · vertex–breech in 30–40%
  · breech–vertex or breech–breech in 8–12%.

Key implications

Cerebral palsy is nearly three times more common and perinatal mortality is four times higher in twins compared with singleton pregnancies. Perinatal mortality is 2–3 times higher in monochorionic twins compared with dichorionic twins due to presence of placental vascular anastomoses. Monochorionic diamniotic twins carry a 25% risk of twin-to-twin transfusion syndrome (TTTS) [1]. The main reasons for high perinatal mortality in twin pregnancy are:

- Prematurity.
- Intrauterine growth restriction.
- Congenital malformations.
- Complications due to placental vascular connections.
- Umbilical cord prolapse.

Maternal morbidity is high due to:

- Hyperemesis gravidarum.
- Antepartum haemorrhage.
- Anaemia.
- Preeclampsia.
- Placental abruption.
- Placenta praevia.
- Postpartum haemorrhage.

Obstetric and Intrapartum Emergencies, ed. Edwin Chandraharan and Sabaratnam Arulkumaran. Published by Cambridge University Press. © Cambridge University Press 2012.

Complications of internal podalic version and breech extraction of second twin include:

Fetal

- Skeletal injury (femur, humerus, hips, skull).
- Visceral injury (kidney, liver, spleen).
- Neural injury (facial nerve palsy).
- Hypoxic cerebral damage.
- Cord prolapsed.
- Hand prolapsed.

Maternal

- Uterine rupture.
- Placental abruption.
- Vaginal and perineal trauma.
- Postpartum haemorrhage.
- Puerperal sepsis.

Key pointers

- Dizygotic twin rate has increased by about 50% over the past two decades due to the wide use of ovarian stimulation regimes in the treatment of subfertility.
- Exaggerated symptoms in early pregnancy with symphysio-fundal height greater than period of amenorrhoea or the presence of multiple fetal parts should arouse the suspicion of multiple pregnancy in a low-resource setting where recourse to a routine ultrasound scan in early pregnancy is not available.
- Preterm labour.

Key diagnostic signs

Diagnosis can be made by ultrasound in the first trimester and the chorionicity has to be assessed before 14 weeks [2].

Inspect the placental base of the membrane separating the two sacs.

- Thick 'Lambda' shape – dichorionic diamniotic twins.
- Thin 'T' shape – Monochorionic diamniotic twins.

Colour Doppler can be used to demonstrate a functional artery-to-artery anastomosis which provides definitive proof of monochorionicity. Doppler ultrasound is also useful in monitoring fetal compromise in twins in late pregnancy. Current evidence suggests that use of Doppler reduces the risk of perinatal deaths and results in fewer obstetric interventions.

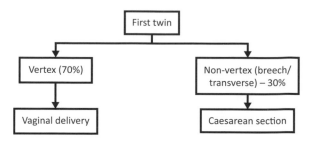

Figure 13.1 Delivery of the first twin.

Monozygotic twins have a 50% increase in structural abnormalities per baby and therefore a 20 weeks' gestation anomaly scan is very important in the management of twin pregnancy. Serial growth scans are necessary to monitor fetal growth.

Key actions

Timing of delivery

There is no evidence to show that elective delivery of twins at 37 weeks or after by induced labour or caesarean section is beneficial.

During labour

Delivery should be done in a hospital where facilities are available for immediate caesarean section if needed (Figure 13.1).

Continuous cardiotocograph (CTG) monitoring of both twins is mandatory.

An epidural analgesia is preferable, especially if additional manoeuvres are required during the second stage of labour.

An intravenous cannula should be inserted and oxytocin augmentation should be considered, if first stage is delayed.

Blood should be cross-matched.

Time interval between twin births

There is no ideal time interval between delivery of the first and second twin.

Continuous electronic fetal monitoring of the second twin is mandatory, after the birth of the first twin.

Cord prolapse is more common after the delivery of the first twin and this should be anticipated. If there is evidence of cord prolapse, delivery of the second twin should be expedited.

The risk of hypoxia and acidosis of the second twin increases with increasing interval between births,

Figure 13.2 Delivery of the second twin.

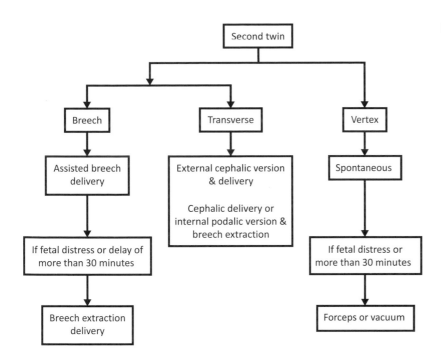

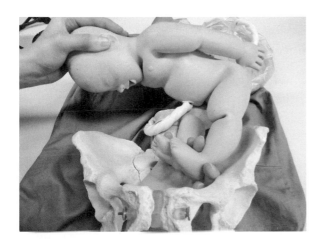

Figure 13.3 Identifying the heel and holding the ankle in internal podalic version.

especially in monochorionic twins. In general, if the inter-twin delivery interval exceeds 30 minutes, then delivery should be expedited. However, if facilities for continuous electronic fetal heart rate monitoring are available, a longer inter-twin interval is acceptable, if the fetal heart rate of the second twin is normal.

Descent of the presenting part of the second twin should be carefully monitored (Figure 13.2).

When the presenting part of the second twin is breech or transverse, internal podalic version and

breech extraction should be attempted. There is no evidence to show caesarean delivery is more beneficial in this situation [3, 4].

Internal podalic version

This is best performed with the patient in the lithotomy position. Urinary bladder should be catheterised. The clinician's hand should be introduced carefully into the uterus via the vagina to identify the fetal heel (Figure 13.3). If the membranes have not ruptured, this procedure should be carried out through the intact membranes so that the membranes can be ruptured as late as possible. The fetal foot should be grasped and gently pulled down into the vagina by applying gentle continuous traction (Figure 13.4). This procedure is relatively easy when the transverse lie is with the back superior or posterior. If the back is inferior (Figure 13.5) or if the limbs are not easily recognised a quick abdominal ultrasound scan to identify the fetal limbs will be helpful. At this stage the other leg will automatically come down, and if not, it should be pulled down in the same manner. As the breech is visible at the introitus, an assisted breech delivery should be performed. If there is evidence of acute fetal compromise of the second twin, after the delivery of the first twin, a breech extraction may be performed (Figure 13.6). This is the only indication for breech extraction in modern obstetric practice.

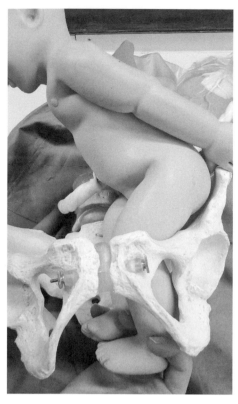

Figure 13.4 Applying a gentle traction to bring the legs into the vagina.

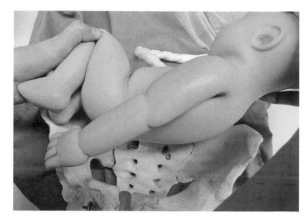

Figure 13.5 Transverse lie of the second twin with 'dorso-inferior'.

Third stage

- Syntometrine 1 vial should be administered with delivery of the second twin after making sure that there is no undiagnosed triplet.
- After delivery of the placenta commence oxytocin infusion (40 units in 500 ml of normal saline at the rate of 10 units/hour) to avoid uterine atony and postpartum haemorrhage.
- Patient should be examined for perineal and birth tract trauma, especially if internal podalic version, vacuum or forceps delivery has been performed.
- Close monitoring should continue for 24 hours to ensure there is no postpartum haemorrhage.
- Diclofenac sodium suppositories are effective for pain relief when the epidural is wearing off.

Key pitfalls

- Failure of continuous electronic monitoring of second twin.
- Failure to anticipate postpartum haemorrhage.
- Failure to examine the mother for perineal and birth tract trauma.
- Failure to double clamp the umbilical cord of the first twin may lead to unrecognised haemorrhage from the second twin.
- Failure to keep adequate records, including time keeping, and documentation of cord gases.
- Locked twins – possibility exists when the first twin is presenting by breech, although incidence is very low at 1 in 645. The most common form of interlocking is chin to chin, when the first twin presents by the breech and the second by the vertex. When arrest in the descent of the first twin occurs in the late second stage after delivery of the shoulders, interlocking should be suspected. Delivery can be achieved by extraction of the second twin past the first using forceps, especially if the twins are very preterm. Delivery of the first twin can then be completed. An alternative method of delivery is to apply forceps to the head of the second twin and to deliver both infants simultaneously by flexion. Interlocking of twins is very rare at term as there is insufficient space for both fetal heads to occupy the pelvic cavity.
- Conjoined twins are very rare and occur in around 1 in 100 000 pregnancies. This is usually due to incomplete separation of the developing embryo, development of co-dominant axes or embryonic fusion. Prenatal diagnosis is important and delivery should be by caesarean section. Dystocia and uterine rupture have been reported in undiagnosed cases.

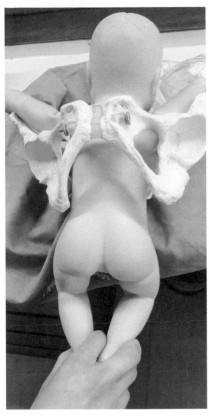

Figure 13.6 Breech extraction in cases of acute fetal compromise of the second twin.

Key pearls

- Active management of the third stage is important to reduce postpartum haemorrhage.
- Exclude an undiagnosed triplet by ultrasonography after delivery of the second twin.
- Inform other team members well in advance and an anaesthetist and a neonatologist should be present at delivery.
- Operating theatre should be kept informed when the woman is fully dilated so as to ensure staff are ready if an urgent caesarean section becomes necessary. In many centres, a woman with twin pregnancy is transferred to the operating theatre, when she is fully dilated and delivery of twins is conducted in the theatre.
- There is no evidence to show that prolonged bed rest in pregnancy reduces the incidence of preterm birth in twins and this should be discouraged.

Management in low-resource settings

Vaginal delivery is always preferable to caesarean delivery in low-resource settings when the first twin is vertex. When the second twin is non-vertex internal podalic version and breech extraction should be the aim over emergency caesarean delivery, if there are no other contraindications for vaginal birth. Obstetricians should undergo drills and should be trained in the manoeuvre. In situations where epidural anaesthesia is not available maternal sedation with intravenous pethidine 50 mg with naxolone 10 mg is effective. In this situation, clinicians should ensure that naloxone is available at hand if neonatal respiratory depression does occur after birth.

References

1. Royal College of Obstetricians and Gynaecologists. *Monochorionic Twin Pregnancy, Management.* Green-top Guideline No. 51. London: RCOG, 2008.

2. Chudleigh T, Thilaganathan B (Eds.). *Obstetrics Ultrasound – How, When and Why.* Edinburgh: Elsevier, Churchill Livingstone, 2004.

3. Howell C, Grady K, Cox C. *Managing Obstetric Emergencies and Trauma – the MOET Course Manual.* Second Edition. London: RCOG, 2007.

4. Webster SNE, Loughney AD. Internal podalic version and breech extraction. *Obstet Gynaecol* 2011; 13: 7–14.

Chapter

14

Instrumental vaginal delivery

Vikram Sinai Talaulikar and Sabaratnam Arulkumaran

Key facts

Definition: Use of obstetric forceps or ventouse (vacuum) to expedite vaginal delivery of a fetus.

Types: Either of the two instruments, forceps or ventouse, may be chosen for the delivery. The procedures are classified as (1) midcavity, (2) low and (3) outlet (Table 14.1) [1].

Incidence: Between 5 and 15% of all vaginal deliveries are assisted by an instrument. Incidence varies depending on population, institution and individuals performing the procedure. In modern obstetrics, use of ventouse has gained popularity as it can be performed with less profound anaesthesia and is associated with lower risk of maternal trauma.

Table 14.1 Classification for instrumental vaginal delivery.

Outlet	Fetal scalp visible without separating the labia Fetal skull has reached the pelvic floor Sagittal suture is in the anterio-posterior diameter or right or left occiput anterior or posterior position (rotation does not exceed 45°) Fetal head is at or on the perineum
Low	Leading point of the skull (not caput succedaneum) is at station plus 2 cm or more and not on the pelvic floor Two subdivisions: • rotation of 45° or less from the occipito-anterior position • rotation of more than 45° including the occipito-posterior position
Mid	Fetal head is no more than 1/5th palpable per abdomen Leading point of the skull is above station plus 2 cm but not above the ischial spines Two subdivisions: • rotation of 45° or less from the occipito-anterior position • rotation of more than 45° including the occipito-posterior position
High	Not included in the classification as operative vaginal delivery is not recommended in this situation where the head is 2/5th or more palpable abdominally and the presenting part is above the level of the ischial spines

Adapted from the American College of Obstetrics and Gynecology, 2000 [1].

Key implications

Caesarean section rates are on the rise and this may be partly due to lack of appropriate training and experience in instrumental deliveries as well as medico-legal issues. Since caesarean section performed in the second stage of labour is associated with increased maternal morbidity, an appropriately performed instrumental vaginal delivery may help avoid the unnecessary risks.

Instrumental vaginal deliveries can be hazardous in inexperienced hands and should be undertaken with due care and supervision. Various intrapartum measures may help reduce the need for assisted vaginal delivery such as use of partogram, upright or lateral maternal position, one-to-one support to the woman in labour, delayed pushing in women having epidural anaesthesia or judicious use of oxytocin in the second stage of labour especially in women with epidural anaesthesia.

Obstetric and Intrapartum Emergencies, ed. Edwin Chandraharan and Sabaratnam Arulkumaran. Published by Cambridge University Press. © Cambridge University Press 2012.

About 27% of fetal head positions diagnosed clinically on digital vaginal examination were found to be incorrect when checked with ultrasonography [2]. This demonstrates the importance of continued training, supervision and review of practice in the area of instrumental deliveries.

On the medico-legal side, clinical negligence claims may arise due to delay in delivery, inappropriate choice of instrument or excessive use of force during delivery and maternal/fetal trauma. In cases of fetal distress it is essential that the instrumental delivery be straightforward as the combination of trauma and hypoxia is potentially damaging to the fetus. Careful documentation of events immediately after delivery is of paramount importance.

Key pointers

Indications for assisted vaginal delivery are:

Maternal

- Exhaustion with non-progressive pushing efforts.
- Medical conditions such as severe cardiac, respiratory, cerebrovascular disease or severe hypertension and where pushing is not possible e.g. paraplegia/tetraplegia or myasthenia gravis.
- Proliferative retinopathy.

Fetal

- Fetal compromise manifest by pathological CTG or cord prolapse in second stage of labour.
- To control after-coming head of breech.

Combined

- Prolonged non-progressive second stage of labour with risk of damage to maternal pelvic floor and risk of trauma and hypoxia to the fetus. Prolonged second stage may be defined as [3]:

  Nullipara: 2 hours without regional anaesthesia and 3 hours with regional anaesthesia.
  Multipara – 1 hour without regional anaesthesia and 2 hours with regional anaesthesia.

However, it is important to recognise that no rigid time limits should be set and the decision to intervene should take into consideration various maternal and fetal factors in labour.

Key diagnostic signs

Before forceps or ventouse are applied, the following prerequisites should be fulfilled.

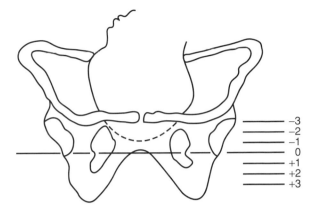

Figure 14.1 Fetal head in relation to the maternal pelvis – 0 station refers to the level of ischial spines. An engaged fetal head will be 2/5th or less palpable on abdominal examination.

These may be summarised as 'F O R C E P S' [4].

F – Fully dilated cervix.

O – Obstruction ruled out (by abdominal and vaginal examination).

Abdominal examination: No more than 1/5th of fetal head should be palpable on abdominal examination. This ensures that the head has descended to at least beyond the ischial spines to +1 station or lower.

Vaginal examination: Station of the fetal head should be identified in cm above or below the ischial spines (Figure 14.1). Ideally the station should be below spines, with descent of the head with contraction and bearing-down effort.

Placement of sutures and fontanelles should be identified. The inverted Y-shaped suture lines or overlapping of parietal bones over the occipital bones in labour help to identify the posterior fontanelle. Anterior fontanelle is felt as a soft diamond-shaped depression at junction of four bones. If the anterior fontanelle is felt easily near the centre of the pelvis it indicates the possibility of a deflexed head.

If the amount of caput succedaneum makes examination difficult, then feel anteriorly for the fetal ear. Care should be taken to feel the pinna and the canal, as the ear can be folded and give a false impression of its position. Also, since the ear is just below the biparietal diameter, it can aid in judging the descent of the head.

Synclitism is assessed by feeling the relationship of the sagittal suture to the transverse plane of the pelvic cavity. Anterior asynclitism, in which the

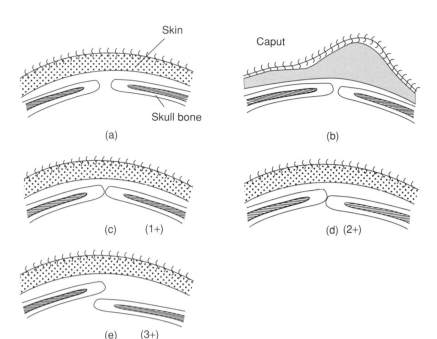

Figure 14.2 Caput succedaneum and moulding. (a) Normal fetal scalp with suture separating the skull bones; (b) Caput succedaneum; (c) Grade 1 moulding with apposition of skull bones; (d) Grade 2 moulding with overlap of skull bones reducible with gentle pressure; and (e) Grade 3 moulding with overlap of skull bones irreducible with gentle pressure.

anterior parietal bone is more easily felt and the sagittal suture is further back in the transverse plane, is normal. Posterior asynclitism however may be a sign of disproportion [5].

Excessive caput succedaneum (soft tissue swelling of fetal scalp) and 'moulding' (over-riding of fetal skull bones) may suggest possibility of cephalopelvic disproportion (Figure 14.2).

Clinical assessment of the bony pelvis has limitations but with experience, obstetricians may be able to judge how well a given fetal head fits the pelvis in particular circumstances to arrive at the decision for a safe instrumental delivery.

R – Membranes should have **R**uptured and instrument checked and assembled correctly.

C – **C**atheterise or ensure that the bladder is empty. **C**onsent the patient appropriately.

E – **E**xplain the procedure, check the need for **E**pidural anaesthesia or other pain relief and whether **E**pisiotomy will be needed.

P – Confirm **P**osition of head and adequate **P**ower (uterine contractions).

S – Determine **S**tation of the fetal skull in relation to ischial spines.

Once it is confirmed that all the above criteria have been met, follow appropriate steps of delivery and repair any perineal tears or episiotomy.

Go back to check the baby's head to confirm the positioning of the instrument used and document the details of delivery completely including indication, discussion, consent, precise description of station, moulding, caput succedaneum, position, degree of flexion of fetal head. Description of procedure should include manoeuvres, rotation, traction, degree of difficulty and number of pulls. The amount of estimated blood loss should be noted. Associated episiotomy or vaginal lacerations and repair should be described in detail.

Key actions

Introduce yourself to the woman and her partner and explain the reason for instrumental vaginal delivery. It is important to document the discussion with the woman as regards options of waiting, assisted delivery or caesarean section.

Carry out thorough abdominal and vaginal assessment and explain the findings and plan of action to the woman. Verbal or written consent must be obtained as appropriate.

Provide adequate analgesia in the form of epidural or spinal anaesthesia, pudendal block or local anaesthetic infiltration (20 ml of 1% lignocaine) of perineum. Amount of anaesthesia required will depend on level of fetal head and need for rotation. Usually ventouse deliveries require less analgesia. In cases of cord prolapse, antepartum bleeding or prolonged deceleration actions should proceed with a brisk speed.

Oxytocin infusion may be considered if uterine contractions are inadequate (fewer than four in 10 minutes and lasting less than 40 seconds each) in the absence of signs of fetal compromise.

Vulva and perineum should be cleansed.

Bladder should be empty.

Lithotomy position (with slight lateral tilt) is the preferred maternal position.

Inform the neonatologist at the start of the procedure.

The choice of instrument will depend on the operator's experience, station of fetal head and position of the vertex. Ventouse should not be used to deliver babies below 34 weeks and those with suspected bleeding tendencies. In general ventouse is preferred when the position is occipito-transverse (OT) or occipito-posterior (OP) to allow for autorotation of the fetal head during traction unless the accoucher is experienced in Kielland's rotational forceps delivery. Where maternal expulsive efforts may be compromised, forceps may be better than ventouse delivery. The failure rates are higher with ventouse as compared with forceps. In most cases the ventouse cup detaches in the lower pelvis almost at the introitus and the delivery is completed by an outlet forceps. Hence the contradiction that with ventouse there are more failed cases but the caesarean deliveries are fewer. If the cup slips higher up use of forceps is not advisable.

Forceps delivery

Commonly used forceps include:

Outlet forceps – Wrigley's.
Mid cavity/low forceps – Simpson's or Neville-Barnes'.

Not so commonly used:

Rotational/Kielland's forceps – considerable experience and skill are required for the safe use of this instrument.
Piper's forceps – for after-coming head of breech.

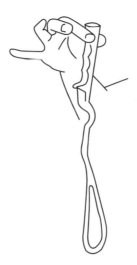

Figure 14.3 Pencil grip of forceps: Left forceps blade held in the left hand with a pencil grip just before application.

Classic forceps like Simpson's forceps and Neville Barnes' forceps are used when the sagittal suture is in direct anteroposterior position or within 45 degrees from the midline (direct OA or OP) while Kielland's forceps are used for rotational deliveries when the occiput is in transverse or posterior position (OT or OP).

Blades of forceps should be assembled and well lubricated. Handle of the left blade is held in the left hand and applied on the left side of maternal pelvis. The handle of the forceps is held with a 'pencil grip' (Figure 14.3). The blade is held parallel to the right inguinal ligament and inserted between the fetal head and the fingers of the right hand which protect the left lateral vaginal wall as the blade is inserted in a circular movement to negotiate the cephalic and pelvic curves (Figure 14.4). In a similar manner, the right blade is held in the right hand, parallel to the left inguinal ligament and the toe of the blade inserted between the right vaginal wall and the head while negotiating the cephalic and pelvic curves. The shanks and the handles of the blades should sit horizontally: if one is at an angle or above the other blade, check for malposition or asynclitism. Slight inwards or downward movements of the handles may be needed to gently bring the blades into position. If the blades were applied correctly, the handles should lie horizontally and lock easily. Correct application is ensured by noting that (a) the sagittal suture in the middle is equidistant from the two blades and perpendicular to the plane of shanks, (b) there is equal space – about one fingerbreadth between the fetal head and heel of the

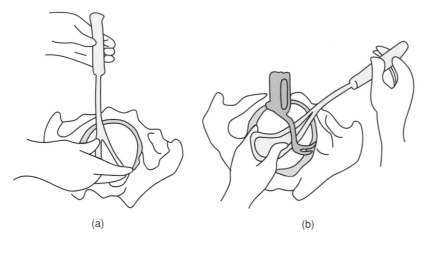

Figure 14.4 Insertion of forceps blades. (a) Left forceps blade introduced under the guidance of right thumb and fingers; (b) Insertion of right forceps blade.

(a)   (b)

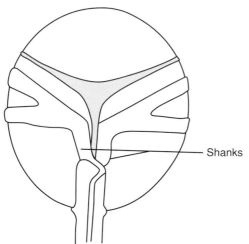

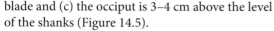
Shanks

Figure 14.5 Correct application of forceps. The sagittal suture is perpendicular to the plane of shanks; there is equal space – about one fingerbreadth between the fetal head and heel of the blade; and the occiput is 3 to 4 cm above the level of the shanks.

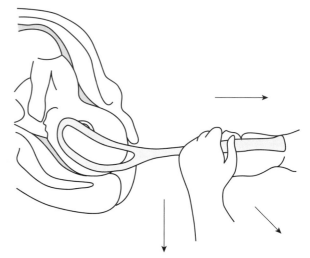

Figure 14.6 Direction of traction. Dominant hand applies traction along the axis of the forceps blades while the other hand applies downward pressure on the shanks of the blades. The net direction of traction is in line with the pelvic axis (Pajot's manoeuvre).

blade and (c) the occiput is 3–4 cm above the level of the shanks (Figure 14.5).

Steady downwards and backwards traction should be given coordinated with uterine contraction and maternal effort to negotiate the pelvic curve (curve of Carus). Traction should not be carried out by gripping the handles but rather with the first and second fingers on the finger guards.

The heel of the other hand may be used to exert downward pressure on the shanks (Pajot's manoeuvre) to ensure that the traction is along the axis of pelvic curve (Figure 14.6).

As the head descends and begins to crown, the direction of pull arches upwards to gently deliver

the head and face over the perineum by extension. An episiotomy may be performed at this stage if there is considerable resistance felt at the perineum or possibility of multiple vaginal/perineal tears.

One may remove the handles of the forceps at this point and assist final spontaneous delivery by flexing the head and pushing the perineum over the head.

For outlet forceps deliveries, the direction of traction may be slight downward traction and as the maximal parietal diameter emerges, a direct upward pull along the direction of the terminal part of the pelvic curve.

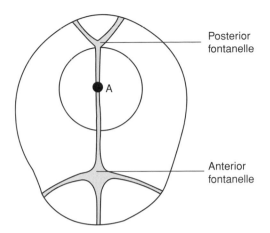

Figure 14.7 Flexion point: correct application of ventouse over the flexion point (A) 3 cm in front of the posterior fontanelle.

Ventouse delivery

Two types of vacuum cups are in common use:

- Anterior cups – where both the suction and traction attachments are close to the middle of the cup. These are mainly designed for occipito-anterior (OA) well flexed head.
- Posterior cups – these have a peripheral vacuum port and are useful in cases of deflexed occipito-posterior (OP) or occipito-transverse (OT) positions. This design permits the cup to be slipped between the head and the vaginal wall to allow placement over the flexion point.

Concept of 'flexion point'

The principle of flexion point is central to effective and safe application of ventouse or forceps delivery.

In the term infant, the distance between the anterior and posterior fontanelles is approximately 9 cm. The flexion point is 3 cm in front of the posterior fontanelle. When placing the centre of a 6 cm vacuum cup over the flexion point, the anterior edge of the cup will be 3 cm behind the anterior fontanelle (Figure 14.7). When the cup is placed over the flexion point, the most favourable diameter of fetal head is presented at the time of delivery. If the cup is placed more anteriorly it will cause deflexion and present a larger diameter of fetal head. If the cup is placed more to one side of the sagittal suture than the other, the application will be paramedian and again present a larger diameter because of the asynclitism produced (Figure 14.8) [4].

The ventouse cups may be made of metal, soft silicon or plastic and come in 4–6 cm sizes. Once the cup is satisfactorily applied over the flexion point, a small amount of vacuum is created.

Vacuum may be created by a hand-held pump or a mechanical suction device to 0.2 bars or 150 mmHg or 0.2 kg/cm^2 negative pressure.

Finger checks need to be done around the periphery of the cup to ensure that no maternal tissue is included. Once this has been confirmed, increase the vacuum to 0.8 bars or 500–600 mmHg or 0.8 kg/cm^2 negative pressure (green mark on the measuring bar of the hand-held 'Omnicup' device).

Traction should be applied in synchrony with the uterine contractions and maternal bearing-down effort at a right angle to the cup as much as possible to avoid the cup slipping (Figure 14.9). The direction of pull should follow the pelvic curve of Carus and changed gradually as the head descends. From downwards and backwards in mid pelvis, it should

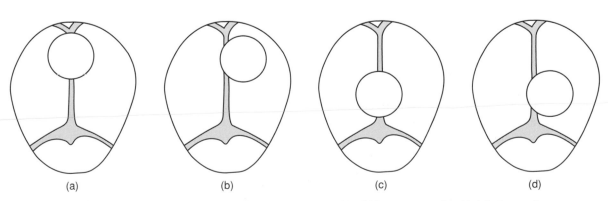

(a) (b) (c) (d)

Figure 14.8 Correct and incorrect ventouse cup applications. (a) Flexing median; (b) flexing paramedian; (c) deflexing median; and (d) deflexing paramedian.

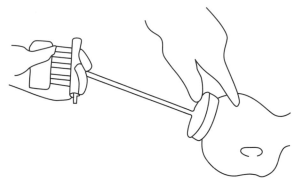

Figure 14.9 Technique of ventouse delivery: traction is applied with the dominant hand while the thumb and index finger of the other hand are placed against the cup and fetal scalp respectively. Traction should be perpendicular to the cup where possible to prevent the cup from slipping.

progressively become downwards and finally downwards and forwards. The descent of the head with flexion promotes autorotation of the head to a favourable occipito-anterior position from an occipito-transverse or occipito-posterior position.

During traction with the right hand, keep the left thumb on the top of the vacuum cup and left index finger on the scalp to see whether the bony part of the head is descending rather than just the scalp. The two hands work in combination, with the thumb over the cup providing counter traction against the pulling hand.

If the vacuum cup slips (pops off), a very careful reappraisal should occur and one further application may be justified.

With either forceps or ventouse, 'one pull' equals two or three traction efforts synchronising with the maternal bearing-down effort during one uterine contraction.

As a general rule, delivery should occur with three pulls of any of the instruments or it should be clear that the head has descended to justify continuing with the delivery. In the case of ventouse delivery, if the cup pops off, consideration may be given to the use of forceps to complete delivery if the head is at the low/outlet level and very favourable. However if there was failure to achieve descent with ventouse at the mid cavity level, it may be best to complete the delivery by a caesarean section. The risk of fetal trauma is greatest on sequential use of both instruments (ventouse followed by forceps) when they are performed at the mid cavity level.

Higher rates of failure of instrumental delivery may be associated with:

- Maternal body mass index over 30.
- Estimated fetal weight over 4000 g or clinically big baby.
- Occipito-posterior position.
- Mid-cavity delivery or when 1/5th of the fetal head is palpable per abdomen.

The procedure must be abandoned if there is no evidence of progressive descent with each pull or where delivery is not imminent following three pulls in spite of correct application by an experienced operator.

Paired cord blood samples should always be processed at the time of delivery for acid–base analysis. Ventouse delivery causes an elevated circular soft tissue swelling called chignon on the fetal scalp. This soft tissue swelling settles in the next 2–3 days and it is important to reassure parents about this after the delivery.

Appropriate postpartum bladder care and thromboprophylaxis should be instituted as per the hospital protocol.

Complications of instrumental delivery

Maternal complications are higher with forceps whilst neonatal complications are more common with the use of ventouse.

Maternal: Vaginal/cervical lacerations, third or fourth degree tears, postpartum haemorrhage.

Fetal: Superficial bruising and abrasions of scalp and face, transient facial nerve palsy, neonatal jaundice, cephalhaematoma. Rarely subgaleal haemorrhage with lethal hypovolaemia after ventouse delivery, retinal haemorrhage, subdural and cerebral haemorrhages, serious cranial injury such as depressed skull fracture.

Key pitfalls

- Failure to anticipate difficult delivery and involve senior clinicians.
- Failure to call for help/communicate in difficult situation.
- Failure to avoid excessive or inappropriate traction.
- Failure to abandon the procedure in time and proceed to caesarean section.

- Failure to anticipate shoulder dystocia and postpartum haemorrhage (PPH).
- Failure to recognise and repair perineal trauma.
- Failure to document appropriately.

Key pearls

- In most cases it will be clear that the head is in a low or outlet position and that assisted delivery will be accomplished with ease. However in those cases in which the fetal head is arrested in between spines to +1 station it is often prudent to declare 'a trial of instrumental delivery'. This should be performed in an operating theatre with facilities and personnel available to perform a caesarean section. If difficulties are encountered during the delivery the obstetrician can immediately abandon the procedure and proceed to caesarean section. This takes away the pressure from the obstetrician to persist with an attempt at vaginal delivery and minimises risks to both mother and fetus [5].
- During ventouse delivery it is important not to change the direction of pull sooner than necessary or else it often results in cup detachment. It is wise to wait until the vacuum cup and the biparietal diameter are beyond the vulval outlet, prior to applying traction upwards.
- Recognising potential difficulties and making the timely decision to abandon any further attempts at vaginal delivery form an important part of learning the art of an instrumental delivery.
- All staff performing instrumental vaginal deliveries should undergo annual skills and drills training involving use of ventouse and forceps for assisted vaginal delivery.
- Learning points emerging from adverse incidents related to use of ventouse or forceps should be discussed at an appropriate risk management forum and disseminated amongst the entire labour ward team to facilitate continued learning.

Management in low-resource settings

In developing countries, caesarean section may not be universally available due to lack of resources. It is important for practising obstetricians and midwives to be familiar with common operative procedures applicable in their set-up to improve maternal and fetal outcome. At all instrumental vaginal deliveries, someone in attendance should be capable of performing neonatal resuscitation. Although instrumental delivery is a service provided in both basic and comprehensive essential (or emergency) obstetric care, it is under-used in low-resource settings [6]. There is a definite need for instrumental vaginal deliveries to be made widely available. This in turn will require specific interventions to increase the availability of both the necessary equipment and the operators skilled in its use. Political will and increasing international advocacy will play a major role in implementation of country-specific interventions to ensure provision of equipment and trained operators to areas where they are currently unavailable.

Training and assessment

Training is central to patient safety. There are increased levels of neonatal trauma associated with initial unsuccessful attempts at operative vaginal delivery by inexperienced operators. The Royal College of Obstetricians and Gynaecologists (RCOG) recommends that obstetricians should achieve experience in spontaneous vertex delivery before commencing training in operative vaginal delivery. Competency in instrumental deliveries under supervision should be achieved before conducting unsupervised deliveries and should be monitored regularly thereafter. An experienced operator, competent at mid cavity deliveries, should be present from the outset for all attempts at rotational or mid cavity operative vaginal delivery [7]. The RCOG also recommends dedicated consultant sessions on the labour ward to facilitate better training and supervision of trainees. Assessment of clinical competence should be carried out using the Objective Structured Assessment of Technical Skills (OSATS) form designed for operative vaginal delivery by the RCOG [http://www.rcog.org.uk/files/rcog-corp/uploaded-files/ED-CORE-OSATS-OP-Vag-Delivery_0.pdf]. Local and specialist courses in labour ward management can contribute to the development and maintenance of operative delivery expertise. In general, the supervising obstetrician should make a full assessment as to whether the indication for instrumental delivery is appropriate and choice of instrument correct. During traction he or she should confirm that the descent is occurring and not wait until three pulls have been completed, as this will lead to abandoning of any further attempt and also risk use of excessive force.

After delivery, an adequate review of overall conduct of the delivery, perineal repair and postpartum care should follow.

References

1. American College of Obstetricians and Gynecologists. *ACOG Practice Bulletin No. 17: Operative Vaginal Delivery*. Washington, DC: ACOG, 2000.

2. Howell C, Grady K, Cox C. *Managing Obstetric Emergencies and Trauma – the MOET Course Manual*. Second Edition. London: RCOG, 2007.

3. Baskett TF, Calder AA, Arulkumaran S. Assisted vaginal delivery. In *Munro Kerr's Operative Obstetrics*. Eleventh Edition. Edinburgh: Elsevier, 2007, pp. 91–125.

4. Chandraharan E, Arulkumaran S. Operative delivery, shoulder dystocia and episiotomy. In Arulkumaran S, Penna LK, Bhasker Rao K (Eds.), *The Management of Labour*. Second Edition. Orient Longman (India), 2006, pp. 137–162.

5. Baskett TF, Arulkumaran S (Eds.) Assisted vaginal delivery. In *Intrapartum Care for the MRCOG and Beyond*. London: RCOG, 2002, pp. 63–74.

6. Ameh C, Weeks A. The role of instrumental vaginal delivery in low resource settings. *Br J Obstet Gynaecol* 2009; 116 (Suppl. 1): 22–25.

7. Royal College of Obstetricians and Gynaecologists. *Operative Vaginal Delivery*. Green-top Guideline No. 26. London: RCOG, 2011.

Chapter

15

Emergency caesarean section

Chitra Ramanathan and Leonie Penna

Key facts

Definition

A caesarean section (CS) is an operation where a laparotomy (abdominal incision) is undertaken to allow a uterine incision to deliver one or more fetuses, alive or dead after period of viability (usually 24 weeks' gestation).

Depending on the urgency, caesarean sections are categorised as follows [1]:

- Grade 1 – for indications that are an immediate threat to the life of mother or fetus (about 16% of all) e.g. massive abruption with fetal bradycardia. These caesareans are often described as 'crash'. Perimortem CS done for a woman with cardiac arrest not responding to resuscitation falls within this category.
- Grade 2 – for indications where there is no immediate but likely compromise to the mother (e.g. bleeding) or fetus (pathological CTG) where urgent delivery is required, plus slow progress in the first stage of labour with a reassuring fetal heart pattern (about 32% of all).
- Grade 3 – for indications where there is a need for early delivery for a fetal or maternal reason but there is no acute compromise (18% of all) e.g. planned next-day delivery for a 34-week fetus with growth restriction and deteriorating Dopplers. These caesareans are often described as 'semi-planned'.
- Grade 4 – for non-urgent indications where delivery is timed to suit the mother and the healthcare provider (31% of all) e.g. pre-labour delivery at 39 weeks for two previous caesarean

sections. These caesareans are also called 'elective' or planned.

Grades 1–3 are all types of emergency CS with differing degrees of urgency.

There are few recommendations made on time-scales for different grades, as even within the grades the exact urgency of the indication is variable. The RCOG advises that the urgency of CS should be considered as a 'continuum of risk' pointing out that whilst in some grade 1 indications decision to delivery intervals (DDI) of as little as 15 minutes can be achieved, studies have shown that this is not invariably the case and also that evidence shows that a DDI of up to 75 minutes is not associated with an increased risk of neonatal compromise compared with a shorter DDI [1]. They also point out that in some cases even delivery within 30 minutes cannot prevent a poor neonatal outcome adding argument for the need to treat each case individually. Overall they conclude that the urgency of CS should be individualised based on the risk to the fetus and the safety of the mother. They recommend that in cases of acute fetal compromise a target DDI of 30 minutes is used but with the caveat that in some cases delivery needs to be undertaken even more rapidly to try to reduce the risk of a poor outcome.

Incidence

The World Health Organization recommends that the total CS rates (combination of elective and emergency procedures) should be 10–15% but makes no assessment of appropriate emergency CS rates within this total rate. Additionally it has recently acknowledged that these rates are not being achieved, with most developed countries reporting rates well in excess of

Obstetric and Intrapartum Emergencies, ed. Edwin Chandraharan and Sabaratnam Arulkumaran. Published by Cambridge University Press. © Cambridge University Press 2012.

these levels and commenting that 'there is no empirical evidence for an optimum percentage' [2, 3]. There are no studies that have assessed what the optimal rate of CS should be and it is likely that this would vary significantly depending on population demographics. A study of 620 604 births in English hospitals in 2008 showed a rate of 23.8% but that rates varied between 13.6% and 32.1% in different hospitals and that the variation in the rate of emergency CS was even greater than the rates for elective CS [4].

Key implications

Benefits

- To prevent threat to the mother's long-term health or life. This benefit is rarely in doubt as the clinical signs allow a firm diagnosis of a situation with serious risk.
- To prevent intra-uterine fetal demise or damage usually due to hypoxia. It is not always possible to confirm that a fetus is at risk and so this benefit may be based on a situation with a high likelihood of risk.

Maternal risks

Emergency caesarean section has risks for both mother and baby. The risks are greater than those associated with planned CS (24% versus 16%) [5].

Maternal morbidity:

- Operative and postpartum haemorrhage.
- Infection and wound problems.
  Wound, urinary tract, endometritis, chest (if general anaesthetic).
  Wound dehiscence.
  Burst abdomen.
  Visceral injury.
  Bladder and ureteric injury.
  Bowel injury.
- Thromboembolism.
- Deep vein thrombosis and pulmonary embolism.
- Anaesthetic risks.
  Major – total spinal or aspiration pneumonia.
  Minor – post spinal headaches.
  Long-term risks.
  Increased risk of future caesarean section.
  Increased risk of complications during future abdominal surgery.

Increased risk of placenta praevia and morbidly adherent placenta.
Reduced future fertility.
Small increase in the risk of stillbirth in future pregnancies.
Development of adhesions and incisional hernias.

All these risks are common to both elective and emergency CS but many of the typical indications for emergency CS further increase the risk of the possible complications associated with CS:

- Infection more likely in ruptured membranes and in cases where multiple repeated vaginal examinations were performed.
- Haemorrhage more likely as prolonged labour predisposing to uterine atony and greater risk of tears in the lower segment due to deeply engaged fetal head.
- Anaesthesia may be more complicated as the woman is less well prepared or may have a risk factor related to the indication for CS.
- Thromboembolism more likely in prolonged labour and preeclampsia.
- Surgical complications more likely in cases with deeply engaged (or even impacted) head and with CS in advanced rather than early labour (33% incidence of complications at 9–10 cm dilation versus 17% at 1 cm or less) [5].
- Both anaesthesia and surgery are more likely to be undertaken by a less-experienced clinician than planned surgery, increasing blood loss, anaesthetic and surgical complications.

Mortality

Although rare, the risk of maternal death is increased following CS. In the UK the risk of death for the woman during/following CS is three times that related to vaginal birth. However, this figure includes CS for all indications and in women with comorbidities. The true risk will depend on the absolute indication with the risk of certain operations being much greater than others. The absolute risk for a healthy woman for simple indications such as fetal distress has never been calculated but in all probability is not much higher than the risk with vaginal birth.

Fetal risks

- A scalp or buttock laceration (2%).
- Trauma.

- Skull, femoral or humeral fracture.
- Increased risk of respiratory distress syndrome (RDS) and transient tachypnoea of the newborn (TTN) when compared with equivalent gestation infants delivered vaginally.
- Iatrogenic prematurity with early delivery.
- Neonatal prematurity-related complications.

Key pointers

- All unnecessary emergency caesarean sections should be avoided to limit maternal risks [6].
- Consider the use of syntocinon in cases of slow progress in labour.
- Undertake fetal blood sampling in cases of suspected fetal distress wherever clinically possible.
- Involve a senior obstetrician in the decision for all emergency caesarean sections.
- Avoid induction of labour unless clinically indicated.
- The indication for all caesarean sections should be carefully considered with any borderline indications reviewed using a full assessment of the risk and benefit.
- It is essential to avoid carer bias by remaining 'open minded' when taking care of women in labour and not to become overly focused on risk factors that are known to increase the risk of emergency CS but are not in themselves an indication to recommend emergency CS (examples include increased BMI, increased maternal age, previous delivery by CS). These factors should be reviewed in the context of the usual obstetric indications for CS.

Indications for emergency caesarean section

Suspected fetal compromise

- Cord prolapse or transverse lie/oblique lie in labour.
- Suspected uterine rupture.
- Suspected fetal distress – either a pathological fetal heart rate pattern (without fetal blood sampling) or fetal blood sample showing pH < 7.20.

Serious maternal compromise

- Severe antepartum haemorrhage due to major placenta praevia or abruption, causing fetal compromise or maternal compromise in spite of aggressive resuscitation.
- Severe hypertension requiring delivery with contraindication to induction.
- Perimortem caesarean section.

Failure to progress in labour

- Failed induction.
- Failure to progress in first stage.
- Failure to progress in second stage.
- Failed instrumental deliveries.

Peri-operative preparation

Consent

Proper consent requires that the risks and benefits of the proposed caesarean section be discussed with the mother. It is good practice to obtain written consent for emergency CS wherever possible [7]. In extreme emergency situations like fetal bradycardia or massive abruption with fetal compromise (grade 1 CS) verbal consent is acceptable, however a rapid and clear explanation of the operation is still required.

Anaesthesia

It is important to communicate the grade of the CS to the anaesthetist to help the decision about appropriate anaesthesia for the situation. Regional anaesthesia is appropriate for the majority of cases but general anaesthesia maybe needed in a grade 1 CS. No anaesthesia is required for a perimortem CS.

Antibiotics

Prophylactic antibiotics are recommended for all women undergoing CS as they significantly reduce the risk of postoperative infective morbidity. The antibiotic should be broad spectrum and cover Gram-negative organisms and anaerobes. A combination of a cephalosporin and metronidazole (single dose) given immediately prior to skin incision is the recommended regimen [8]. Although there is no evidence of specific neonatal issues antibiotics have previously been administered after the cord has been clamped to avoid placental transfer but current evidence suggests maternal benefit of early antibiotics outweighs any possible theoretical neonatal issue. In women at higher risk of infective complications (for example preexisting conditions such as BMI > 35) the dose of cephalosporin should be adjusted for weight and the option of continuing antibiotics into the postnatal period should be considered. This should also be considered when the intraoperative haemorrhage is more than 1000 ml as the risk of infection is increased. Although intravenous antibiotics are often prescribed these have no advantage over oral antibiotics for prophylaxis following the loading dose in a woman who is eating and drinking and oral administration avoids the need for prolonged cannulation.

Thromboprophylaxis

A risk assessment should be undertaken immediately after delivery in all women to decide on the duration of prophylactic measures. However, a group of universal precautions is recommended for all cases:

- Peri-operative pneumatic calf compression.
- Thromboembolic deterrent stockings (TEDS) until fully mobile (usually discharge from hospital).
- Ensuring early mobilisation and good hydration.
- Low molecular weight heparin (LMWH): all women undergoing emergency CS should be prescribed a prophylactic dose of LMWH such as enoxaparin 30–80 mg depending on their weight for the first 7 days after surgery. Very high-risk women should be prescribed LMWH for 6 weeks.

Premedication

Improving gastric emptying and reducing the acidity of stomach contents reduces the risk of aspiration and damage to lung parenchyma if it occurs.

Women who are considered to be more likely to have delivery by emergency CS (such as poor progress between vaginal examinations in spite of oxytocin) should be prescribed premedication as a precaution (usually metoclopramide 10 mg and ranitidine 150 mg orally). If premedication has not been administered previously it should be prescribed as soon as the decision to perform CS is made, in this situation metoclopramide 10 mg and ranitidine 50 mg can be given intravenously. Sodium citrate 10–15 ml as a single oral

dose should also be administered immediately prior to transfer to theatre.

Catheterisation

All women should have a catheter inserted in the bladder prior to the skin incision regardless of the need for rapid delivery. This is essential to reduce the risk of bladder injuries during entry to the uterus.

Personal protective equipment (PPE)

For all caesarean sections it is good practice to wear visor masks to avoid splashes of body fluids. This is recommended as part of the standard precautions that should be adopted for all surgical cases even if the woman is known to be low risk for infections such at HIV or hepatitis B.

Double gloving has not been shown to reduce the risk of needle stick injuries but does reduce the risk of skin contamination due to micro-glove puncture. It is not recommended where high-quality gloves are in use but may be required where poor-quality gloves are used.

Surgical techniques

Skin incision and abdominal entry

Most obstetricians adopt a preferred technique that combines a number of described techniques, but a low transverse incision (10–12 cm) is recommended, as these are associated with shorter operating times and reduced postoperative febrile morbidity.

- Joel Cohen incision: transverse straight incision 3 cm above the symphysis pubis with subsequent tissue layers opened bluntly or if required with Mayo scissors.
- Pfannensteil incision: transverse curved incision approximately 2 cm above the symphysis pubis with sharp dissection of fascia and peritoneum. This is associated with less postoperative pain and an improved cosmetic effect compared with midline incision.
- Midline incision: a midline incision should only be used if required for access usually where an upper segment uterine incision may be required (for example massive lower segment fibroids) as they are associated with greater postoperative morbidity. Midline incisions are still commonly used for CS in developing countries although a

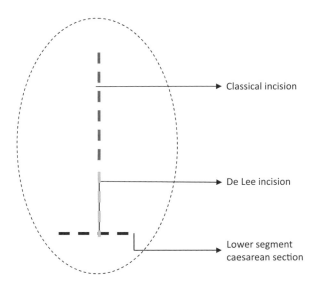

Figure 15.1 Schematic representation of uterine incisions for caesarean section.

lower segment incision is made on the uterus. If repeat CS is required a new transverse incision is usually preferable to the use of the old midline incision but should be discussed with the woman prior to surgery. A midline incision may be chosen for perimortem CS since for a skilled operator it may give quicker access than a transverse incision.

- Paramedian incisions are rarely used in obstetrics unless some surgical comorbidity is suspected.

Uterine incision (see Figure 15.1)

The need for a non-standard uterine incision should be anticipated from the clinical history.

- Lower segment transverse incision: This is the commonest incision used and is associated with the lowest intra operative haemorrhage as the lower segment is thin at this level. It has the disadvantage that the options for extending the incision to improve access are limited as lateral extension may not be possible if the lower segment is narrow without significant risk of bleeding from the uterine artery. This is especially true in preterm deliveries where the lower segment may be very poorly formed. This incision can be extended by blunt dissection (digitally) or by sharp dissection (Mayo scissors).
- De Lee incision: This is vertical lower segment incision and is recommended when the lateral extension of a transverse incision is more likely

such as in a preterm delivery where the lower segment is assessed as narrow. This incision has the advantage that it can be extended upwards to give the required access. However, it is associated with more haemorrhage and there is also a risk of the incision extending to bladder and vagina. This incision needs to be extended by sharp dissection with either a blade or Mayo scissors.

- Classical incision: This is a rarely used vertical incision in the upper segment of the uterus. It has the advantage of providing excellent access, avoiding the lower segment and thus any structures in that part of the uterus. It has the disadvantage that the myometrium is very thick (often several centimetres) and vascular, resulting in more operative haemorrhage and a more complex surgical procedure with a three-layer uterine closure required. Additionally the risks of classical incisions in future pregnancies are uncertain with the risk of rupture in labour being significantly greater than for a lower segment incision and cases of spontaneous dehiscence in the third trimester reported.

Needles/sutures

Vicryl no. 1 on a blunt needle for uterine closure and Vicryl no. 1 on a sharp needle for rectus sheath are commonly used sutures. However, as there is no good evidence to guide choice it largely depends on the surgeon's preference.

Drains

A tube (Robinson) drain can be used in the pelvis or a suction drain (Redi-vac) for the sub-rectus space if there are concerns about haemostasis. Routine drainage is not recommended, as it does not decrease the risk of wound infection or haematoma. Drains should be removed as soon as possible when no longer draining significantly (usually less than 100 ml in 24 hours).

Uterine closure

Two layers is recommended as although a single layer is associated with shorter operating time it increases the risk of uterine dehiscence in future pregnancies. A locked continuous suture is commonly used for the first layer to improve haemostasis.

Skin closure

The suture used for skin closure depends on operator preference with no strong evidence of the benefit of one material over another. Subcuticular Prolene (requires removal) or Monocryl (absorbable) are commonly used. Skin staples or gluing techniques are less commonly used alternatives.

A subcutaneous suture should be used where the wound gapes by 2 cm or more as this reduces the risk of postoperative wound disruption.

Difficulties during delivery

Deeply impacted fetal head

This is very common in second stage caesarean sections especially after failed instrumental delivery with deflexed occipito-posterior position. The risk of deep impaction can often be predicted from the clinical circumstances and the findings on vaginal examination (excessive caput succedaneum and moulding) and anticipated.

Techniques to assist delivery:

- Anticipate and ensure appropriately skilled surgeon.
- Request an assistant to 'push' the head up into the abdomen from pelvis by performing a vaginal examination. It is important that this role is not delegated to a junior clinician as the procedure requires skill to flex the head so that minimal upward force is required to assist the surgeon in achieving dis-impaction. The application of excessive upward force will increase the risk of skull fracture and uterine tears.
- Extension of the incision in the shape of a 'J' on one side or in the midline to an inverted 'T' incision.
- Releasing the rectus sheath and muscle by extending the incisions already made. If rectus muscle is partially cut a formal repair is not usually required as it heals very well spontaneously.
- Internal podalic version and breech extraction has been described in the literature. This works on the principle that flexion of the body is greater compared with flexion at the neck in a deeply engaged head. With emergence of the legs and breech outside the uterus the head ascends to the uterine incision from the pelvis.

Extension of the angles

This occurs more commonly with second stage caesarean section and in any situation where the head is deeply impacted or deflexed.

Techniques for management:

- Anticipate and ensure appropriately experienced operator.
- Ensure flexion of presenting part to reduce the diameters of the head during delivery. Make the uterine incision slightly higher on the uterus to avoid tearing down into the vagina and avoid making an incision at or below the cervix. This has to be carefully balanced against the difficulty this may create if the head is deeply engaged.
- If a tear occurs then haemorrhage will often be a problem and haemostasis should be secured immediately using a non-crushing clamp (Green Armytage) to reduce blood loss whilst the full extent of the tear is assessed.
- Blind suturing of a tear should not be undertaken as this has the risk of inadvertent ureteric occlusion. The course of the ureter must be identified in a complex tear.
- Request the assistance of a second experienced surgeon early if a problematic tear occurs.

Other considerations [9]

Delivery of the placenta

Manual separation of the placenta before spontaneous separation increases the blood loss during CS and also the risk of postoperative endometritis. An oxytocin (5 IU syntocinon intravenously) should be administered after delivery of the baby and controlled cord traction performed following signs of separation. Uterine massage or compression can be employed to speed up separation. Manual removal of the placenta should be reserved for cases where separation does not follow in a timely manner or where other circumstances require that the placenta is delivered quickly (e.g. bleeding from the angles).

Perimortem caesarean section [10]

Current resuscitation guidelines recommend that the fetus be delivered after 4 minutes of maternal cardiac arrest that is not responding to standard measures of resuscitation. The intention is to improve the chances of successful maternal resuscitation and not to deliver a viable fetus (although this may occur) thus caesarean section should be undertaken regardless of gestation and the expected condition of the fetus.

The procedure for caesarean section should aim for delivery as rapidly as possible. A full instrument set is not required (A&E and labour ward resuscitation trolley equipment lists should include a disposable scalpel for use in this situation), skin cleaning is only undertaken if this is immediately available and surgical technique is adapted to allow the most rapid entry and delivery.

A midline incision in skin and uterus is appropriate if the operator is confident with this approach but a transverse supra-pubic with a Joel-Cohen incision is an alternative rapid entry with which many obstetricians may feel more comfortable in this very stressful situation. Bleeding is not a problem during perimortem CS as the maternal hypotension results in a virtually bloodless field.

Standard closure technique should be adopted. If resuscitation is successful there is possibility of haemorrhage when the blood pressure normalises or with disseminated intravascular coagulation (DIC) that occurs as a sequela to the cardiac arrest. A widebore pelvic drain and a sub-rectus suction drain are prudent and will assist ongoing care in the intensive care unit.

Sterilisation at emergency caesarean section

Sterilisation should only be undertaken at the time of emergency CS if this has been discussed during an antenatal appointment prior to the onset of labour as the incidence of regret is known to be higher if it is undertaken as an emergency without time for reflection. It is therefore good practice to ensure that the option of sterilisation is broached and documented in any woman who may wish this (for example multigravid women who enquire about interval sterilisation during pregnancy) even if their risk of emergency CS would appear to be low.

Postnatal debrief

All women who have undergone a traumatic labour and delivery including emergency CS should be debriefed, ideally by the doctor undertaking surgery (or if this is not possible by another senior obstetrician) on the first postoperative day. This should include an explanation of the reasons why a CS was required on this occasion and a recommendation for mode of delivery in future pregnancies. Women often think that all future deliveries will require CS when in reality most emergency deliveries are as a result of non-recurrent factors and thus the recommendation for delivery after one emergency CS for most women is to plan for vaginal birth (VBAC).

For the majority of women no further consultation will be required but a further discussion should be arranged if requested either before discharge or as an interval outpatient consultation. Referral for specialist counselling should be considered in women who display signs of a posttraumatic stress disorder.

Modified Early Obstetric Warning System (MEOWS) charts

After CS, women should be observed on a one-to-one basis by a trained healthcare professional until they have regained airway control (if a general anaesthetic was given), have cardiorespiratory stability and are able to communicate their needs.

Observations (respiratory rate, pulse, blood pressure, pain score and consciousness) should be measured every 30 minutes for 2 hours, and hourly until stable when 4-hourly observations are recommended. All the observations should be recorded on a MEOWS chart, which uses trigger scoring to allow the early identification of developing complications. If observations are unstable, more frequent observations and medical review are required.

Emergency caesarean section in low-resource settings

Emergency CS is much less common in low-resource settings but unfortunately the extreme indications that occur increase maternal morbidity considerably.

Indications such as neglected obstructed labour increase the risk of haemorrhage and infective morbidity. The lack of antenatal care worsens comorbidities such as anaemia. The choice of resources such as antibiotics and suture materials may be limited, forcing compromises from optimal management.

Emergency CS for fetal reasons is less common as comprehensive fetal monitoring is not ubiquitous. Fetal demise may have occurred in cases of prolonged obstructed labour. The option of a destructive procedure should be considered if the fetus has died; however, in practice this often cannot be achieved safely in most cases as the presenting part is too high or there are concerns about infection or uterine rupture.

Anaesthetic support is often limited with the available spinal anaesthetic using only local anaesthetic; this gives a shorter duration of anaesthesia thus operative technique needs to be rapid and precise. The use of a Joel-Cohen transverse incision (with avoidance of a midline incision) and uterine exteriorisation are recommended to shorten operative time [11]. Prophylactic antibiotic administration is essential (ampicillin or a cephalosporin) and in most situations should be continued for at least 24 hours postoperatively [12].

The limited availability of suture material may result in the use of a single-layer uterine closure. However, this is associated with an increase in the risk of scar rupture in future pregnancies and this is very important, as subsequent labours may not be in hospital thus the adaptation of technique to achieve a two-layer closure with a single suture is recommended rather than a single-layer closure. A single-layer closure can be considered in women who are undergoing tubal ligation at the time of the CS.

The option of tubal ligation should be discussed with any women of high parity having emergency CS or where the indication is suspected uterine rupture. However it is essential that proper consent for this is obtained as an interval procedure is preferable if there is any doubt about understanding or agreement.

Prolonged catheterisation in women who have had long, obstructed labours is recommended as although it prolongs hospital stay it will reduce the risk of bladder dysfunction and fistula formation.

Careful postnatal observations are essential with aggressive treatment of any postoperative fever.

Counselling about future pregnancies is essential with the advice to seek antenatal care and delivery in a hospital in all cases.

References

1. Royal College of Obstetricians and Gynaecologists. *Classification of Urgency of Caesarean Section – a Continuum of Risk*. RCOG Good Practice Guideline No. 11. London: RCOG, 2010.

2. World Health Organization. Appropriate technology for birth. *Lancet* 1985; 2: 436–437.

3. World Health Organization. *Monitoring Emergency Obstetric Care – A Handbook*. Geneva: WHO, 2009.

4. Bragg F, Cromwell D, Edozien L *et al.* Variation in rates of caesarean section among English NHS trusts after accounting for maternal and clinical risk: cross sectional study. *Br Med J* 2010; 341: c506.

5. Royal College of Obstetricians and Gynaecologists. *Caesarean Section Consent Advice No. 7*. London: RCOG, 2009.

6. Thomas J, Paranjothy S, RCOG Clinical Effectiveness Support Unit. *The National Sentinel Caesarean Section Audit Report*. London: RCOG, 2001.

7. Royal College of Obstetricians and Gynaecologists. *Obtaining Valid Consent*. Clinical Governance Advice No. 6. London: RCOG, 2008.

8. National Collaborating Centre for Women's and Children's Health. *Caesarean Section*. Clinical Guideline. London: RCOG, 2011.

9. National Collaborating Centre for Women's and Children's Health. *Caesarean Section*. Clinical Guideline. London: RCOG Press, 2004.

10. Howell C, Grady K, Cox C. *Managing Obstetric Emergencies and Trauma – the MOET Course Manual*. Second edition. London: RCOG, 2007.

11. Abalos E. *Surgical Techniques for Caesarean Section: RHL Commentary*. The WHO Reproductive Health Library. Geneva: World Health Organization, 2009.

12. Cecatti JG. *Antibiotic Prophylaxis for Caesarean Section: RHL Commentary*. The WHO Reproductive Health Library. Geneva: World Health Organization, 2005.

Chapter 16

Unintended trauma and complications during caesarean section

Osama Abu-Ghazza and Edwin Chandraharan

Key facts

The incidence of caesarean section (CS) is rising and the average rate of CS (including both elective and emergency) across England and Wales is about 24.8% [1]. In some maternity units this rate is even higher, reaching 32.1%, even after adjusting for complex variables [2], contributing to increased morbidity and mortality. Several variables affect the outcome of caesarean section; these include patient characteristics (body mass index, previous abdominal surgery, congenital malformations), fetal characteristics (lie, presentation, position, size and number), presence or absence of uterine contractions (advanced labour with deeply engaged head), need for rapid delivery and the experience of the operator. Due to these interactions of complex variables, unintended trauma and complications do occur during both elective and emergency CS.

Unintended trauma and complications during CS include:

- Difficult delivery of the fetus.
- Fetal injuries.
- Bleeding.
- Bladder and/or ureteric injuries.
- Small or large bowel injuries.

Key implications

- Maternal: Longer surgical procedure; conversion from regional to a general anaesthetic; multiple blood transfusions and additional procedures; delay in bonding with the newborn; a longer

hospital stay; intermediate effects – prolonged urinary catheterisation; colostomy bag; sepsis due to unrecognised bowel complication which may lead to death – sepsis is the leading cause of maternal deaths in the UK according to the recent **CMACE** report [3].
- Fetal: Fetal injuries; delay in delivering the fetus may result in peripartum hypoxia leading to hypoxic brain injury; neonatal admission for convulsions and multi-organ support; long-term neurological outcomes (learning difficulties, cerebral palsy); and very rarely, intrapartum stillbirths and early neonatal death.
- Medico-legal: clinical negligence claims due to failure to recognise unintended complications intra-operatively and inappropriate management of complications.

Key pointers

- Difficulty in delivering a fetus during CS: deeply engaged head (late second stage of labour); failed attempt of instrumental vaginal delivery prior to caesarean section; occipito-posterior position and macrosomia; oligohydramnios in non-cephalic presentation; abnormal lie (oblique or transverse); and increased maternal BMI.
- Unexpected bleeding: sources of bleeding may vary. Bleeding may occur from uterine hypotonia, unexpected coagulopathy, abnormal placental site, as well as from uterine angular extensions, vesical venous plexus or broad ligament tears. Other possible unintended sources of bleeding include damage to inferior epigastric vessels during forcible separation of rectus abdominis muscles, and bleeding from greater omental vessels after

Obstetric and Intrapartum Emergencies, ed. Edwin Chandraharan and Sabaratnam Arulkumaran. Published by Cambridge University Press. © Cambridge University Press 2012.

division of omental adhesions. Risk factors include: previous history of postpartum haemorrhage; prolonged labour; excessive use of syntocinon; uterine over-distension (multiple pregnancies, polyhydramnios, macrosomia); uterine inversion; uterine fibroids; and conditions associated with coagulation failure (placental abruption, preeclampsia, retained dead fetus or preexisting coagulation abnormalities).

- Bladder or ureteric injuries: failure to deflect the bladder before making lower uterine segment incision; previous caesarean section; failure to empty the bladder prior to caesarean section; presence of adhesions between bladder and lower uterine segment; and CS at full cervical dilation (failure to recognise altered anatomy).
- Small or large bowel injuries: any previous abdominal surgery; adhesions due to inflammatory bowel disease (e.g. Crohn's disease); and endometriosis.

Key actions

Difficulty in delivering the fetus

Clinicians should remain calm and not lose confidence and identify the possible reason for experiencing difficulty. This could be due to increased maternal BMI, inadequate surgical incision, presence of dense adhesions or abnormal lie of the fetus.

If inadequate access is the identified issue, then attempts at delivery should be stopped immediately and the surgical incision should be enlarged, using the surgeon's fingers as a 'guard' to avoid any injury to the fetus. A transverse rectus muscle cutting incision (Maylard's) may be useful, if rapid delivery is warranted (e.g. fetal compromise). If abnormal lie poses difficulty for delivery, feet may be grasped by passing one hand into the uterine incision whilst the other hand placed over the uterus could aid rotation (i.e. a combination of internal podalic version and external cephalic version). In rare cases, especially if there is fetal compromise or neglected shoulder presentation, if internal podalic version is proving difficult an 'inverted T' incision may be required.

If the fetal head is deeply impacted, this should be pushed up to disengage the head from the pelvis, prior to commencing CS. During CS, an assistant may be asked to push the fetus's head up in between uterine contractions, by placing a hand through the vagina. In occipito-posterior position, the head should be first disengaged by flexion and rotated to occipito-transverse position, prior to delivery. If the head is not deeply engaged, but difficulty is experienced during delivery, a Wrigley's forceps or a Kiwi cup (hand-held ventouse 'OMNI' cup) could be applied to facilitate delivery. If these measures fail, a breech extraction may be attempted.

Top tip: Consider 'acute tocolysis' [4] to abolish uterine contractions and to relax the myometrium and improve utero-placental blood flow, whilst awaiting senior help.

Bleeding

Always remember the 4 Ts as the causes of bleeding (Tone, Tissue, Trauma, Thrombin).

Management of uterine hypotonia

Always alert the anaesthetist, check uterine cavity for retained products and commence direct uterine massage and administer uterotonic drugs (intravenous oxytocin at 10 units/hour, intramuscular prostaglandin E2 (Haemabate) 250 mcg every 15 min or rectal Misoprostol 600 mcg). Monitor response to treatment. Algorithms such as HAEMOSTASIS may aid management (see Chapter 5, this volume) [5]. If bleeding continues despite these first-line measures, consider informing experienced obstetricians and attempt uterine compression sutures such as B-Lynch, vertical or horizontal compression sutures and commence systematic pelvic devascularisation (bilateral uterine artery ligation and ligation of both uterine and tubal branches of uterine arteries – 'quadruple ligation'). Uterine tamponade by packing the uterine cavity with a ribbon gauze or hydrostatic balloon should also be considered, if appropriate. Massive Obstetric Haemorrhage Protocols such as 'Code Blue' should be activated when the bleeding exceeds 2 litres (or earlier, if continued bleeding is anticipated) to ensure multidisciplinary input, to alert experienced clinicians and to facilitate timely administration of blood and blood products.

Further measures include internal iliac artery ligation, interventional radiology for pelvic arterial embolisation and hysterectomy as the last resort [6].

Extension of lower segment uterine incision

Deep and angular extension of lower segment incisions must be followed to visualise the apex. Care should be

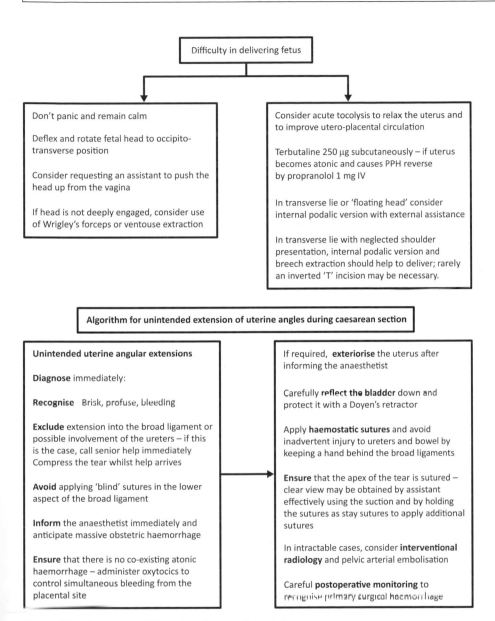

Figure 16.1 Algorithm for difficulty in delivering a fetus during a caesarean section.

taken to avoid inadvertent injury to adjacent structures (ureters and bladder) and these extensions should be secured with haemostatic sutures (see algorithm in Figure 16.1). Failure to do so would result in continuous haemorrhage or secondary postpartum haemorrhage [7]. Rarely, pelvic arterial embolisation may be required [5].

Injury to inferior epigastric vessels

The inferior epigastric artery arises from the external iliac artery, immediately above the inguinal ligament and it curves forward in the sub-peritoneal tissue and then ascends obliquely along the medial margin of the abdominal inguinal ring, continuing its course upward to pierce the transversalis fascia and pass in front of the linea semicircularis. It ascends between the rectus abdominis muscle and its sheath and lies on the posterior surface of this muscle, close to its lateral border. Sharp dissection to get into abdominal cavity or cutting the rectus abdominis muscle can injure inferior epigastric vessels. Knowledge of anatomy should help avoid injury to these blood vessels, which if not recognised may result in a haematoma or intra-abdominal bleeding. Inferior epigastric vessels are notorious for retraction and hence prompt recognition of injury and immediate repair is mandatory to avoid primary surgical haemorrhage and return to theatre. Deep haemostatic sutures should be applied.

Omental vessels

Bleeding from omental vessels occurs after releasing omental adhesion without securing them with Vicryl ties. Care should be taken to clamp, cut and ligate omental vessels whilst performing adhesiolysis.

Bleeding from upper abdominal organs

Rupture of liver or spleen may be encountered during CS [8]. Although these are not directly related to CS, failure to recognise and institute immediate management may result in increased maternal morbidity and mortality. Any unexplained haemoperitoneum during CS should alert the clinician to consider a source from the upper abdomen and the general surgical team should be alerted.

Thrombin

Any coagulation defects or low platelet counts or disorder must be corrected after liaising with the haematologist prior to CS.

Bladder injuries

It is good practice to always check for bladder injuries after closure of the uterine incision and before closing the peritoneal cavity. In cases of uncertainty, the bladder can be filled through an indwelling Foley's catheter with methylene blue in 500 ml of normal saline. This test could also be performed to check the integrity of the repair. Bladder injuries not involving the trigone can be repaired in two layers using continuous vicryl (polygalactic acid) sutures. However, it is recommended that urological opinion should be sought during surgery for medico-legal purposes, even if the size of bladder injury is small. Large bladder lacerations and suspected ureteric injuries require intra-operative urology input and planning of follow-up.

Small or large bowel injuries

Previous abdominal surgery can lead to adhesions between the anterior abdominal wall and loops of bowel. Possibility of bowel adhesions should always be considered during CS, even if a woman has not had any previous surgery, as congenital peritoneal adhesions or adhesions due to unrecognised peritoneal infections may be present. Parietal peritoneum should be lifted using two Spencer Wells forceps and incised carefully, during entry into the abdominal cavity. A finger may be inserted to 'feel' for adherent bowel loops prior to enlarging the incision. If bowel injury is suspected or confirmed, the surgical team should be contacted. Small bowel injuries in the 'anti-mesenteric border' are usually closed in two layers transversely, using a delayed absorbable suture like polygalactic acid (Vicryl) to avoid postoperative strictures.

Injuries to the mesenteric part of the small bowel can disturb its blood supply and may lead to bowel ischaemia and bowel perforation after a few days of surgery. These often require bowel resection and anastomosis.

Small bowel injury within 10–12 cm from the ileo-caecal junction, where the terminal ileum is usually supplied by end arteries with less collateral circulation, may be managed by anastomosis of the ileum to the transverse colon.

In the case of large bowel or right colon injury, bacterial colonisation of this part of the bowel is relatively low therefore local repair is feasible if the damaged section is not over 1 cm, depending on the blood supply of the injured area and the condition of the rest of the right colon. If optimal wound healing is anticipated, primary local repair is preferable. Otherwise, resection of the right colon with anastomosis of the ileum to transverse colon is safest, staying at least 10–12 cm proximal to the ileo-caecal junction. Injuries to the transverse colon can be locally repaired if the wound edges have a good blood supply and are suitable for primary wound healing. If this is not the case, then resection and two-layer anastomosis is preferable.

The rectum is rarely injured during CS. The sigmoid colon is at a higher risk of injury. Primary repair or the use of colostomy and end-to-end repair may be required.

Complete the '3 Es' after every obstetric emergency

Examine – for possible organ damage and integrity of any repair after organ damage.
Explain the delivery events, possible reasons, complications and future plan of care to the patient (i.e. debrief).

Escalate – Complete the incident reporting form and inform senior colleagues and the team to identify learning points to continuously improve patient care.

Key pitfalls

- Failure to anticipate organ damage or to recognise unintended injury during CS.
- Failure to call for help/communicate clearly in an emergency.
- Failure to involve a multidisciplinary team.
- Failure to keep adequate records, including time keeping, and documentation of type, site and extent of injury.
- Failure to debrief the patient and to provide explanation, apology and support.

Key pearls

- Obstetricians should be able to recognise organ damage and repair the injury in low-resource settings.
- Lessons learned from adverse incidents due to damage to internal organs should be disseminated to the entire team through the 'maternity dashboards' and clinical governance seminars.

References

1. Health and Social Care Information Centre. *Hospital Episodes Statistics, Maternity Data 2009–10.* http://www.hesonline.nhs.uk.

2. Bragg F, Cromwell DA, Edozien LC *et al.* Variation in rates of caesarean section among English NHS trusts after accounting for maternal and clinical risk: cross sectional study. *Br Med J* 2010; 341: c5065.

3. Centre for Maternal and Child Enquiries (CMACE). *Saving Mothers' Lives: Reviewing Maternal Deaths to make Motherhood Safer – 2006–2008. The Eighth Report on Confidential Enquiries into Maternal Deaths in the United Kingdom. Br J Obstet Gynaecol* 2011; 118 (Suppl. 1): 1–208.

4. Chandraharan E, Arulkumaran S. Acute tocolysis. *Curr Opin Obstet Gynecol* 2005; 17: 151–156.

5. Mishra N, Chandraharan E. Postpartum haemorrhage. In Warren R, Arulkumaran S (Eds.), *Best Practice in Labour and Delivery.* Cambridge: Cambridge University Press, 2008.

6. Chandraharan E, Arulkumaran S. Surgical aspects of postpartum haemorrhage. *Best Pract Res Clin Obstet Gynaecol* 2008; 22 (6): 1089–1102.

7. Abu-Ghazza O, Hayes K, Chandraharan E, Belli AM. Vascular malformations in relation to obstetrics and gynaecology: diagnosis and treatment. *Obstetric Gynaecol* 2010; 12: 87–93.

8. Kaluarachchi A, Krishnamurthy S. Post-cesarean section splenic rupture. *Am J Obstet Gynecol* 1995; 173 (1): 230–232.

Chapter

17

Acute puerperal uterine inversion

Hemantha Senanayake, Probhodana Ranaweera and Mohamed Rishard

Key facts

Acute puerperal uterine inversion is
a rare, potentially life-threatening complication
of pregnancy. It usually follows vaginal delivery
but, very rarely, it may follow caesarean section
[1]. It is defined as 'the turning inside out of the
fundus into the uterine cavity' [2]. It may occur
either before or after the delivery of the placenta.

Its incidence is quoted between 1 in 2000 to
1 in 23 000 pregnancies [36]. It is estimated that
most maternity units in the UK would
experience one uterine inversion once in every
decade [4, 5]. The incidence may be higher in
developing countries [6].

Since its reported mortality rate could be as
high as 15% [7] and because it may occur
suddenly and unpredictably, it is imperative that
every practitioner providing maternity care is
familiar with the management of this
potentially catastrophic event. However, due to
its rarity, it is unlikely that obstetricians would
be able to become experienced in its
management. Successful management is largely
dependent on accurate diagnosis but its rarity
and variation in the severity of clinical features
may allow it to go undetected in its initial
phases [8]. Failure to institute prompt treatment
could lead to haemorrhage, rapid development
of shock and death.

Aetiology

While 50% of cases of inversion of the uterus have
no identifiable risk factors [9, 10], mismanagement
of the third stage (applying traction on the umbilical cord before contraction of the uterus and fundal
pressure) is considered as the prime cause [4].Other
recognised predisposing factors include uterine atony,
fundal implantation of a morbidly adherent placenta,
manual removal of the placenta, precipitate labour, a
short umbilical cord, placenta praevia and connective
tissue disorders (Marfan syndrome and Ehlers–Danlos
syndrome) [5, 11]. It has also been reported to follow
sudden increases in intra-abdominal pressure such as
coughing, sneezing before contraction of uterine muscles [12], delivery of a baby with cord round the neck,
giving birth in sitting or erect position, precipitated
labour [8] and very rarely during caesarean section [1].

Even though individual risk factors do commonly
occur, rarity of the condition indicates that these factors have to act in an orchestrated manner to culminate
in an inversion of the uterus [13].

Key implications

A dilated cervix with a relaxed uterus and simultaneous downward traction on the fundus are the possible
factors leading to inversion of the uterus [14]. Proper
retraction of the uterus would therefore be the primary
factor that prevents acute inversion of the uterus. There
are many accounts of uterine inversion in the literature from times when fundal pressure was the method
used for expulsion of the placenta [15–17]. Thus, the
introduction of active management of the third stage
of labour has been a major contributor to the current
low incidence of the condition [11].

The inverted fundus becomes trapped within the
cervix creating progressive oedema and congestion
due to interruption of venous and lymphatic drainage

[3]. This becomes a vicious cycle, which makes repositioning of the uterus more difficult with time elapsed since the inversion.

As the inversion progresses, the round and infundibulo-pelvic ligaments and ovaries become indrawn into the inverting uterine fundus, which forms a depression in it. The extent to which the ligaments and ovaries get drawn into it will obviously depend on the degree of inversion. The in-drawing of the peritoneum, the ligaments and the ovaries will result in significant pain and stimulation of the autonomic nervous system, resulting in the neurogenic shock which accounts for the picture that is typical of the early course of the condition [18]. The degree of shock observed is out of proportion to the bleeding that is observed [19]. Significant haemorrhage due to poor retraction and congestion of the inverted uterus and partial separation of the placenta will follow and amplify these effects.

Key diagnostic signs

Inversion of the uterus is classified according to the time elapsed from the time of birth and depending on how far the fundus of the uterus has inverted.

It is classified as acute if the inversion has occurred within 24 hours of birth, subacute between 24 hours and 4 weeks of delivery and chronic if it occurs after 4 weeks of delivery or in a non-pregnant state [20].

The uterine fundus that has inverted and lies within the endometrial cavity without extending beyond the external os is referred to as a first-degree uterine inversion. An inverted fundus that has extended beyond the external os and remains within the vagina is a second-degree inversion. These two categories are collectively referred to as incomplete inversions. When the inverted fundus extends down to or beyond the vaginal introitus it is classified as a third-degree or complete inversion. When the vagina also inverts with the uterus it is classified as a fourth-degree or total inversion [8, 14, 18]. Second-degree uterine inversion is the commonest presentation [18].

Key pointers

Clinical signs and symptoms form the basis of diagnosis of uterine inversion. Its most dramatic presentation is as a uniform mass appearing at the introitus with the cervix felt around its base [18]. The placenta may or may not be attached to the mass. Initially, the inversion may feel to palpation like a fetal head and appear as a pinkish-white mass. With time the mass will become oedematous and bluish in colour [8].

When there is complete inversion, the diagnosis is most easily made by palpating the inverted fundus at the cervical os or vaginal introitus and the inability to palpate the uterus abdominally. In incomplete inversion, the uterus may appear to be normal or a fundal dimple may be palpable if the woman is thin.

However, the vast majority of the cases present with haemorrhage (94%) with or without cardiovascular collapse [5]. The blood loss depends on the inversion–reversion interval and can lead to serious haemodynamic instability [21].

Typically shock appears early and initially this is neurogenic, producing signs that are out of proportion to the severity of blood loss. However, within a short period of time marked haemorrhage ensues, leading to hypovolaemic shock [1, 3]. Acute inversion of the uterus must be excluded in all cases of postpartum collapse with or without haemorrhage.

Severe and sustained hypogastric pain in the third stage of labour, profuse bleeding, absence of the uterine fundus with or without an obvious defect of it on abdominal palpation, as well as evidence of shock with severe hypotension are important diagnostic clues which point to a diagnosis of uterine inversion [22].

Key actions

Early diagnosis, early involvement of experienced personnel and teamwork play a major role in the successful treatment of uterine inversion. Management of shock and repositioning of the uterus as soon as possible are the key aims of management. These have to be pursued aggressively and run concurrently [5]. Delays would result in progressive oedema of the inverted uterus and its entrapment within the cervix, a combination that is self-propagating and one that makes repositioning increasingly difficult.

Adherence to basic principles of managing an emergency situation (calling for help, multidisciplinary approach, etc.) will improve the outcome.

Management of shock

While the cause of the initial shock is neurogenic (bradycardia, hypotension), hypovolaemia will follow due to haemorrhage [23]. Some studies quote the incidence of postpartum haemorrhage to be as high as 94% [24] with an average blood loss of about 1250 ml [19]. Aggressive resuscitation is needed. Resuscitation of an obstetric patient is described in Chapter 2 in this volume.

The best way to manage the neurogenic component would be to reposition the uterus [25]. Providing adequate analgesia while this is being attempted would help mitigate some of the effects of vagal stimulation.

Repositioning of uterus

Non-surgical methods

Manual replacement of uterus

Manual repositioning of the uterus should be attempted without delay once the diagnosis is established. This first-line procedure which is commonly used for repositioning of the uterus is referred to as Johnson's manoeuvre as it was first described by AB Johnson in 1949 [26]. The rationale behind this manoeuvre is that lifting the uterus into the abdomen will increase tension on the ligaments causing the uterus to reposition itself.

The operator introduces two-thirds of a forearm into the vagina and extends the hand at the wrist to place the palm on the inverted fundus and fingertips at the utero-cervical junction. Lifting the uterus above the level of the umbilicus creates adequate tension for the cervical ring to dilate and for the fundus to revert to its normal position. The chance of successful repositioning is between 43 and 88% with earlier attempts at repositioning resulting in higher success rates [5].

The uterus should be held in position for a few minutes after reduction and uterotonic drugs should be administered to aid contraction of the uterus and thus prevent re-inversion [27]. Administration of an appropriate antibiotic is essential to prevent infection [5].

The placenta should only be removed after repositioning of the uterus and complete correction of the inversion, in order to avoid shock and torrential bleeding [28].

With delay the formation of a contraction ring and oedema of the uterus will make the procedure more difficult, resulting in more bleeding [29].

If this initial method fails or cannot be performed due to an already oedematous uterus with a contraction ring, hydrostatic reduction should be attempted in an operating theatre.

Hydrostatic reduction

JV O'Sullivan described the method of hydrostatic reduction in 1945 [30]. In this procedure the lower genital tract is made to distend by filling it with isotonic saline under pressure. The distension created in the vagina first and then in the cervical ring will help the uterus to reduce into its normal position. The operator places a hand across the introitus, in order to create a water seal. A continuous infusion of isotonic saline using a tube introduced into the vagina via the first interdigital space is used to create hydrostatic pressure. This should be done in an operating theatre after excluding uterine rupture, with the patient in the lithotomy position. The fluid should be warm and there should be a pressure head of 150 cm above the vagina to generate adequate distension. The main problem with this technique is the maintaining of a tight water seal at introitus by hand. The wider tubing used for delivery of distending media in resectoscopic procedures will circumvent the problem of maintaining a water seal over standard intravenous sets.

In a further attempt to overcome this difficulty, a modification to this procedure by using a silicon ventouse cup has been described [31]. A point to remember is that the cup should be directed towards the posterior fornix and care must be taken to avoid the fundus of the uterus so that the vagina can be distended. This is required first to overcome spasm of the cervical ring. Even with this modification, the operator's hand at the introitus may be needed. The main drawback of this method is that it may be time consuming when a quick resolution of the problem is required.

It is recommended that about 4–5 litres of fluid are used for infusion. Possible complications would be infection, the theoretical risk of fluid overload [32] and pulmonary oedema. However, to date there are no reported cases of the latter two complications in the literature.

There are reported cases of using the SOS Bakri balloon catheter [33] and Rusch balloon catheter [34] to create hydrostatic pressure. These have been used in instances where the placenta is already separated. An additional advantage in this method is that after repositioning the uterus the balloon will help prevent re-inversion and reduce postpartum haemorrhage.

Tocolytics

Use of tocolytics in a situation where postpartum haemorrhage is a common accompaniment is fraught with danger. The cardiovascular effects of these drugs may further compromise the patient who is already in danger of cardiovascular instability. However, in the presence of a tight constriction ring repositioning of the uterus may be difficult and the use of a tocolytic will help relax it and facilitate repositioning of the uterus. Tocolysis in this situation may therefore offset the dangers of uterine atony causing a worsening of haemorrhage.

Terbutaline is the drug of choice due to its rapid onset of action and short half-life [10]. Many other drugs have been used including magnesium sulphate [35], nitroglycerin [36] and betamimetic drugs [37, 38]. The recommended doses are as follows [5]: terbutaline (0.25 mg intravenously slowly); magnesium sulphate (4–6 g intravenously over 20 minutes); nitroglycerin (100 μg intravenously slowly, achieving uterine relaxation in 90 seconds).

The place for tocolysis in a conscious patient is very limited. When repositioning has failed or is presumed difficult, it is advisable not to re-attempt the procedure in the delivery suite using tocolytics [5].

General anaesthesia

When manual reduction fails or seems difficult, it is necessary to transfer the patient to an operating theatre. Indeed, moving the patient to the operating theatre at the appropriate time forms an important part of modern management of postpartum haemorrhage. Administration of general anaesthesia is recommended for management of uterine inversion [10]. The main advantages are pain relief for the patient and possible relaxation of uterine muscles, aiding repositioning. Halothane used to be recommended for uterine relaxation [39] but due to its profound effects of hypotension it is now not used [5].

Surgical methods

The need to resort to surgery for management of uterine inversion by surgical methods is rare. There are a few techniques which have been used during surgery to reduce the inverted uterus.

Huntingdon's operation [40]

After a laparotomy the indrawn uterine cup is identified near the region of the cervix with the tubes and round ligaments pulled into the cup. By the use of two Allis forceps the uterus is pulled out of the constriction ring in a progressive fashion and restored to its normal position. The serosa of the uterus will invariably sustain lacerations and these are repaired with absorbable sutures.

Haultain's operation [41]

In this procedure the constriction in the region of cervix is incised posteriorly using a longitudinal incision. As in the Huntingdon's method two Allis forceps are used to pull the uterus to its normal position. Two fingers are inserted through the incision to push the inverted fundus upwards. The incision is repaired with interrupted sutures. Uterotonics are given to maintain contraction of the uterus.

During laparotomy, use of a silastic cup from above to pull the uterine fundus has been reported [42].

A case has been reported where acute inversion of the uterus was managed under laparoscopic guidance [22]. The risk of creating a pneumoperitoneum in a haemodynamically unstable patient should be considered.

Hysterectomy

When all the above methods fail, a hysterectomy will become the only viable option.

Recurrence during the puerperium and in future pregnancies

Regardless of the method used for repositioning, the risk of re-inversion is common following the procedure. This is due to occurrence of uterine atony and sometimes due to use of tocolytic drugs for facilitation of reduction [3].Close monitoring of the patient after repositioning is essential.

It is recommended to use an uterotonic drug in the initial phase of management after repositioning. Oxytocin infusion, misoprostol per rectum or prostaglandins can be used for this purpose. In instances where magnesium sulphate had been used as a tocolytic, calcium gluconate could be administered to reverse the effect [3].

Patients should be educated regarding the possibility of recurrent inversion in subsequent deliveries; even though the incidence is presumed to be low there are no published data available regarding the incidence. Van Vugt et al., in their case series of 172 cases, report cases with recurrences in subsequent pregnancies but do not give an incidence [43]. The more recent review in 2002 by Baskett did not record any recurrences in the subsequent 26 deliveries of the 40 cases of uterine inversions drawn from 125 081 births over 24 years [11].

Key pitfalls

- The rarity of the condition and variability of its presentation often lead to delayed diagnosis which impacts on the outcome.
- Acute uterine inversion often occurs without warning and it is imperative that practitioners are aware of the possibility of acute inversion, in every case of postpartum maternal collapse.

Key pearls

- Inversion of the uterus represents a potentially lethal complication of pregnancy.
- Prompt recognition, early repositioning of the inverted uterus and resuscitation of the mother will result in a better outcome.
- The early involvement of experienced personnel and a multidisciplinary approach are vital.

References

1. Emmott RS, Bennett A. Acute inversion of the uterus at cesarean section. *Anaesthesia* 1988; 43: 118–120.

2. Sivasuriya M, Maharoof HM. Chronic complete puerperal inversion of the uterus treated by Kustner operation. *Ceylon Med J* 1974; 19(2): 100–101.

3. O'Grady JP. Malposition of the uterus 2011. Available from: http://emedicine.medscape.com/article/272497-overview#aw2aab6b7.

4. Calder AA. Emergencies in operative obstetrics. *Baillieres Best Pract Clin Obstet Gynaecol* 2000; 14: 43–45.

5. Bhalla R, Wuntakal R, Odejinmi F, Khan RU. Acute inversion of the uterus. *Obstetric Gynaecol* 2009; 11: 13–18.

6. Mehra U, Ostapowicz F. Acute puerperal inversion of the uterus in a primipara. *Obstet Gynecol* 1976; 47: 30–32.

7. Hostetler DR, Bosworth MF. Uterine inversion: a life-threatening obstetric emergency. *J Am Board Fam Pract* 2000; 13 (2): 120–123.

8. Silva DNKP, Jayaweera BA. Acute puerperal inversion of the uterus. *Ceylon Med J* 1966; 11 (3): 111–114.

9. Adesiyun AG. Septic postpartum uterine inversion. *Singapore Med J* 2007; 48 (10): 943–945.

10. Abouleish E, Ali V, Joumaa B, Lopez M, Gupta D. Anaesthetic management of acute puerperal uterine inversion. *Br J Anaesth* 1995; 75 (4): 486–487.

11. Baskett TF. Acute uterine inversion: a review of 40 cases. *J Obstet Gynaecol Can* 2002; 24 (12): 953–956.

12. Kitchin JD, Thiagarajah S, May HV, Thomton WN. Puerperal inversion of the uterus. *Am J Obstet Gynecol* 1975; 123: 51–58.

13. Peña-Martí G, Comunián-Carrasco G. Fundal pressure versus controlled cord traction as part of the active management of the third stage of labour. *Cochrane Database Syst Rev* 2007; 4: CD005462.

14. Kellog FS. Puerperal inversion of the uterus. Classification for treatment. *Am J Obstet Gynecol* 1929; 18: 815.

15. Galloway DC. Subacute inversion of the uterus treated with Aveling's repositor. *Br Med J* 1952; 197.

16. McHenry AG. Management of acute inversion of the uterus. *Obstet Gynaecol* 1960; 16 (6): 671–673.

17. Lee WK, Baggish MS, Lashgari M. Acute inversion of the uterus. *Obstet Gynaecol* 1978; 51 (2): 144–147.

18. Samathar JG. Acute inversion of the uterus: a case report. *Jaffna Med J* 1980; 15: 20–22.

19. Beringer RM, Patteril M. Puerperal uterine inversion and shock. *Br J Anaesth* 2004; 92 (3): 439–441.

20. Baskett TF, Calder AA, Arulkumaran S. Acute uterine inversion. In *Munro Kerr's Operative Obstetrics*. Eleventh Edition. Edinburgh: Elsevier, 2007, pp. 243–250.

21. Rudloff U, Joels LA, Marshall N. Inversion of the uterus at cesarean section. *Arch Gynecol Obstet* 2004; 269: 224–226.

22. Vijayaraghavan R, Sujatha Y. Acute postpartum uterine inversion with haemorrhagic shock: laparoscopic reduction: a new method of management? *Br J Obstet Gynaecol* 2006; 113 (9): 1100–1102.

23. Hussain M, Jabeen T, Liaquat N, Noorani K, Bhutta SZ. Acute puerperal uterine inversion. *J Coll Physicians Surg Pak* 2004; 14 (4): 215–217.

24. Watson P, Besch N, Bowes WA Jr. Management of acute and subacute puerperal inversion of the uterus. *Obstet Gynecol* 1980; 55: 6–12.

25. O'Grady JP. Malposition of the uterus. Available at: http://emedicine.medscape.com/article/272497-overview

26. Johnson AB. A new concept in replacement of the inverted uterus and report of nine cases. *Am J Obstet Gynecol* 1949; 57: 557–562.

27. Catanzarite VA, Moffitt KD, Baker ML *et al*. New approaches to the management of acute puerperal uterine inversion. *Obstet Gynecol* 1986; 68 (3 Suppl.): 7S–10S.

28. Kochenour NK. Intrapartum obstetric emergencies. *Crit Care Clin* 1991; 7 (4): 851–864.

29. Nazneen K, Ferdousi I, Fatematul Z, Mollika R. Early recurrent inversion – a case report. *Bangladesh J Obstet Gynaecol* 2008; 23 (1): 35–37.

30. O'Sullivan J. Acute inversion of the uterus. *Br Med J* 1945; 2: 282–283.

31. Ogueh O, Ayida G. Acute uterine inversion: a new technique of hydrostatic replacement. *Br J Obstet Gynaecol* 1997; 104 (8): 951–952.

32. Ward HR. O'Sullivan's hydrostatic reduction of an inverted uterus: sonar sequences recorded. *Ultrasound Obstet Gynecol* 1998; 12: 283–286.

33. Majd HS, Pilsniak A, Reginald PW. Recurrent uterine inversion: a novel treatment approach using SOS Bakri balloon. *Br J Obstet Gynaecol* 2009; 116 (7): 999–1001.

34. Azubuike U, Bolarinde O. Complete uterine inversion managed with a Rusch balloon catheter. *J Med Cases* 2010; 1 (1): 8–9.

35. Grossman RA. Magnesium sulfate for uterine inversion. *J Reprod Med* 1981; 26 (5): 261–262.

36. Bayhi DA, Sherwood CD, Campbell CE. Intravenous nitroglycerin for uterine inversion. *J Clin Anesth* 1992; 4 (6): 487–488.

37. Thiery M, Delbeke L. Acute puerperal uterine inversion: two-step management with a beta-mimetic and a prostaglandin. *Am J Obstet Gynecol* 1985; 153(8): 891–892.

38. Clark SL. Use of ritodrine in uterine inversion. *Am J Obstet Gynecol* 1985; 151 (5): 705.

39. Soto RG, McCarthy J, Hoffman MS. Anaesthetic management of uterine inversion. *J Gynecol Surg* 2002; 18: 165–166.

40. Huntington JL, Irving FC, Kellogg FS, Mass B. Abdominal reposition in acute inversion of the puerperal uterus. *Am J Obstet Gynaecol* 1928; 15: 34–38.

41. Haultain FW. Abdominal hysterotomy for chronic uterine inversion. *Proc R Soc Med* 1908; 1 (Obstet Gynaecol Sect): 279–290.

42. Antonelli E, Irion O, Tolck P, Morales M. Subacute uterine inversion: description of a novel replacement technique using the obstetric ventouse. *Br J Obstet Gynaecol* 2006; 113 (7): 846–847.

43. van Vugt PJ, Baudoin P, Blom VM, van Deursen CT. Inversio uteri puerperalis. *Acta Obstet Gynecol Scand* 1981; 60 (4): 353–362.

Chapter 18

Sudden postpartum maternal collapse

Karolina Afors and Amarnath Bhide

Key facts

- Definition: Maternal collapse is an acute event involving the cardiorespiratory system and/or brain, resulting in a reduced or absent consciousness level (and potentially death), in the immediate period following delivery and up to 6 weeks after delivery.
- Aetiology: It represents an acute illness with multiple aetiologies which can be potentially life threatening particularly if unrecognised.
- Incidence: The true incidence of postpartum collapse is difficult to quantify due to the large variety of presentations and differences in definitions. The true rate of maternal collapse lies somewhere between 0.14 and 6/1000 maternities [1]. In the UK, the maternal mortality rate for 2006–08 was 11.39 per 100 000 maternities [2].

Causes of sudden postpartum maternal collapse

Figure 18.1 and Table 18.1 elucidate causes of sudden maternal collapse.

Consequences

- Maternal: increase in deaths related to genital tract sepsis, particularly group A streptococcal disease. Sepsis is now the leading cause of direct maternal mortality in the UK, and has increased from 0.85 to 1.13 per 10 000 maternities [2].
- Fetal: peripartum hypoxia secondary to maternal hypotension resulting in intra-uterine death or

long-term neurological morbidity (learning difficulties, cerebral palsy).
- Medico-legal: clinical negligence claims due to delay in recognising signs and symptoms of critical illness.

Key differences in resuscitation due to pregnancy changes

The pregnant woman undergoes many physiological changes that accelerate the development of hypoxia and acidosis and make ventilation more difficult.

- Supine hypotension and aorto-caval compression – can significantly reduce cardiac output by 30–40%, and reduce the efficacy of chest compressions during resuscitation.
- Increased oxygen consumption, alterations in lung function and diaphragmatic splinting make the pregnant woman become hypoxic more readily and make ventilation more difficult.
- Difficult intubation is more likely in pregnancy. This is due to fluid retention leading to narrower airways and increase in breast size limiting the working space.
- Pregnant women are at an increased risk of aspiration due to slowing of gastric emptying, compression on the gut by enlarging uterus and smooth muscle relaxation related to high levels of progesterone.
- Increased cardiac output and vascularity of the genital tract in pregnancy make rapid rate of blood loss possible. Healthy pregnant women tolerate blood loss remarkably well. Clinical deterioration is late to set in, but quick to progress with continued loss.

Obstetric and Intrapartum Emergencies, ed. Edwin Chandraharan and Sabaratnam Arulkumaran. Published by Cambridge University Press. © Cambridge University Press 2012.

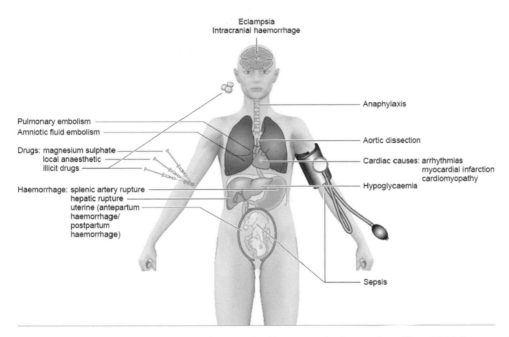

Eclampsia
Intracranial haemorrhage

Anaphylaxis

Pulmonary embolism
Amniotic fluid embolism

Aortic dissection

Drugs: magnesium sulphate
local anaesthetic
illicit drugs

Cardiac causes: arrhythmias
myocardial infarction
cardiomyopathy

Hypoglycaemia

Haemorrhage: splenic artery rupture
hepatic rupture
uterine (antepartum
haemorrhage/
postpartum
haemorrhage)

Sepsis

Figure 18.1 Diagrammatic representation of causes of sudden maternal collapse. Adapted from *RCOG Green-top Guideline No. 56* [1].

Key pointers

- Early recognition of acutely unwell women by healthcare professionals. The use of an Early Warning Score system modified for pregnancy (MEOWS) is being encouraged.
- Early involvement of medical specialists and intensive care support in the event of clinical deterioration.
- Prompt resuscitation whilst considering underlying cause and initiation of appropriate treatment.
- Aetiology: Non-critical causes of postpartum collapse include hyperventilation and vaso-vagal syncope, events which are typically self limiting and reversible with simple interventions such as position change. Critical causes of collapse can be further divided into obstetric and non-obstetric to facilitate recall.

Key diagnostic signs

- Concise history taking from patients or relatives including obstetric, relevant past medical history and drug history. These key pieces of information may aid in identifying risk factors and arriving at a diagnosis. See Table 18.1.

- Examination of patient including cardiorespiratory system.
- Organising appropriate investigation whilst commencing resuscitation of patient. Basic investigations including pulse oximetry, electrocardiogram, cardiac monitoring, and automated blood pressure recording should be initiated and urinary catheter inserted. Specific investigations such as blood tests, arterial blood gas analysis, and portable chest X-ray if appropriate can then be organised.

Key actions (see Figure 18.2)

- Awareness of potential barriers which may impede resuscitation.
- See above for key differences in resuscitation due to pregnancy changes.
- Structured approach to resuscitation as recommended by the Resuscitation Council, UK [3].
- Initial assessment is carried out by primary survey consisting of A, B, C, D and E which are addressed in this order. Senior staff should be involved and other members of staff alerted (including senior obstetrician, anaesthetist and experienced midwives).

Table 18.1 Common conditions responsible for maternal collapse.

Cause	Incidence	Risk factors	Clinical symptoms/signs	Specific management
Obstetric causes:				
Massive haemorrhage	3.7/1000	Placenta praevia	Tachycardic, hypotensive, ↑cap refill time	Replacement with blood and blood products
Includes:		Placenta accreta/percreta	Pallor, loss of consciousness	Stop bleeding: surgery, uterotonic drugs, UAE
PPH, uterine rupture				Anticipate DIC consider use of factor VII
Placental abruption	1.7 in 100	Smoking, multiparity, preeclampsia	Uterine tenderness, pallor, tachycardia	Bleeding may be concealed. Risk of DIC
Placenta praevia/accreta		Antepartum haemorrhage, previous CS		Delivery by CS. Multidisciplinary team approach with involvement of interventional radiologist and haematologist
Uterine inversion	1 in 2000	Fundal placenta, cord traction before separation	Tachycardia, hypotension, incomplete third stage with mass in vagina	Manually replace, intravaginal hydrostatic pressure, consider laparotomy – Huntington procedure
Eclampsia	1 in 2000	Preeclampsia	Tonic–clonic seizure, postictal	Magnesium sulphate, lower blood pressure. Monitor renal/liver for complications
			Hypertension, hyper-reflexive	
Amniotic fluid embolism	1 in 8000– 80 000	Ruptured membranes, induction	Dyspnoea, hypotension, cardiac arrest	Oxygenation, maintenance of cardiac output + blood pressure
Non-obstetric:				
Cardiovascular				
Aortic dissection	1 in 5000	Marfan syndrome	Back pain	Urgent cardiothoracic involvement
Cardiomyopathy	1 in 1000– 4000	Family history, multiple pregnancies, myocarditis	Tachycardia, cardiac wheeze, oedema	Supportive + early involvement of cardiologist
Myocardial infarction	1 in 10 000	Maternal age, prior/family history	Chest pain	Urgent cardiology review
Pulmonary embolism	1 in 1000	Pregnancy, LSCS, ↑ BMI, thrombophilia	Chest pain, breathlessness, tachycardia	Anticoagulation if any clinical suspicion
Septic shock	1 in 800	HIV positive, ↑ BMI	Pyrexia, tachycardia, tachypnoeic	Cultures – blood, urine, sputum to identify organism
Includes meningitis, swine flu, genital tract		Comorbidites e.g. asthma		Broad spectrum antibiotics + supportive treatment
Neurological CVA	1 in 500	Hypertension	Headache, photophobia, neurological deficit	CT/MRI imaging + urgent neurology review
Metabolic				
Hyponatraemia	rare	Oxytocin infusion	Headache, N+V, lethargy, confusion, seizure	Discontinue oxytocin infusion + fluid restrict
Drugs				
Anaphylaxis	rare	Previous allergic reaction, asthma	Pruritus, erythema, angioedema, laryngeal oedema, bronchospasm, hypotension	Stop administration of drug, give adrenaline, consider antihistamines and corticosteroids
Local anaesthetic, illicit drugs		Previous drug history		Supportive treatment
Anaesthetic				
Regional: high block	rare	↑ BMI, prior epidural, large LA dose	Hypotension, bradycardia, resp compromise	Oxygenation, secure airway, vagolytic e.g. atropine
General: aspiration pneumonia		Recent meal, no use of H_2 antagonists or metoclopramide	Tachycardic, tachypnoeic, hypoxic	Pre-oxygenation, rapid sequence induction with cricoid pressure

UAE, uterine arterial embolisation; DIC, disseminated intravascular coagulation; LSCS, lower segment caesarean section; BMI, body mass index; CT/MRI, computed tomography/magnetic resonance imaging; N + V, nausea plus vomiting; LA, local anaesthetic.

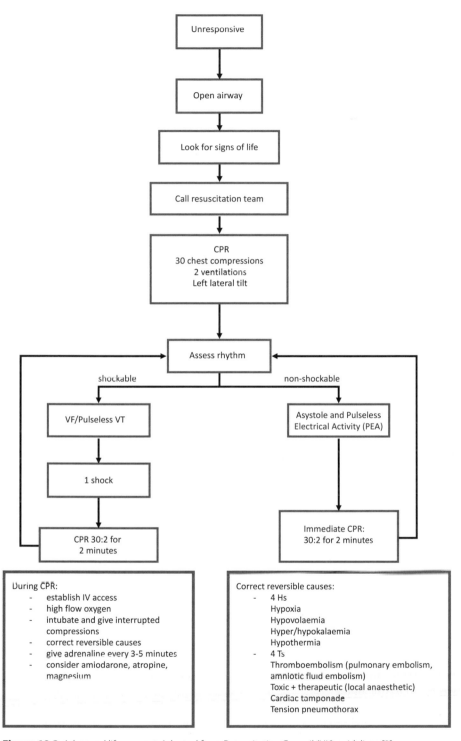

Figure 18.2 Advanced life support. Adapted from Resuscitation Council (UK) guidelines [3].

- **A – Airway:** A clear patent airway must be established and maintained. This can be achieved using either the head tilt jaw thrust or head tilt chin lift. Suction can be used to clear the airway of secretions or vomit and the airway maintained by inserting either oropharyngeal or nasopharyngeal airway.
- The patient should be put in the left lateral tilt position to displace the gravid uterus and high-flow oxygen administered at a rate of 12–15 litres/min.
- **B – Breathing:** Breathing should be monitored by observing, listening and feeling. Intermittent positive pressure ventilation should be commenced if there is inadequate breathing. Typically two rescue breaths are given either by mouth, pocket face mask or 100% oxygen and a reservoir bag. Intermittent ventilation should be continued until the airway is more adequately protected with tracheal intubation.
- **C – Circulation:** The rate of cardiac arrest in pregnancy is rare with an incidence of $1:30\,000$. Circulatory arrest is diagnosed by absence of a palpable carotid or femoral pulse and resuscitation with external chest compressions should be commenced immediately. A ratio of 30 compressions to 2 breaths should be maintained and external monitoring to assess cardiac rhythm attached. Recent changes to resuscitation guidelines suggest that chest compression alone may be sufficient. Physiological barriers such as flared ribs, raised diaphragm, obesity and breast hypertrophy can make effective chest compressions difficult to achieve. Compression of the inferior vena cava by the gravid uterus can impair venous return and cardiac output. Therefore, all pregnant patients should be placed in the left lateral position to displace the uterus from its anatomical position. This tilt position can be achieved using an object such as the Cardiff resuscitation wedge. Alternatively, the patient can be tilted on to an assistant's knees. Priority is resuscitation of the mother and the fetal heart should not be auscultated until the mother has been stabilised. In instances of circulatory arrest emptying of the uterus via caesarean section should be considered to provide more effective resuscitation.

Circulatory collapse secondary to haemorrhagic shock is one of the leading causes of postpartum collapse. Blood loss may be concealed or underestimated and healthy young pregnant women may not initially show signs of hypovolaemic shock. Persistent tachycardia, pallor, increased capillary refill and hypotension may only develop once one-third of the patient's total circulating blood volume is lost. As part of the primary survey two large-bore intravenous cannulas should be sited and bloods taken for the following investigations if deemed necessary:

- Full blood count and coagulation screen. Cross match 6 units.
- Urea and electrolytes, liver function test, CRP, blood glucose and blood cultures. Fluid replacement should be given in the form of crystalloid or colloid and the need for blood and blood products assessed. The source of bleeding should be identified and controlled as soon as possible. Heart rate, blood pressure and urine output should be regularly recorded to assess response to resuscitation.

- **D – Disability:** Glasgow Coma Scale can be used as an objective assessment of patient's level of consciousness. It provides a method of monitoring any deterioration of patient's neurological status and may be of particular benefit in cases of suspected neurological causes of collapse such as CVA.
- **D – Defibrillation and Drugs:** Automated external defibrillators or external monitors to assess cardiac rhythm should be applied as per advanced life-support guideline. If a shockable rhythm of either ventricular fibrillation or pulseless ventricular tachycardia is observed a shock may be administered. Primary assessment of A, B, C, D should recommence immediately and following adrenaline given every 3–5 minutes. In cases of unexplained collapse magnesium toxicity should be monitored and serum levels measured as this may contribute to circulatory collapse. Tachyarrhythmias as a result of bupivacaine toxicity should also be noted and may be treated with electric cardio-version.
- **E – Exposure:** Once initial resuscitation has been initiated the patient should be adequately exposed.

This will ensure no injuries or signs of illness (i.e. rashes) are missed. Bair huggers to avoid hypothermia should be applied and measurement of patient's glucose level should not be forgotten. Once a cause for maternal collapse has been determined, involvement and admission to either a high dependency unit or intensive care should be considered. Early involvement of relevant specialists should be encouraged to maintain high standards of care and reduced maternal morbidity and mortality.

Key pitfalls

- Failure to recognise acutely unwell patient.
- Failure to notice gradual but progressive deterioration.
- Failure to appreciate physiological and anatomical changes in pregnancy affecting resuscitation.
- Failure to involve necessary specialist teams.
- Failure in organising high dependency unit or intensive care bed promptly.

Key pearls

- Modified Early Obstetric Warning System (MEOWS) – to prompt anticipation, early referral and recognition for medical review.
- Multidisciplinary team training with acute clinical scenarios.
- Ensure practitioners are up to date with resuscitation guideline.
- Work with simulators.

References

1. Royal College of Obstetricans and Gynaecologists. *Maternal Collapse in Pregnancy and the Puerperium.* Green-top Guideline No. 56. London: RCOG, 2011.

2. Centre for Maternal and Child Enquiries (CMACE). *Saving Mothers' Lives: Reviewing Maternal Deaths to make Motherhood Safer – 2006–2008. The Eighth Report on Confidential Enquiries into Maternal Deaths in the United Kingdom. Br J Obstet Gynaecol* 2011; 118 (Suppl. 1): 1–208.

3. Resuscitation Council, UK. http://www.resus.org.uk

Chapter 19

Retained placenta

Kapila Gunawardane

Key facts

- Definition: The definition of retained placenta is arbitrary and based on the length of time that elapses between the birth of the baby and the expected delivery of the placenta. The most widely accepted definition is the retention of the placenta in utero for more than 30 minutes. The management is influenced by whether or not significant bleeding is occurring. This bleeding may be visible or manifest only by the increasing size of the uterus. In the absence of any evidence of placental detachment, consider the diagnosis of complete placenta accreta or a variant. This condition may be present with bleeding if a portion of the placenta detaches.

- Types: (1) Detached (placenta has separated completely and is retained inside); (2) Partially detached (placenta has partially separated and is retained inside); (3) Non-detached (placenta has not separated at all) (Figure 19.1).

- Incidence: Retained placenta affects 0.5–3% of women following delivery and is a cause of maternal death from postpartum haemorrhage (PPH) and puerperal sepsis. About 25% of maternal deaths in African and Asian countries are due to haemorrhage during pregnancy, delivery or the postpartum period. Of these, almost 30% are caused by PPH. About 15–20% of these PPH maternal deaths are due to retained placenta. In less developed countries, it affects about 0.1% of deliveries and has a 10% case fatality

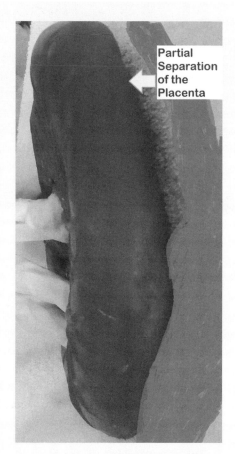

Figure 19.1 Illustration of partial separation of placenta.

rate. In developed countries, it is more common (about 3% of vaginal deliveries) but is very rarely associated with mortality. A systematic review of observational studies

---

Obstetric and Intrapartum Emergencies, ed. Edwin Chandraharan and Sabaratnam Arulkumaran. Published by Cambridge University Press. © Cambridge University Press 2012.

show that the median rate of retained placenta at 30 minutes was higher in developed countries (2.67% vs. 1.46%, p < 0.02), as was the median manual removal rate (2.24% vs. 0.45%, p < 0.001). In addition to this, there appears to have been a rise in rate of manual removal in the UK from a mean of 0.66% in the 1920s to 2.34% in the 1980s (p < 0.0001) [1]. The retained placenta is the second major indication for blood transfusion in the third stage of labour. Appropriate management of the third stage of labour can help to reduce retained placenta and it is a potentially preventable cause of PPH. Incidence of retained placenta varies according to the management practices of the third stage of labour [2].

Key implications

- Maternal: postpartum haemorrhage, shock, sepsis, perforation, retained products, uterine inversion, trauma, rhesus-isoimmunisation, anaesthetic complications, severe maternal morbidity and maternal deaths.
- Medico-legal: clinical negligence claims due to delay in removing the placenta or inappropriate management.

Key pointers

- Morbid adherent placenta.
- Placenta accreta.
- Placenta increta.
- Placenta percreta.
- Uterine abnormality, uterine scars.
- Constriction ring or reforming cervix.
- Full bladder.
- Inappropriate active management of third stage of labour.
- Uterine atony.
- Age above 35 years.
- Following induction of labour.
- Past history of retained placenta.
- Preterm labour.

Key diagnostic signs

Failure of the expulsion of the placenta and its membranes or absence of signs of placental separation after 30 minutes of vaginal delivery of the baby.

Key actions

Many interventions are in practice for the management of retained placenta. The choice of intervention will depend on the clinical scenario, the available facilities, skill and experience of the doctor. If the patient is stable and presents no evidence of active bleeding there is no necessity to rush and proceed to every available intervention at once. An expectant management for a period of an hour (arbitrary time period) will be useful. Meanwhile the bladder will be emptied and the patient has to be observed carefully for bleeding and signs of separation of placenta. In trapped placenta ultrasound can be performed to confirm separation and use controlled cord traction with or without a short-acting tocolytic such as glyceryl trinitrate. Sometimes when it is trapped in the cervical canal and in the vagina it can be removed easily during vaginal examination with or without anaesthesia.

The role of systemic oxytocics in the management of retained placentas is controversial. Oxytocics given prophylactically at the time of delivery increase the number of placental deliveries at 20 and 40 minutes but have no effect on the number of placentas that eventually need manual removal [3]. As an alternative to all of the above, intra-umbilical vein oxytocin injection can be tried. Use of tocolytics, either alone or in combination with uterotonics, may be of value in minimising the need for manual removal of the placenta in the theatre under anaesthesia. The following drugs can be useful during the procedure: nitric oxide donors, beta-adrenergic stimulants, calcium channel blockers, halogenated anaesthetics and magnesium sulphate. One randomised controlled trial (involving 24 women) compared the use of nitroglycerin tablets versus placebo after the treatment with oxytocin had failed. There was a statistically significant reduction in the need for manual removal of placenta (risk ratio (RR) 0.04, 95% confidence interval (CI) 0.00 to 0.66). There was also a statistically significant reduction in mean blood loss during the third stage of labour (mean difference (MD) −262.50 ml, 95% CI −364.95 to −160.05). Sublingual nitroglycerin caused some haemodynamic changes as it lowers the systolic blood pressure and diastolic blood pressure by a mean of 6 and 5 mmHg respectively. The pulse rate increased by a mean of two beats per minute [4]. Although sublingual nitroglycerin appears to be an effective and safe drug that can be used to manage retained placenta, its routine use cannot be recommended because of the small study sample size.

If there is significant bleeding, it should be managed as a primary postpartum haemorrhage and manual removal of the placenta should be done without delay. The time allowed to lapse before manual removal varies, but many authorities suggest a delay of 30–60 minutes in the absence of haemorrhage. This is because there is no increase in haemorrhage until at least 30 minutes postpartum, and because of the finding that between 30 and 60 minutes a further 40% of placentas will spontaneously deliver with an average blood loss of only 300 ml.

Suggested algorithm

We have classified the interventions into 'first line' (SP) and 'second line'. The latter should be used when the first-line interventions fail and are associated with increased maternal morbidity. Therefore, an experienced medical officer's presence is recommended during the performance of second-line interventions.

First-line procedure

Use of intra-umbilical vein oxytocin injection

Much interest has been aroused by the notion that oxytocin may be delivered directly to the retro-placental myometrium by injecting it into the placental bed via the umbilical vein. This allows the treatment to be directed specifically at the area with the contractile failure. If there is no active bleeding, consider intra-umbilical uterotonic agents before resorting to a more invasive procedure such as manual removal.

S
<u>S</u>hout for help (experienced medical officer, anaesthetist and alert the blood bank) as soon as possible.
<u>S</u>top unnecessary handling of the uterus. Do not pull on the cord: it can avulse.
<u>S</u>cribe – assign someone to alert the blood bank and to monitor the patient.

P
<u>P</u>rocedure – The Pipingas technique has shown to be effective in delivering drugs to the placental bed [5]. A size 10 nasogastric tube is passed along the umbilical vein until resistance is felt, under aseptic conditions, then retracted about 5 cm, and prostaglandin $F_{2\alpha}$ (20 mg diluted in 20 ml of normal saline) or oxytocin (30 IU diluted in 20 ml of normal saline) is injected through the catheter [6]. There is some evidence that the umbilical vein injection of normal saline with uterotonic drugs like oxytocin to induce uterine contractions seems to have promising results [7]. Umbilical vein injection of normal saline alone compared with expectant management has no significant difference in the incidence of manual removal of placenta (RR: 0.97; 95% CI: 0.83 to 1.14). Umbilical vein injection of saline solution plus oxytocin compared with expectant management showed a reduction in manual removal, although this was not statistically significant (RR: 0.86; 95% CI: 0.72 to 1.01). Saline solution with oxytocin compared with saline solution alone showed a significant reduction in manual removal of the placenta (RR: 0.79; 95% CI: 0.69 to 0.91) (number needed to treat: 8; 95% CI: 5 to 20). No discernible difference was detected in the length of the third stage of labour, blood loss, haemorrhage, haemoglobin, blood transfusion, curettage, infection, hospital stay, fever or abdominal pain.

Second-line manoeuvres

Manual removal of placenta

When expectant and other methods have failed, the manual removal of the placenta will be attempted. In adherent placenta if there is active bleeding manual removal may be necessary. In the past the most common treatment for retained placenta has been manual removal of the placenta under spinal, epidural or general anaesthesia in the operating theatre.

The placenta may be trapped in the uterus by a localised contraction of circular muscles of the uterus. Administration of oxytocics especially ergometrine in the active management of the third stage of labour is an important cause. The ring should be made to relax by anaesthesia and then a cone-shaped hand is introduced along the umbilical cord and the already separated placenta can be removed easily. However, if the placenta is partially separated or not separated the accoucher must proceed to do manual removal of the placenta. It must be reiterated that in the absence of haemorrhage there is no urgency to resort to manual removal when less invasive alternatives are available.

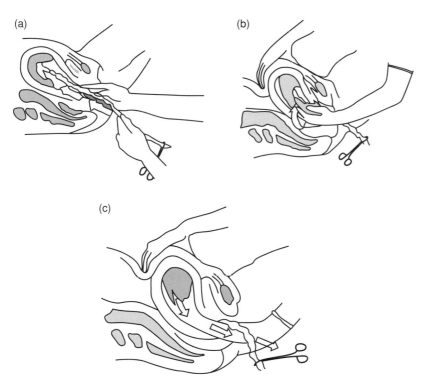

(a)

(b)

(c)

Figure 19.2 Procedure for manual removal of placenta. Please see text for details.

S

Shout for help (experienced medical officer, anaesthetist and alert the blood bank) as soon as possible.

Stop unnecessary handling of the uterus. Do not pull on the cord: it can avulse.

Scribe – assign someone to alert the blood bank and to monitor the patient.

P

Position – Lithotomy position

Procedure – Aseptic conditions are maintained. Bladder is emptied by using an indwelling catheter. When possible, an elbow-length glove is worn and the cut end of the cord is held by the gloved left hand and the cone-shaped gloved right hand is introduced into the uterine cavity along the cord (Figure 19.2a). Once the right hand touches the point of insertion of the cord then the fingers are outstretched to identify the edge of the placenta. While the uterine fundus is stabilised by the left hand and by using the ulnar border or the fingers of the right hand, separation of the placenta will be commenced by starting from the edge of placenta or partially separated edge by gently developing a space between the placenta and uterus to shear off the placenta (Figure 19.2b). The placenta is pushed to the palmar aspect of the hand and wrist; when it is entirely separated, the hand is withdrawn with the whole placenta (Figure 19.2c). Ensure that an oxytocin 20–40 IU in normal saline infusion is running rapidly as the hand is withdrawn in order to encourage strong uterine contraction, and then perform uterine massage. Care must be taken to tease out the membranes. Once uterine contraction is established, examine the placenta and membranes to determine whether the placenta is complete and the uterus must be explored to make sure it is empty, to decide on further exploration or whether curettage is necessary. The administration of antibiotics following manual removal is advised although the evidence is limited; a single, small, randomised trial supports this practice.

If the placenta is found to be accreta when manual removal is attempted, there are a number of management options available. Under the circumstances, a senior experienced obstetrician must be available in the operating theatre. Often partial removal is achieved manually and curettage is used to remove as much as possible of the remaining tissue. So long as haemorrhage is controlled with this method and the uterus remains well contracted, it is usually adequate to prevent continued haemorrhage. The remaining trophoblast is usually reabsorbed spontaneously, although levels of β-HCG take longer to return to normal [8]. Further curettage may be needed if haemorrhage continues. In the case of placenta percreta, blood will continue to flow through the area of invasion (even after the bulk of the placenta is removed) due to the absence of the myometrial 'living ligature' action which would normally stop the flow. However, a hysterectomy is usually required due to severe haemorrhage. If the diagnosis of placenta percreta can be made before any of the placental tissue is removed then the patient may be treated conservatively. This involves delivering the baby as normal but leaving the placenta in situ. Systemic methotrexate may be beneficial in this situation [9].

Complete the '3 Es' after every obstetric emergency

Examine – For maternal trauma (genital tract trauma, PPH) and the general condition.

Explain – the events that took place, possible reasons, complications and future plan of care to the patient (i.e. debrief).

Escalate – Discuss at the morbidity meeting with the team to identify learning points to continuously improve patient care.

Key pitfalls

- Failure to identify the risk factors for retained placenta.
- Failure to manage the third stage properly.
- Failure to call for help/communicate clearly in an emergency/involve experienced clinicians.
- Excessive or inappropriate handling of the uterus and the placenta leading to uterine inversion and retained placenta.
- Failure to observe strict aseptic condition during the manual removal of the placenta.
- Failure to anticipate postpartum haemorrhage (PPH).
- Failure to recognise vaginal, cervical and uterine trauma after the procedure.
- Failure to keep adequate records, including time keeping, and documentation of the events.

Key pearls

- All staff providing intrapartum care should undergo annual skills and drills training on the management of retained placenta.
- Regular fire drills on management of retained placenta should be conducted in the labour ward.
- Lessons learned from adverse incidents due to retained placenta should be disseminated to the entire team through the 'maternity dashboards' and clinical governance seminars.
- All new staff should have hands-on training on the management of retained placenta as part of their training.

Management in low resource settings

One third of all pregnant women in developing countries deliver at home. At home or in the community these deliveries are assisted either by relatives or trained/untrained traditional birth attendants (TBA). In communities where home deliveries are common, women and birth attendants should be educated about retained placenta and the need for prompt transfer in such cases.

At primary-care level doctors and nursing staff should be trained to use intra-umbilical vein injection of saline and oxytocin for the management of retained placenta [10]. If trained staff are not present women with retained placenta should be transferred to secondary care without delay. The importance of minimal handling of the uterus and the placenta must be stressed in order to avoid a partial separation of the placenta during the transfer that may lead to postpartum haemorrhage. At secondary-level care, blood transfusion and operating-theatre services for manual removal of placenta should be available for the appropriate management of retained placenta. During manual removal of the placenta, the woman is exposed to anaesthetic risks as well as to the risk of infections that comes from inserting a hand into the uterus. Both risks are higher in developing countries where the prevalence of infections is high due to improper aseptic procedures and personnel skilled in obstetrics anaesthesia are in short supply.

If there are no facilities to transfer to, medical treatment with the prostaglandin analogue misoprostol or prostaglandin E2 (sulprostone) can be tried. The orally active prostaglandin E1 analogue misoprostol is inexpensive and does not need to be stored in a refrigerator. Therefore, it is of potential use in low-resource countries. Misoprostol has an effect similar to that of an oxytocin infusion, producing an increase in both background tone and contraction strength for around 90 minutes [11].

References

1. Cheung WM, Hawkes A, Ibish S, Weeks AD. The retained placenta: historical and geographical rate variations: *J Obstet Gynaecol* 2011; 31 (1): 37–42.

2. Daftary SN, Nanawati MS. Management of postpartum haemorrhage. In Buckshee K, Patwardhan VB, Soonawala RP (Eds.), *Principles and Practice of Obstetrics and Gynaecology for Postgraduates. FOGSI Publication.* New Delhi: Jaypee Brothers Medical Publishers, 1996.

3. Prendiville WJ, Elbourne D, McDonald S. Active versus expectant management of the third stage of labour. *Cochrane Database Syst Rev* 2000; 3: CD000007. Update in 2009; 3: CD000007

4. Abdel-Aleem H, Abdel-Aleem MA, Shaaban OM. Tocolysis for management of retained placenta. *Cochrane Database Syst Rev* 2011; 1: CD007708.

5. Pipingas A, Hofmeyr GJ, Sesel KR. Umbilical vessel oxytocin administration for retained placenta: in vitro study of various infusion techniques. *Am J Obstet Gynecol* 1993; 168: 793–795.

6. Bider D, Dulitzky M, Goldenberg M *et al.* Intraumbilical vein injection of prostaglandin F2α in retained placenta. *Eur J Obstet Gynecol Reprod Biol* 1996; 64: 59–61.

7. Nardin JM, Weeks A, Carroli G. Umbilical vein injection for management of retained placenta. *Cochrane Database Syst Rev* 2011; 5: CD001337.

8. Reyes FI, Winter JSD, Falman C. Postpartum disappearance of chorionic gonadotrophin from the maternal and neonatal circulations. *Am J Obstet Gynecol* 1985; 153: 486–489.

9. Arulkumaran S, Ng CSA, Ingemarsson I, Ratnam SS. Medical treatment of placenta accreta with methotrexate. *Acta Obstet Gynecol Scand* 1986; 65: 285–286.

10. Purwar MB. Injection into umbilical vein for management of retained placenta: RHL practical aspects (last revised: 15 January 2002). *The WHO Reproductive Health Library.* Geneva: World Health Organization.

11. Danielsson KG, Marions L, Rodriguez A *et al.* Comparison between oral and vaginal administration of misoprostol on uterine contractility. *Obstet Gynecol* 1999; 93: 275–280.

Chapter

20

Perineal trauma

Stergios K. Doumouchtsis

Key facts

- Perineal trauma may occur during vaginal birth spontaneously or when the accoucher makes a surgical incision (episiotomy) to increase the vaginal opening.
- Perineal trauma can cause short- and long-term morbidity such as urinary or faecal incontinence, pelvic organ prolapse, pain and sexual dysfunction.
- The current classification of perineal trauma according to RCOG guidance is presented in Table 20.1 [1].

Table 20.1 Classification of perineal trauma [1].

First degree: laceration of the vaginal epithelium or perineal skin only

Second degree: involvement of the perineal muscles but not the anal sphincter

Third degree: disruption of the anal sphincter muscles. This should be further subdivided into:
    3a: < 50% thickness of external sphincter torn
    3b: > 50% thickness of external sphincter torn
    3c: internal sphincter also torn

Fourth degree: a third degree tear with disruption of the anal epithelium as well

Buttonhole tears are isolated tears of the anal mucosa and the vaginal epithelium without involvement of the sphincters

- In the UK more than 85% of women sustain perineal trauma during vaginal delivery [2].
- Several factors may affect this incidence including episiotomy rates. The rate of episiotomy in the USA has decreased from 60.9% in 1979 to 24.5% in 2004 [3].

- In centres where mediolateral episiotomies are practised, the rate of obstetric anal sphincter injuries (OASIS) is 1.7% (2.9% in primiparae) compared with 12% (19% in primiparae) in centres practising midline episiotomy [4].
- The rates of OASIS vary widely between countries, e.g. 0.4% (Italy) to 9.2% (Sweden) [5] and from one hospital to another (1.3–4.7% in Norway) [6].
- The true incidence of OASIS in primiparae using endoanal and 3D ultrasound is 11–35.4%.

Key implications

- Between one-third and two-thirds of women who sustain a recognised third-degree tear during delivery subsequently suffer from faecal incontinence.
- The prevalence of anal incontinence (including flatus as a sole symptom) and faecal incontinence (with or without flatus) following end-to-end repair ranges between 15–61% (mean = 39%) and 2–29% (mean = 14%) respectively. In addition faecal urgency can affect a further 6–28% [4].
- Persistent sonographic anal sphincter defects are identified in 34–91%.
- Following OASIS, anal incontinence during coitus affects about 17% of women.
- Compared with women with a minor (Grade 3a/3b) tear, those with a major (Grade 3c/4) one have a significantly poorer outcome with respect to defecatory symptoms and quality of life (QoL),

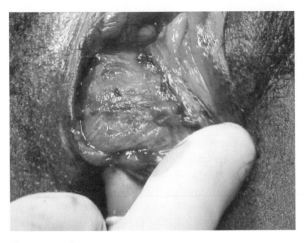

Figure 20.1 Tear.

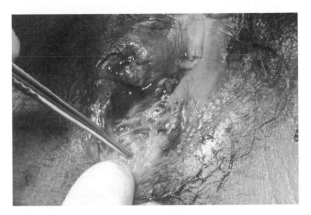

Figure 20.2 Tear with the forceps pointing at the exposed IAS.

as well as anal manometry. Women with major tears are significantly more likely to have an endosonographic isolated internal anal sphincter (IAS) or combined IAS and external anal sphincter (EAS) defect. Combined defects are associated with a higher risk of faecal incontinence and lower anal canal pressures [7].

- Compared with controls, more women with OASIS report stress urinary incontinence (33 vs 14%; p = 0.002; odds ratio (OR) 3.06; CI = 1.54–6.07) and overall urinary incontinence (21.2 vs 38%, p = 0.005) and have worse QoL scores. At 10 weeks after delivery the adjusted OR for stress urinary incontinence (SUI) is 2.65 (1.22–5.74) [8].

Long-term implications:

- Subjective and objective anal function after anal sphincter injury deteriorates further over time and with subsequent vaginal deliveries. A thin perineal body and internal sphincter injury seem to be important predictors of continence and anal pressure.
- Women who sustained OASIS have no further deterioration in urinary or sexual symptoms 18 years after delivery [9].

Key pointers

- Instrumental delivery, nulliparity, birth weight, shoulder dystocia, persistent occipito-posterior position and midline episiotomy are major risk factors.

- The angle of mediolateral episiotomy is significantly narrower in women who sustain OASIS.
- The perineal length is significantly shorter in women who sustain perineal tears, and OASIS.

Key diagnostic signs

- Following informed consent, a vaginal and rectal examination is performed with adequate analgesia (Figures 20.1 and 20.2).
- Visual inspection of the genitalia is followed by digital vaginal examination to establish the extent of the vaginal tear(s) and the apex. With the labia parted, assessment of the anal sphincter and exploration for buttonhole tears is undertaken by a digital examination of the anal canal and the rectum.
- With the index finger in the anal canal and the thumb in the vagina, the EAS can be palpated circumferentially and the extent and the depth of the tear further ascertained.
- Clinical diagnosis of OASIS can be suboptimal. Studies with endoanal ultrasound have shown that 'occult' OASIS is common after vaginal delivery, ranging between 20 and 41%.
- However, are these injuries truly occult or unrecognised at delivery? In women having their perineum re-examined by an experienced person clinically and/or by endoanal ultrasound the prevalence of OASIS increases over two-fold.
- Most sphincter defects considered as 'occult' injuries are actually injuries that should have been

139

clinically diagnosed but were missed. Although 98.8% of OASIS can be detected clinically at the time of delivery, the use of endoanal ultrasound shows that midwives can miss 87% of injuries and doctors 28% [10].

- However, as endoanal ultrasound is a technique that requires equipment and expertise, the diagnosis rests on clinical assessment and in practice, postpartum anal endosonography is of limited value.

Key actions (management algorithm)

The following surgical principles should be followed when performing perineal repairs:

- Check equipment and count swabs and instruments before and after the repair.
- The woman should be placed in a comfortable position with proper lighting for adequate exposure of the perineum.
- Ensure the woman has effective anaesthesia.
- 10–20 ml of lignocaine 1% is injected into the perineal wound. If the woman has an epidural, it may be 'topped-up'.
- In cases of extensive tears or OASIS general or regional anaesthesia will ensure muscle relaxation for proper evaluation and repair of the injury.
- The injury should be evaluated in lithotomy position and graded according to the recommended classification.
- The repair should be undertaken under aseptic conditions.
- Polyglactin 910 (Vicryl®, Ethicon Ltd, Edinburgh, UK) and a more rapidly absorbable polyglactin 910 material (Vicryl Rapide®) are the two most common absorbable synthetic suture materials used for perineal repair. The tensile strength of Vicryl Rapide® is reduced in 10–14 days and it is completely absorbed in 42 days. Vicryl Rapide® is associated with a significant reduction in the need for suture removal up to 3 months postpartum.

Repair of episiotomy, first- and second-degree tears

- First-degree tears and labial lacerations can be left unsutured, unless there is excessive bleeding or concerns about the anatomical alignment and

healing. In unsutured bilateral labial lacerations there is a risk of labial adhesions and voiding difficulties.

- The trauma should be repaired using a continuous non-locking technique to re-approximate all layers (vagina, perineal muscles and skin).
- First, a continuous layer is inserted to close the vaginal trauma, commencing above the vaginal apex of the wound and finishing at the level of hymen with a loop knot.
- The needle is then inserted into the vaginal skin and emerges through the perineal muscles to reconstruct the fourchette.
- The perineal muscles are reconstructed with continuous non-locking suturing. If the trauma is deep, the perineal muscles can be closed in two layers (a deep interrupted layer may be required).
- At the inferior end of the wound, the suturing direction is reversed and continuous sutures are applied in the subcutaneous tissue. The repair is then completed with a loop or Aberdeen knot at the level of the hymenal remnants. The skin may also be closed using interrupted transcutaneous sutures.
- Optimal alignment of the muscles avoiding undue tension ensures re-approximation of the perineal skin edges. Leaving the perineal skin unsutured may reduce superficial dyspareunia.

Repair of OASIS

- The most common techniques of primary repair following OASIS have been by 'end-to-end' approximation with interrupted sutures [11] and overlap repair of the EAS with separate end-to-end repair of the IAS; the latter showed promising results when introduced with a reduction of anal incontinence from 41% to 8% compared with matched historical controls who had an end-to-end repair [12].
- Several studies have evaluated the two techniques with varying results and a Cochrane review concluded that 'compared to primary end-to-end repair, overlap repair appears to be associated with lower risks for faecal urgency and anal incontinence symptoms but it would be inappropriate to recommend one type of repair in

favour of another, as the experience of the surgeon has not been addressed' [13].

- Repair of OASIS should be conducted in the operating theatre with assistance, good lighting, equipment and aseptic conditions.
- A 'buttonhole' tear without injury of the anal sphincter is repaired transvaginally using interrupted Vicryl sutures in layers including repair of the rectovaginal fascia to reduce the risk of healing defects and rectovaginal fistula.
- In fourth-degree tears, the torn anal epithelium is repaired with interrupted Vicryl 3/0 sutures with the knots tied in the anal lumen to reduce the suture material within the tissue.
- The sphincter muscles are repaired with 3/0 PDS as monofilament sutures carry lower risks of infection. Complete absorption of PDS takes longer than Vicryl, with 50% tensile strength lasting more than 3 months compared with 3 weeks. However, a randomised controlled trial revealed no differences in suture-related morbidity between Vicryl and PDS at 6 weeks postpartum [14].
- The IAS should be identified and, if torn, repaired by an end-to-end repair with interrupted or mattress 3/0 PDS sutures.
- As the torn ends of the EAS tend to retract they should be identified with Allis forceps and overlapped using PDS 3/0 sutures.
- If the EAS is only partially torn (grade 3a/3b), an end-to-end repair is technically more feasible using two or three mattress sutures similar to IAS repair.
- After repair of the sphincter, the vaginal skin and the perineal muscles should be sutured and the perineal skin approximated with a Vicryl 3/0 subcuticular suture.
- After completion of the procedure a vaginal and rectal examination should confirm haemostasis and a complete repair, ensure that all instruments and swabs have been removed and exclude inadvertent insertion of sutures through the rectal mucosa.
- The woman should be informed of the injury and given instructions about analgesia, hygiene, the importance of diet and avoidance of constipation and about pelvic floor exercises. She should be given contact details if she develops any symptoms during the postnatal period, with access to a perineal specialist or clinic.
- A detailed documentation with a diagram should be included in the case notes.
- Intra-operative and postoperative antibiotics following repair of OASIS for 5–7 days are essential to minimise risks of infection and wound breakdown, which may result in incontinence or fistula formation.
- An indwelling urethral catheter should be left in situ for about 24 hours as perineal pain and regional anaesthesia may cause voiding difficulty or reduced bladder sensation.
- The degree of pain following perineal trauma is related to the extent of the injury.
- Analgesia such as diclofenac is effective and its excretion in breast milk is negligible.
- In extensive perineal tears or OASIS, stool softeners (lactulose and a bulking agent e.g. Fybogel) for 10–14 days should be prescribed, to avoid constipation and wound disruption.
- Women who sustain OASIS should be assessed in a perineal clinic by a senior obstetrician or a specialist midwife 6–8 weeks after delivery. A pelvic examination is performed, to look for healing defects, scarring, granulation tissue and tenderness. Subsequently women should be scheduled for anal manometry and endoanal ultrasonography.
- The women are advised to continue pelvic floor exercises supervised by a pelvic floor physiotherapist.

Management of subsequent pregnancies

- Women who sustain OASIS should be counselled regarding their management in a subsequent pregnancy. The main risks are those of recurrence and anal incontinence.
- Women with previous OASIS who have no antenatal evidence of objective compromise of anal sphincter function can be reassured that a vaginal delivery is not associated with any significant deterioration in function or QoL.
- In women who had vaginal deliveries following previous OASIS the rate of anal incontinence is 56% compared with 34% in those who did not

subsequently deliver (RR 1.6; 95% CI 1.1–2.5) [15].

- Anal incontinence is significantly more common in women who had sustained fourth-degree tears compared with those with third-degree tears. Symptoms of worse bowel control are 10 times higher in women who sustained fourth- as opposed to third-degree tears.
- Of all the asymptomatic women after the first vaginal delivery who have a large 'occult' sonographic anal sphincter defect (> one quadrant) or anal squeeze pressures of less than 20 mmHg, 75% may become symptomatic after the second vaginal delivery. By contrast, only 5% with less extensive defects become symptomatic [16].
- All women who are symptomatic should be referred for anorectal physiology and endosonography and should be counselled for CS.
- Asymptomatic women who have minimal compromise of their anal sphincter function should be allowed to have a vaginal delivery. These women have a 95% chance of not sustaining recurrent OASIS or developing de novo anal incontinence following delivery [16].
- However, the delivery should be conducted by an experienced accoucher. A mediolateral episiotomy should be performed if necessary.
- A caesarean section should be considered in the presence of additional risk factors such as fetal macrosomia, shoulder dystocia, prolonged labour, or anticipated difficult instrumental delivery.
- Women with anal incontinence whose symptoms are controlled by conservative management (biofeedback and electrical muscle stimulation, dietary advice with avoidance of gas-producing foods, low-residue diet and constipating agents such as loperamide) are offered caesarean sections in subsequent pregnancies to avoid further compromise to anal sphincter function.
- Those women where conservative measures have failed should be offered incontinence surgery and caesarean section in future pregnancies.
- However, women with faecal incontinence who desire further pregnancies may opt for a vaginal delivery and anal sphincter surgery at a later date.

Prevention of perineal trauma

- Restrictive episiotomy policies compared with policies based on routine episiotomy are associated with less posterior perineal trauma, less suturing and fewer complications, no difference for most pain measures and severe vaginal or perineal trauma, but there is an increased risk of anterior perineal trauma with restrictive episiotomy [17].
- Antenatal perineal massage reduces the likelihood of perineal trauma (mainly episiotomies) and of ongoing perineal pain [18].
- Delivery technique that is unrushed and controlled may help reduce obstetric trauma in normal, spontaneous vaginal births [19].

Key pitfalls (things to avoid)

- An end-to-end repair can result in incomplete apposition if it does not include the full thickness of the muscle.
- Non-absorbable monofilament sutures such as nylon or Prolene (polypropylene), although used by some colorectal surgeons when performing secondary sphincter repairs, are best avoided as they may require removal due to abscesses and chronic pain.
- When suturing a vaginal tear, the suture insertion points should not be too wide, to avoid narrowing of the vagina.
- Sutures should not be over-tightened, as tissue ischaemia may cause healing complications.
- Codeine-based preparations are best avoided, as they may cause constipation, leading to excessive straining and possible wound breakdown.

Key pearls (things to remember)

- Perineal trauma is one of the major causes of postpartum haemorrhage.
- When performing a mediolateral episiotomy, the angle should be between 45 and 60° from midline at crowning of the fetal head.
- Continuous suture techniques compared with interrupted sutures for perineal closure are associated with less pain postpartum, requirements for analgesia, dyspareunia and suture removal, but there are no significant

differences in the need for re-suturing of wounds or long-term pain.

- Dead space in the vagina or perineum should be closed for haemostasis and prevention of haematoma.
- Repair of OASIS should be conducted only by a doctor who has been formally trained (or under supervision).
- Combined defects (EAS and IAS) are associated with poorer outcome and it is therefore important to identify the full extent of injury and to pay particular attention to repair of IAS defects.
- As the inherent tone of the EAS can result in retraction of the torn muscle ends, adequate muscle relaxation is important to enable retrieval of the ends of the EAS and repair without tension.
- More experienced assistance should be summoned if the trauma is beyond the operator's expertise.
- Good anatomical alignment and consideration to the cosmetic results is essential.
- In cases of labial tears it is important to advise the woman to part the labia daily during bathing to prevent adhesions.

Management in low-resource settings

- The steps described in the management of perineal tears are applicable in most settings.
- If specialist perineal services are not available, women with OASIS should be given instructions about signs of infection, wound dehiscence, incontinence of stool or flatus and contact details for follow-up and further management by an obstetrician or midwife.
- If there are no facilities for anal manometry and endosonography, asymptomatic women with previous OASIS without clinical evidence of compromise of the anal tone could be allowed to have a vaginal delivery in a subsequent pregnancy.

References

1. Royal College of Obstetricians and Gynaecologists. *The Management of Third and Fourth Degree Perineal Tears*. Green-top Guideline No. 29. London: RCOG, 2007.

2. McCandlish R, Bowler U, van Asten H *et al.* A randomised controlled trial of care of the perineum during second stage of normal labour. *Br J Obstet Gynaecol* 1998; 105 (12): 1262–1272.

3. Frankman EA, Wang L, Bunker CH *et al.* Episiotomy in the United States: has anything changed? *Am J Obstet Gynecol* 2009; 200 (5): 573, e1–7.

4. Sultan A, Thakar R, Fenner D. *Perineal and Anal Sphincter Trauma*. London: Springer, 2007.

5. Prager M, Andersson KL, Stephansson O *et al.* The incidence of obstetric anal sphincter rupture in primiparous women: a comparison between two European delivery settings. *Acta Obstet Gynecol Scand* 2008; 87 (2): 209–215.

6. Valbo A, Gjessing L, Herzog C *et al.* Anal sphincter tears at spontaneous delivery: a comparison of five hospitals in Norway. *Acta Obstet Gynecol Scand* 2008; 87 (11): 1176–1180.

7. Roos AM, Thakar R, Sultan AH. Outcome of primary repair of obstetric anal sphincter injuries (OASIS): does the grade of tear matter? *Ultrasound Obstet Gynecol* 2010; 36 (3): 368–374.

8. Scheer I, Andrews V, Thakar R *et al.* Urinary incontinence after obstetric anal sphincter injuries (OASIS) – is there a relationship? *Int Urogynecol J Pelvic Floor Dysfunct* 2008; 19 (2): 179–183.

9. Otero M, Boulvain M, Bianchi-Demicheli F *et al.* Women's health 18 years after rupture of the anal sphincter during childbirth: II. Urinary incontinence, sexual function, and physical and mental health. *Am J Obstet Gynecol* 2006; 194 (5): 1260–1265.

10. Andrews V, Thakar R, Sultan AH, Jones PW. Occult anal sphincter injuries – myth or reality? *Br J Obstet Gynaecol* 2006; 113 (2): 195–200.

11. Sultan AH, Kamm MA, Hudson CN, Bartram CI. Third degree obstetric anal sphincter tears: risk factors and outcome of primary repair. *Br Med J* 1994; 308 (6933): 887–891.

12. Sultan AH, Monga AK, Kumar D, Stanton SL. Primary repair of obstetric anal sphincter rupture using the overlap technique. *Br J Obstet Gynaecol* 1999; 106 (4): 318–323.

13. Fernando R, Sultan AH, Kettle C *et al.* Methods of repair for obstetric anal sphincter injury. *Cochrane Database Syst Rev* 2006; 3: CD002866.

14. Williams A, Adams EJ, Tincello DG *et al.* How to repair an anal sphincter injury after vaginal delivery: results of a randomised controlled trial. *Br J Obstet Gynaecol* 2006; 113(2): 201–207.

15. Poen AC, Felt-Bersma RJF, Strijers RLM *et al.* Third-degree obstetric perineal tear: long-term clinical and functional results after primary repair. *Br J Surg* 1998; 85 (10): 1433–1438.

16. Fynes M, Donnelly V, Behan M, O'Connell PR, O'Herlihy C. Effect of second vaginal delivery on

anorectal physiology and faecal continence: a prospective study. *Lancet* 1999; 354 (9183): 983–986.

17. Carroli G, Mignini L. Episiotomy for vaginal birth. *Cochrane Database Syst Rev* 2009; 1: Art. CD000081.

18. Beckmann MM, Garrett AJ. Antenatal perineal massage for reducing perineal trauma. *Cochrane Database Syst Rev* 2006; 1: Art. CD005123.

19. Albers LL, Sedler KD, Bedrick EJ, Teaf D, Peralta P. Factors related to genital tract trauma in normal spontaneous vaginal births. *Birth* 2006; 33 (2): 94–100.

Chapter

21

Palpitations during pregnancy

Niraj Yanamandra and Edwin Chandraharan

Key facts

The physiological state of pregnancy is associated with significant haemodynamic changes associated with adaptation of the cardiovascular system to deal with the metabolic requirements of the mother and her growing fetus. Consequently, maternal heart rate increases by 25%; thus sinus tachycardia, particularly in the third trimester, is not uncommon. Premature atrial beats ('ectopic beats') and non-sustained arrhythmia are encountered in more than 50% of pregnant women.

Palpitations are unpleasant sensations of irregular and/or forceful beating of the heart. They can occur in women with no known heart disease or rhythm abnormalities. Palpitations, dizziness, pre-syncope and even syncope frequently occur during pregnancy. The reasons for these palpitations remain unknown. In others, palpitations result from abnormal heart rhythms (arrhythmias). Palpitations are most often caused by cardiac arrhythmias or anxiety. Cardiac arrhythmias can be identified on Holter recordings in up to 60% of normal people under the age of 40 years. It is, therefore, not uncommon to see women complaining of palpitations while pregnant.

Arrhythmias refer to heartbeats that could either be slow, too fast, irregular or too early. Palpitations can result from many arrhythmias, including any bradycardia and tachycardia, premature ventricular and atrial contractions, sick sinus syndrome, advanced arterio-venous block or ventricular tachycardia. Episodes of ventricular tachycardia and supraventricular tachycardia may be perceived as palpitations but also can be asymptomatic or lead to syncope [1].

- Rapid arrhythmias (greater than 100 beats per minute) are called tachycardias.
- Slow arrhythmias (slower than 60 beats per minute) are called bradycardias.
- Irregular heart rhythms are called fibrillations.
- When a single heartbeat occurs earlier than normal, it is called a premature contraction, and this can cause the sensation of a forceful heartbeat.
- Abnormalities in the atria, the ventricles, and the electrical conducting system (the sino-atrial (SA) node and the atrio-ventricular (AV) node) of the heart can lead to arrhythmias that cause palpitations.

Non-arrhythmic cardiac problems, such as mitral valve prolapse, pericarditis and congestive heart failure, and non-cardiac problems, such as hyperthyroidism, vaso-vagal syncope and hypoglycaemia, can cause palpitations. Palpitations also can result from stimulant drugs, over the counter and prescription medications. No cause for palpitations can be found in up to 16% of patients.

A common sensation of palpitation in the absence of concomitant cardiac arrhythmias may also be related to physiological changes occurring during pregnancy, such as increased heart rate, decreased peripheral resistance and increased stroke volume.

Obstetric and Intrapartum Emergencies, ed. Edwin Chandraharan and Sabaratnam Arulkumaran. Published by Cambridge University Press. © Cambridge University Press 2012.

A study looking at the incidence of arrhythmias in normal pregnancy and relation to palpitations, dizziness and syncope demonstrated a high incidence of arrhythmias, mostly ventricular ectopic activity, in young healthy women presenting with symptoms of palpitations, dizziness or syncope during their pregnancy [2].

Increased sympathetic activity during pregnancy has been proposed as a mechanism for increased incidence of arrhythmias.

Key implications

Identifying the underlying cause is essential for management of palpitations in pregnancy. Differential diagnoses for palpitations are:

- Cardiac conditions.
  - Arrhythmic disorders.
    - Sinus tachycardia.
    - Atrial fibrillation.
    - Premature ventricular contractions.
    - Ventricular tachycardia.
  - Non-arrhythmic disorders.
    - Mitral valve prolapse.
    - Pericarditis.
    - Congestive heart failure.

- Non-cardiac conditions.
  - Hyperthyroidism.
  - Vaso-vagal syncope.
  - Hypoglycaemia.
  - Inflammation.
  - Infection.
  - Anaemia.
  - Hypovolemia.
  - Metabolic – hyperthyroidism.

- Drugs.
  - Alcohol.
  - Caffeine.
  - Prescription drugs e.g. digitalis, phenothiazine, beta-agonists.
  - Street drugs (e.g. cocaine).
  - Tobacco.

- Psychiatric and emotional illnesses e.g. anxiety, panic and somatisation disorders.
- Idiopathic – seen in up to 16% of patients.

Key pointers

Before initiating therapy, it is important to correctly diagnose the type and mechanism of the underlying arrhythmia so that proper therapeutic modalities can be implemented. A detailed history including family history is important to identify those who may have genetic predisposition for heart disease. It is also important to take history of other relevant medical conditions (non-cardiac) such as thyroid disorders, infection, possible inflammation or pulmonary embolism – although other symptoms such as shortness of breath may be more prominent in the latter.

Aims of management:

- Diagnosing the cause of palpitation/arrhythmia.
- Identifying any associated heart disease.
- Rule out non-cardiac condition causing palpitations.

Important elements in management:

- Accurate and detailed history.
- Examination with careful exclusion of other systemic conditions.

Investigations

- Resting electrocardiogram (ECG): Appropriate in all patients complaining of palpitations. In the event of the patient having palpitations at the time of ECG, diagnosis of arrhythmia can be confirmed.
- Prolonged ECG recording: This is usually indicated if the aetiology of palpitations cannot be determined from the patient's history, physical examination and resting ECG. When palpitations occur unpredictably or do not occur daily, an initial 2-week course of continuous closed-loop event recording is indicated. If symptoms occur on a daily basis then a 24-h or 48-h Holter may be sufficient. It is crucial for the woman to keep an accurate diary so any symptoms can be related to any abnormality on the Holter. It is important that the woman continues with her normal activity while wearing the device and keeps a diary of her symptoms, which can be related to the recorded rhythm.

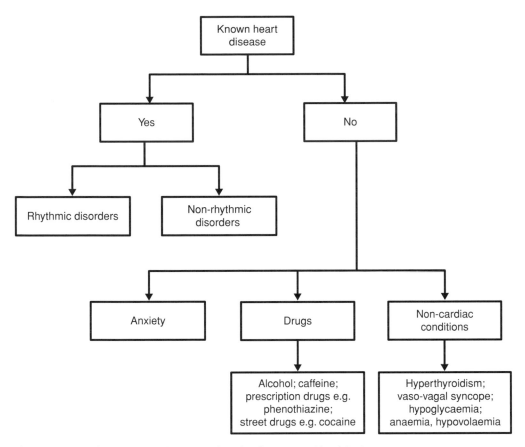

Figure 21.1 Key diagnostic signs. Diagnostic algorithm for women with palpitations.

- Echocardiography: This should be considered an integral part of the investigation of any pregnant patient with proven arrhythmia to diagnose structural and functional heart disease.
- Tilt-table testing: In some cases, the patient will be strapped to a tilt table lying flat and then tilted or suspended completely or almost completely upright (as if standing). The test ends either when the patient faints or develops other significant symptoms, or after a set period. A tilt-table test is considered positive if the patient experiences symptoms associated with a drop in blood pressure or cardiac arrhythmia. This test should be delayed until after pregnancy, where possible.
- Pharmacological testing: A pharmacological challenge may provide important diagnostic information. Flecainide and adenosine have been widely used in pregnancy.
- Electrophysiological studies: Usually done after pregnancy and rarely required while pregnant.

Key pitfalls
- Attributing the symptoms of palpitations to probable physiological changes may lead to delay in diagnosis. Prompt attempts at investigating and determining the underlying cause are essential to avoid missing any significant cardiac lesion.
- There are no obvious contraindications to performing the usual diagnostic modalities (see above) used to diagnose arrhythmias.

Key pearls
- Cardioversion is safe during all trimesters of pregnancy and can be used if necessary.
- Women who have had repair of their congenital heart defects have an increased risk of arrhythmias during pregnancy.
- A multidisciplinary team approach with cardiologists, obstetricians and anaesthetists

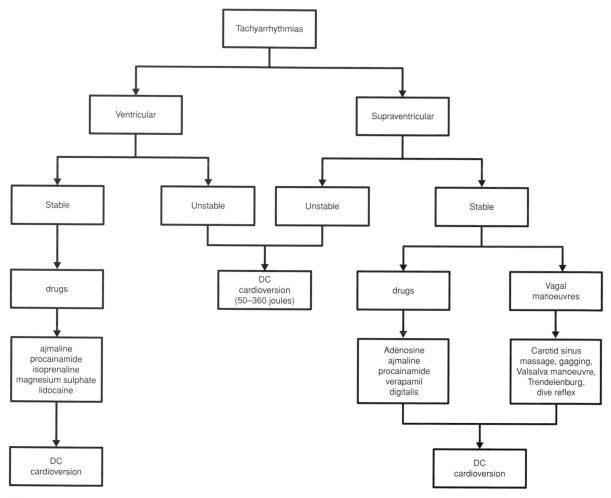

Figure 21.2 Key actions (management algorithm). Treatment algorithm for pregnant patients with tachyarrhythmias [4]. DC, direct current.

during pregnancy, delivery and the postpartum period is recommended.

- Physiological changes during pregnancy influence the pharmacology of antiarrhythmic drugs. Serum concentration is reduced and changes in protein-binding affinity are present, influencing the pharmacology of antiarrhythmic drugs.

- A common sensation of palpitation in the absence of concomitant cardiac arrhythmias may also be related to physiological changes occurring during pregnancy, such as increased heart rate, decreased peripheral resistance, and increased stroke volume. Most often palpitations are caused by cardiac arrhythmias or anxiety [3].

- The majority of arrhythmias that occur during pregnancy are benign. Hence, advice about appropriate actions during symptomatic episodes,

together with reassurance, is usually all that is required. In the remaining minority of cases, judicious use of antiarrhythmic drugs will be needed for a safe and successful outcome for both mother and baby.

- A high incidence of arrhythmias, mostly ventricular ectopic activity, is noted in young healthy women presenting with symptoms of palpitations, dizziness or syncope during their pregnancy [2]. The cause for palpitations in most cases remains unclear and their presence during normal pregnancy is not predictive of cardiac arrhythmia.

- Palpitations are potentially more serious when they are associated with dizziness, near-syncope, or syncope because they suggest tachyarrhythmia.

- No cause can be found in up to 16% of patients.

- Pharmacological therapy of rhythm disorders should be reserved for arrhythmias resulting in maternal or fetal haemodynamic compromise and for arrhythmias with intolerable symptoms.

References

1. Abbott AV. Diagnostic approach to palpitations. *Am Fam Phys* 2005; 71: 743–750.

2. Shotan MDA, Ostrzega MDE, Mehra MDA *et al.* 1997. Incidence of arrhythmias in normal pregnancy and relation to palpitations, dizziness, and syncope. *Am J Cardiol* 1997; 79: 1061–1064.

3. Mabie WC, Freire CM. Sudden chest pain and cardiac emergencies in the obstetric patient. *Obstet Gynecol Clin N Am* 1995; 22: 19–37.

4. Trappe H-J. Acute therapy of maternal and fetal arrhythmias during pregnancy. *J Intens Care Med* 2006; 21: 305–315.

Breathlessness

22

Michael Egbor and Hassan Shehata

Key facts

- Definition: Breathlessness is the subjective sensation of shortness of breath, often exacerbated by exertion. The majority of pregnant women are aware of breathlessness before 20 weeks' gestation [1, 2].
- Types:
  - Physiological – physiological dyspnoea is an isolated symptom, which tends to occur early in pregnancy and often improves or plateaus as term approaches.
  - Pathological – when persistent breathlessness interferes with a woman's ability to engage in daily activities. Also, if symptoms of cardiorespiratory disease are present [3].
- Incidence: Commonly reported in 60–75% of healthy pregnant women, it reaches the maximum incidence at 28–31 weeks' gestation.

Key implications

- Maternal: Breathlessness may be a sign of decompensation of underlying heart or lung disorders, therefore requires urgent investigation and appropriate treatment [4–8].
- Fetal: Severe causes could lead to chronic hypoxia which in turn increases the risk of preterm birth, altered fetal growth and mortality.

Key pointers

- Prolonged bed rest, deep vein thrombosis (DVT), thrombophilia, venous stasis, recent air flight, age, parity, drugs, sickle cell disease and recent surgery may suggest pulmonary embolism (PE).
- Smoking, upper respiratory tract infection (URTI), immunosuppression, preexisting lung disease, recent contact with birds drugs (e.g. steroids) and abuse, may predispose to pneumonia.
- Allergens, cold air, emotions, infection, drugs, exercise and stress are related to asthma.
- Exertional dyspnoea, orthopnoea, paroxysmal nocturnal dyspnoea, nocturnal cough, wheeze and peripheral oedema are associated with cardiac failure.
- Acid reflux, polyarteritis nodosa, Churg–Strauss syndrome (vasculitis) and other atopic diseases are also pointers to asthma.

Key diagnostic signs

- Hypotension, a narrow pulse pressure and tachycardia are seen in cardiac failure.
- Cyanosis is present in pulmonary embolism, cardiac failure and pneumonia.
- A raised jugular venous pressure (JVP), hepatomegaly, cardiomegaly, gallop rhythm; murmurs can be seen in cardiac failure. Also pleural effusion, bibasilar crepitations, wheeze and tachypnoea.
- Polyphonic wheeze, diminished air entry or silent chest is common in asthma.

Obstetric and Intrapartum Emergencies, ed. Edwin Chandraharan and Sabaratnam Arulkumaran. Published by Cambridge University Press. © Cambridge University Press 2012.

Table 22.1 Key features in various causes of breathlessness.

Symptom/Sign	Cardiac failure	Asthma	Pulmonary embolism	Pneumonia
Sputum	Nocturnal	Nocturnal	Dry	Productive
Abdominal pain	–	–	+	+/–
Lungs	Bibasilar crepitations	Exp rhonchi ↓ air entry/Silent	–	Rhonchi
Heart sounds	Gallop rhythm	–	3rd HS	–
Blood pressure	Low	–	↓ / N	–
Pulse	↓ Volume, Pulsus alterans	Pulsus paradoxus	N	N
Pulse rate	↑	↑ / N	↑ / N	↑ / N

Table 22.2 Key features seen in commonly performed investigations.

Investigation	Cardiac failure	Asthma	Pulmonary embolism	Pneumonia
Chest X-ray	Hilar shadowing, Kerley B lines, cardiomegaly, pleural effusion	Hyperinflated lungs	Usually N/wedge-shaped infarction, pleural effusion, atelectasis, areas of translucency in underperfused lung	Patchy/consolidation
Electrocardiography	Left ventricular strain/enlargement	N	N/right axis deviation, right bundle branch block, peaked waves in lead II, S_1 Q_3 T_3 pattern	N
Echo	Cardiomegaly, ↓ function, +/– valve abnormally	N	Right-sided strain	N

- Tachypnoea, audible wheeze and hyper-inflated chest are noted in asthma.
- See Table 22.1 for the differentiating signs in the common causes of breathlessness.

Key actions

- A detailed history including previous medical, family and current medications should be obtained to help establish a diagnosis.

  - Abdominal pain is suggestive of pelvic vein thrombosis or diaphragmatic irritation.
  - Syncope may occur with large pulmonary emboli.
  - Cough is a common symptom in pulmonary embolism and pneumonia but usually nocturnal in cardiac failure and asthma.
  - Purulent sputum, rigors are suggestive of pneumonia.
  - Cardiac lesions such as mitral stenosis should be considered in immigrant women.
  - Past medical and family history.

- A thorough physical examination should be undertaken looking for key diagnostic features listed above which will help establish the correct diagnosis.
- Investigations which have previously been shown to be useful in confirming a definitive diagnosis and excluding possible differentials include (also see Table 22.2):

  - Peak flow meter.
  - Pulse oximetry.
  - ECG – $S_1Q_3T_3$ may be normal in pregnancy.
  - Chest X-ray.
  - C-reactive protein – non-specific, suggestive of inflammatory process.
  - Troponin I.
  - B-type natriuretic peptide.
  - Blood and sputum cultures.
  - Arterial blood gases.
  - Echocardiography.
  - Spirometry.
  - Ventilation–perfusion scan.
  - Doppler/venogram for pelvis/lower limbs.

· Impedance plethysmography and thermography.
· Spiral computed tomography (CT).
· Magnetic resonance imaging (MRI).

- Confirm a definitive diagnosis if possible as this will influence the treatment and counselling given to the patient.

Classification of conditions

Conditions that cause breathlessness in pregnancy can be classified into acute, sub-acute and chronic conditions.

- Acute.
  · Hyperventilation/anxiety.
  · Acute asthma.
  · Pulmonary embolism.
  · Acute pulmonary oedema.
  · Foreign body.
  · Pneumothorax.

- Sub-acute.
  · Asthma.
  · Lung parenchymal disease e.g. pneumonia, alveolitis, effusions.

- Chronic.
  · Physiological.
  · Anaemia.
  · Chronic lung disease.
  · Cardiac causes (mitral stenosis, puerperal cardiomyopathy).

Management

These patients are best managed by a multidisciplinary team involving obstetricians, anaesthetist and other relevant subspecialities such as obstetric physicians, cardiologists and respiratory physicians.

General measures

- Ensure a patent airway, monitor breathing and administer oxygen if required.
- Obtain IV access and correct any dehydration if present.
- Severely ill patients may need monitoring in the high dependency/intensive care unit, involve the intensivist early if necessary.
- Offer appropriate analgesia for pain relief.

- Ensure monitoring for fetal well-being.
- Document a clear plan of obstetric management including need and type of delivery if required.

Specific treatment

- Treat any identified underlying condition.
- Intravenous heparin, low molecular weight heparins given subcutaneously, thrombolytic agents and surgical thrombolectomy in pulmonary embolism. Inferior vena cava filter may be inserted in recurrent emboli.
- Paracetamol and tepid sponging to reduce the complications of pyrexia.
- Administration of broad-spectrum antibiotics with advice from the microbiologists in cases where infection is thought to be the underlying cause.
- Treat exacerbating factors e.g. anaemia, thyroid disease and infection. Avoid exacerbating factors e.g. NSAIDS (fluid retention), verapamil (negative inotrope). Patients should stop smoking, reduce salt intake and maintain optimal weight and nutrition.
- With cardiac causes the most commonly used drugs include diuretics, spironolactone, ACE-inhibitor, beta-blockers, digoxin, vasodilators. Heart transplantation remains a rare and last resort when all else fails.
- In severe acute asthmatic attacks, nebulised salbutamol can be administered along with steroids and intravenous aminophylline if required. Patients are best managed in the intensive care unit if intubation is anticipated. Magnesium sulphate has also been used in severe cases with a return to beta-2-agonist and steroid inhalers when patient becomes stable.
- Physiological cause is only a diagnosis of exclusion.

Key pitfalls

- Failure to differentiate physiological breathlessness from that caused by potentially life-threatening conditions.
- Failure to recognise signs and symptoms of severe illness.
- Failure to involve senior input early.

- Failure to manage the patient in a multidisciplinary context incorporating expertise from other specialities.

Key pearls

- All staff should attend appropriate courses in order to update their knowledge and competence in the management of medical conditions in pregnancy including respiratory and cardiovascular problems.
- All staff should attend regular multidisciplinary training on the recognition and management of the very ill woman in obstetrics.

Management in low-resource settings

Breathlessness is commonly encountered in pregnancy and can be due to potentially life-threatening conditions. There is therefore the need for urgent assessment by a carefully obtained history and physical examination in every setting. Many of the investigations listed may not be available in low-resource settings; however a simple chest X-ray and ECG can provide some useful information to guide initial management.

References

1. Nelson-Piercy C. *Handbook of Obstetric Medicine*. Fourth edition. London: Informa Healthcare, 2010.

2. García-Rio F, Pino J, Gomez L *et al.* Regulation of breathing and perception of dyspnoea in healthy pregnant women. *Chest* 1996; 110; 446–453.

3. Graves C. Acute pulmonary complications during pregnancy. *Clin Obstet Gynaecol* 2002; 45 (2): 369–376.

4. Murdock M. Asthma in pregnancy. *J Perinatal Neonatal Nurs* 2002; 15 (4): 27–36.

5. Fabre E. Use of drugs in pulmonary medicine in pregnant women. *Clin Pulmon Med* 2002; 9 (1): 20–32.

6. Rigby FB, Pastorek JG II. Pneumonia during pregnancy. *Clin Obstet Gynaecol* 1996; 39 (1): 107–119.

7. Shehata H, Nelson-Piercy C. Medical diseases complicating pregnancy, including thromboembolism. *Anaesth Intensive Care Med* 2001; 2: 6 225–232.

8. Susanthi I. Respiratory complications in pregnancy. *Obstet Gynaecol Surv* 2002; 57 (1): 39–46.

Chapter 23

Abdominal pain in pregnancy

Archana Krishna and Edwin Chandraharan

Key facts

- Acute abdomen refers to abdominal pain of less than 1 week's duration requiring admission to hospital, which has not been previously treated or investigated.
- Abdominal pain in pregnancy may be secondary to the anatomical and physiological changes of the pregnant state or may be totally unrelated to pregnancy.
- Abdominal pain of any degree is a cause of significant maternal anxiety and constitutes a major reason for hospital attendance during pregnancy.
- The gravid uterus enlarges to almost 20 times its normal 'non-pregnant' size which results in stretching of the supporting ligaments and muscles as well as pressure on the other intra-abdominal structures and layers of the anterior abdominal wall.
- 20% of adnexal torsions occur during pregnancy – this rarely includes torsion of a morphologically normal ovary.

Key implications

- Physiological leukocytosis and raised alkaline phosphatase that are associated with normal pregnancy may contribute to diagnostic difficulty.
- Imaging techniques such as X-rays, magnetic resonance imaging (MRI) or computerised tomography (CT) to diagnose non-obstetric causes of abdominal pain may be delayed, due to the fear of exposing the fetus to radiation.

- Although there is a risk of teratogenesis in the first trimester and possible link to childhood cancers with late fetal exposure to ionising radiation, exposures of less than 0.05 Gy have not been associated with pregnancy loss or fetal malformations [1].
- Due to anatomical changes associated with pregnancy, classic symptoms and signs that are observed in the non-pregnant state may be distorted. For example, certain organs such as the appendix are progressively displaced upwards and laterally with advancing gestation by the enlarging gravid uterus. Hence, the point of maximum tenderness may not be felt around the McBurney's point.

Key pointers

Miscarriage

A combination of pain and vaginal bleeding should alert a clinician to a possible threatened, inevitable, incomplete or septic miscarriage. Pain is typically described as a 'cramping ache'. On examination the uterus corresponds to the period of amenorrhoea and signs of peritoneal irritation are absent. The internal cervical os might be open or closed based on the type of miscarriage. An open os is diagnostic of an inevitable or incomplete miscarriage. Ultrasound examination is helpful to confirm viability, intra-uterine pregnancy and exclude a subchorionic haematoma [2].

Ectopic pregnancy

Pregnancy is rarely located outside the normal endometrial cavity, most commonly in the Fallopian

Obstetric and Intrapartum Emergencies, ed. Edwin Chandraharan and Sabaratnam Arulkumaran. Published by Cambridge University Press. © Cambridge University Press 2012.

tubes. Pain is typically unilateral and colicky. It may be superimposed on 'dull aching pain' and may be associated with dizziness or fainting episodes. On clinical examination, unilateral iliac fossa tenderness, cervical excitation and adnexal tenderness may be elicited. Size of the uterus is often less than the period of amenorrhoea.

Demonstration of an empty uterine cavity on transvaginal ultrasound despite serum beta HCG levels of over 1500 IU/l may help clinch the diagnosis.

Presence of any symptoms including abdominal pain or evidence of significant haemoperitoneum is a contraindication for medical treatment and surgical treatment is indicated. This includes emergency salpingectomy via laparoscopy or laparotomy.

Ovarian cyst 'accidents'

Ovarian cysts complicate 1 in 1000 pregnancies and a vast majority are benign (98%). Pain is often described as intermittent and unilateral. Torsion also occurs more frequently on the right than the left, by a ratio of 3 : 2, owing to the presence of the sigmoid colon on the left that limits the space available for torsion. Clinical examination may confirm tenderness in either iliac fossa and a large cyst may be palpable during abdominal and/or bimanual examination. However, in modern obstetric practice, the cyst is usually detected on ultrasound. Figure 23.1 shows a dermoid cyst complicating pregnancy.

Most torsions and cyst accidents present as an acute abdomen and would warrant surgical treatment. Twenty per cent of adnexal torsions occur during pregnancy –this also includes torsion of a morphologically normal ovary. In early pregnancy, symptomatic 'benign' ovarian cysts may be removed by laparoscopic ovarian cystectomy. In view of the inaccessibility of the adnexae in late pregnancy, a midline or paramedian incision is recommended. Any ovarian cyst that exhibits sonographic features that are suggestive of malignancy should be referred to the oncological team for further imaging and appropriate treatment.

Acute retention of urine

Pain due to retention of urine caused by stretching of, or direct pressure on, the urethra may be due to a retroverted uterus in early pregnancy or rarely due to an impacted pelvic mass such as an ovarian cyst or a

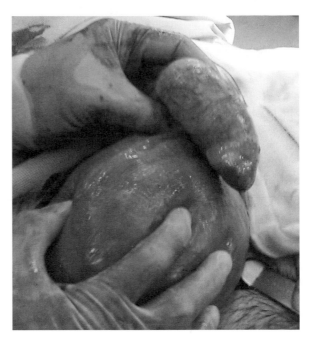

Figure 23.1 Ovarian (dermoid) cyst complicating pregnancy.

fibroid mass. An indwelling catheter to facilitate bladder drainage may help relieve pain. Gentle manual correction of the retroversion and an indwelling catheter should be the conservative management plan until the uterus rises above the pelvis at 12 weeks' gestation.

Musculoskeletal causes

Round ligament pain is a common cause of antenatal attendance in the second and third trimesters. This often presents with pain in one or both iliac fossae. It is believed to be secondary to the stretching of the ligamentous supports of the uterus. The pain is characteristically worse on movement. A support brace and simple analgesia are the mainstays of treatment.

Ovarian hyperstimulation syndrome (OHSS)

This is a systemic condition secondary to the production of vasoactive substances produced by hyperstimulated ovaries. The diagnosis is very straightforward as there is a history of undergoing assisted conception with ovulation induction. Associated symptoms are a result of increased capillary permeability and include headache, vomiting, abdominal distension and rarely oliguria. Based on clinical severity, the initial classification of Schenker and Weinstein [3] has been modified by Golan *et al.* into six grades [4].

Ovarian hyperstimulation syndrome is a potentially life-threatening condition and immediate senior input should be sought and a multidisciplinary care plan should be instituted. Management includes supportive treatment for pain and correction of intravascular dehydration, replacement of albumin, daily weight chart and thromboprophylaxis. Some women may require an urgent laparotomy (multiple cyst rupture) and treatment in an intensive treatment unit.

Gastritis and hyperemesis gravidarum

Gastritis typically occurs up to 16 weeks' gestation and resolves by treatment with fluid replacement, antiemetics and H_2 blockers. Persistent vomiting may rarely lead to Mallory–Weiss tears in the lower oesophagus and resultant haematemesis and abdominal pain. Urgent referral to the upper gastrointestinal surgical team should be made if this condition is suspected for tamponade using a Sengstaken–Blakemore tube.

Fibroid degeneration

Fibroids occur in 1% of all pregnancies and risk of torsion is increased in the pedunculated variety. Red degeneration presents with severe, localised pain and is associated with nausea and vomiting. Ultrasound examination may reveal cystic spaces within the fibroid suggestive of degenerative changes. Conservative management with opiate analgesia and reassurance is required.

Ruptured rudimentary horn

This is extremely rare with a quoted incidence of 1 : 76 000 and presents with persistent severe uterine pain refractory to simple analgesia. This Müllerian tract abnormality typically ruptures in the second trimester and is associated with significant intraperitoneal bleeding. Rarely, it may rupture into the broad ligament (Figure 23.2).

Obstetric complications

Placental abruption

Abruptio placenta refers to the premature separation of a normally situated placenta and it occurs in 0.5–1.5% of all pregnancies.

Abdominal pain may present with or without vaginal bleeding. Fetal heart rate may be absent in severe abruption secondary to utero-placental insufficiency.

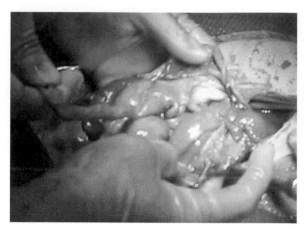

Figure 23.2 Rupture of a pregnancy within the uterine horn at 22 weeks.

There may be varying degrees of haemodynamic compromise secondary to blood loss either vaginally or inside the uterus in the concealed variety [5].

Immediate senior input should be sought and management includes maternal resuscitation, correction of hypovolaemia and coagulation abnormalities through a multidisciplinary approach. Emergency caesarean section should be performed in the event of suspected fetal compromise, once the woman is haemodynamically stable and her coagulation abnormality is corrected.

If an intra-uterine death is confirmed, an amniotomy and oxytocin infusion may be commenced. Haemodynamic instability warrants immediate uterine evacuation to avoid morbidity and maternal mortality.

Acute polyhydramnios

Acute polyhydramnios refers to an amniotic fluid index above the 95th centile for gestational age or the depth of the deepest vertical pool equal to or greater than 8 cm.

Abdominal pain in acute polyhydramnios is secondary to uterine over-distension. Clinical signs include an elevated symphyseal fundal height, difficulty in palpating fetal parts due to a tense and tender abdomen. On examination, a fluid thrill may be elicited on percussion. Confirmatory diagnosis is by ultrasound measurement of amniotic fluid pockets.

Management should involve specialists in fetal medicine and may include immediate amnio-drainage to relieve symptoms and to reduce the risk of preterm labour. Laser ablation of vascular anastomosis (twin-to-twin transfusion syndrome), serial amnioreduction to relieve pressure on the placental bed may be considered at a later stage. Predisposing causes such as congenital malformations and undiagnosed diabetes mellitus should be excluded. Indomethacin may help reduce formation of amniotic fluid but may adversely affect fetal renal function and therefore it is not recommended for prolonged use.

Uterine scar dehiscence

The incidence of intrapartum scar dehiscence is 35 : 10 000 after one caesarean section. Spontaneous rupture of a non-scarred uterus may occur in grand multiparous women with obstructed labour and excessive use of oxytocin or prostaglandins.

Women may present with acute pain between uterine contractions, vaginal bleeding and signs of circulatory collapse. Rarely, if the fetus has been extruded into the peritoneal cavity, fetal parts and uterine asymmetry might be obvious.

The earliest sign of intrapartum scar dehiscence is fetal compromise on the cardiotocograph (CTG). Management involves maternal resuscitation and immediate laparotomy, delivery of the fetus, placenta and repair of the dehisced uterus.

Acute chorioamnionitis

Pre-labour rupture of membranes typically precedes chorioamnionitis. However, infection may be present with intact membranes and leads to severe abdominal pain.

Pain is usually associated with maternal and fetal tachycardia, pyrexia and offensive vaginal discharge. In extreme cases there may be widespread septicaemia/ systemic inflammatory response syndrome (SIRS) and features of septic shock. The recent CMACE report has flagged genital tract sepsis as a leading cause of direct maternal death in the last triennium [6].

Recognising symptoms and signs of sepsis

- Fever with chills and rigors.
- Reduced mental alertness, sometimes with confusion.
- Nausea and vomiting.
- Diarrhoea.
- Increased heart rate, greater than 90 beats per minute.

- Increased respiratory rate, greater than 30 breaths per minute.
- High or low white blood cell count.
- Low blood pressure.
- Altered kidney or liver function.

Aggressive treatment with intravenous, broad-spectrum antibiotics within 1 hour of diagnosis, fluid resuscitation and expediting delivery to remove the focus of infection is essential [7]. Management in accordance with 'Surviving Sepsis Campaign' [8] should be implemented. This includes fluid resuscitation, immediate intravenous broad-spectrum antibiotics, correction of metabolic acidosis initially followed by inotropes, vasopressors, corticosteroids and mechanical ventilation, if required.

Uterine torsion

The uterus rotates axially by 30° to the right in approximately 80% of all pregnancies. Torsion may occur when this rotation extends beyond 90° causing severe abdominal pain, uterine tenderness and urinary retention in the last trimester of pregnancy. Predisposing factors include fibroids, ovarian cysts, Müllerian tract abnormalities and pelvic adhesions. A displaced urethra at catheterisation may lead to the diagnosis. Conservative treatment includes analgesia and change in maternal position with caesarean section being reserved for severe cases [9].

HELLP syndrome

Haemolysis, Elevated Liver enzymes and Low Platelets (HELLP) syndrome often arises following preeclampsia. However, in 20% of women, HELLP syndrome may be the first presentation of preeclampsia. Women often present with acute right upper quadrant or epigastric pain. They may also have other preeclampsia stigmata that include headaches, vomiting, visual disturbances, irritability and altered consciousness. Systemic examination may reveal raised blood pressure. Abdominal examination might note epigastric or right upper quadrant tenderness. Investigations might depict haemolysis (raised lactate dehydrogenase > 500 units/l; bilirubin >12 mg/l), raised liver transaminases (alanine transaminase > 70 units/l) and low platelets (< 10 000/mm³). Management is aimed at stabilising blood pressure, seizure prophylaxis, correction of any coagulation abnormality and delivery.

Rarely, distension of the Glisson's capsule of the liver may lead to hepatic rupture and patients present with features of haemorrhagic shock. Emergency laparotomy with repair of liver laceration and correction of coagulation abnormalities may need to be considered. Resection of the hepatic lobe or hepatic artery ligation may be required as life-saving measures in extreme cases.

Symphysis pubis diasthesis

During pregnancy, the production of progesterone and relaxin causes separation of the symphysis pubis as its supporting ligaments relax. This is functionally essential to facilitate the descent of the fetal head into the pelvis during labour. Exaggeration of this physiological response may result in the separation of the pubic bones causing diasthesis. Patients present with suprapubic pain, which is worse on movement, particularly abduction. Analgesia, reassurance and pelvic support are the available management options. Internal fixation of the symphysis pubis in the postpartum period is rarely undertaken.

Conditions associated with pregnancy

Acute fatty liver of pregnancy (AFLP)

Acute fatty liver of pregnancy occurs in 1 : 10 000 to 1 : 15 000 pregnancies. Women with AFLP present with abdominal pain, nausea and vomiting. There may be rapid deterioration of the clinical condition with hypoglycaemia, renal failure, disseminated intravascular coagulation and hepatic encephalopathy. Impaired liver function, prolonged prothrombin time, leukocytosis and thrombocytopenia are the main laboratory findings. Management should be multidisciplinary with intensivists, renal physicians and obstetricians.

Supportive therapy and correction of deranged metabolic and coagulation abnormalities followed by delivery, when the patient is stable, form the cornerstone of management.

Acute cholecystitis

It is estimated that 3% of pregnant women have asymptomatic gall stones. Acute inflammation is more common owing to biliary stasis, delayed emptying time and increased cholesterol synthesis. The incidence of acute cholecystitis in pregnancy is approximately 1 : 1000. It often presents with a sudden onset right upper quadrant pain, vomiting and jaundice. Murphy's sign (pain on palpation of the gallbladder during deep inspiration) may be elicited. Ultrasound of the gallbladder is a valuable tool in demonstrating a gallbladder distended with stones. Management is conservative and surgical intervention is deferred to the postpartum period unless complications such as empyema or perforation occur.

Rupture of the rectus abdominis

This rare condition occurs mostly in multigravidae due to repeated stretching of the rectus abdominis muscle. This may lead to a haematoma formation following rupture of a branch of the inferior epigastric vessels. Management is conservative with analgesics, unless the resulting haematoma expands. This would warrant surgical exploration and ligation of bleeding vessels.

Urinary tract infections

Structural and immune changes to the urinary tract system during pregnancy predispose to a higher incidence of ascending urinary tract infection. The incidence of asymptomatic bacteriuria in pregnancy is approximately 10%. Symptomatic urinary tract infections can present with abdominal pain, foul-smelling urine, dysuria, increased urinary frequency and vomiting. Infection of the upper urinary tract is associated with symptoms of fever with chills and rigors. Examination may reveal supra-pubic or renal angle tenderness. Urinalysis and mid-stream sample for culture and sensitivities must be obtained and empirical treatment should be commenced whilst awaiting the culture report. Most urinary tract infections in pregnancy are caused by *Escherichia coli*. In clinically suspected pyelonephritis, prompt treatment with intravenous antibiotics is indicated to minimise the risk of a perinephric abscess.

Causes unrelated to pregnancy

Acute appendicitis

The incidence is approximately 1 : 2000 pregnancies. It is the most common obstetrically unrelated surgical emergency in pregnancy. The morbidity and mortality is significantly increased in pregnancy largely due to delays in diagnosis [6].

Abdominal pain, nausea and vomiting are the main clinical features. However, due to the upward and lateral displacement of the caecum and appendix by the enlarging gravid uterus, pain is often felt in the umbilical and hypochondrial regions.

An elevated C-reactive protein, marked leukocytosis and diagnostic ultrasound would support the clinical diagnosis. Magnetic resonance imaging may be indicated in some cases [10]. Laparoscopic appendectomy is usually reserved for the early trimesters. In later trimesters a right paramedian approach is preferred.

Acute pancreatitis

Upper abdominal pain radiating to the back with vomiting are classic symptoms of pancreatitis in pregnancy. A raised serum amylase helps to confirm diagnosis. Hyperglycaemia, hypocalcaemia and electrolyte disturbances may also be associated laboratory findings. Treatment is supportive with electrolyte and fluid replacement, analgesia, antibiotics and thromboprophylaxis. In severe disease nasogastric suction and total parenteral nutrition may need to be considered.

Acute hepatitis

Acute viral or drug-induced hepatitis may present with abdominal pain, vomiting, malaise, fever and jaundice. A full history including travel, blood transfusion and substance misuse must be ascertained. Hepatitis serology and an ultrasound scan of the liver will aid the diagnosis. Management involves supportive therapy in conjunction with the gastro-enterology team.

Peptic ulcer disease

This is rare in pregnancy and most women with peptic ulcer disease will experience remission of symptoms in pregnancy. Increased intra-abdominal pressure and relaxation of the lower oesophageal sphincter may cause gastro-oesophageal reflux.

Pain is typically localised to the epigastric region. Rarely, peptic ulcer disease may present with generalised pain secondary to bleeding or perforation. Management is conservative with antacids except if gastric bleeding or perforation is diagnosed, which would necessitate a laparotomy and repair.

Table 23.1 Key recommended questions for evaluation of acute abdominal pain during pregnancy.

- Onset – How did it start? – Sudden or gradual?
- How would the patient describe the character of the pain? – Is it 'crampy' or 'colicky', 'sharp and stabbing' or 'pricking', 'dull and aching' or 'burning'?
- Site – In which region of the abdomen is it felt? Has this location changed? Does the pain radiate anywhere? If so, from where to where?
- Does anything make the pain worse, or make it better, such as movement, positions, intake of food?
- Was it present prior to pregnancy?
- Any previous history of medical disorder (like peptic ulcer)?
- Was it of sufficient intensity that it awoke the patient from sleep?
- Is it associated with nausea and vomiting; and, if so, did the patient have these symptoms before or after the pain?
- Any unusual symptoms? Shoulder tip pain, feeling faint (intraperitoneal bleeding)?
- Any associated vaginal bleeding or uterine contractions?

Intestinal obstruction

Predisposing factors include intra-peritoneal adhesions and Crohn's disease. Other causes include volvulus, intussusception and hernias. The symptoms include the tetrad of pain, vomiting, distension and constipation. Imaging reveals distended bowel loops with fluid levels. Conservative management includes nasogastric suction, electrolyte replacement, antibiotics and analgesia. If clinical condition deteriorates despite conservative measures, a midline laparotomy may be required to relieve the cause of obstruction.

Sickle cell crisis

Sickle cell disease may present with abdominal or splenic crisis during pregnancy. Abdominal pain, shortness of breath and a low-grade pyrexia are the usual presenting symptoms. On examination there may be pallor and icterus in addition to dehydration. Analgesia, correction of fluid and electrolyte imbalance, blood transfusion, antibiotics, oxygen and thromboprophylaxis are essential in management.

Key pearls

- Asking key questions (Table 23.1) may help arrive at a provisional diagnosis.
- A high degree of clinical suspicion should be exercised to diagnose both common as well as potentially life-threatening causes of acute abdominal pain during pregnancy (Table 23.2).

Table 23.2 Possible causes of abdominal pain during pregnancy.

Pregnancy-related causes	Pregnancy-associated causes	Causes unrelated to pregnancy (incidental)
Early pregnancy (< 24 weeks) • Threatened, septic incomplete or inevitable miscarriage • Rupture of corpus luteum cyst • Ectopic pregnancy • 'Round ligament' strain • Acute urinary retention due to a retroverted gravid uterus **Late pregnancy (>24 weeks)** • Placental abruption • Acute polyhydramnios • Red degeneration of fibroid • Torsion of pedunculated fibroid or an ovarian cyst • HELLP syndrome (haemolysis, elevated liver enzymes, and low platelets) (rarely bleeding into the Glisson's capsule or hepatic rupture) • Uterine rupture (previous uterine scar/spontaneous) • Chorioamnionitis • Pelvic venous thrombosis • Symphysis-pubis dysfunction (SPD)	• Acute cystitis • Acute pyelonephritis • Acute cholecystitis or gall stones • Acute fatty liver of pregnancy (AFLP) • Rupture of rectus abdominis muscle (rare) • Sickle cell crisis (abdominal crisis) • Adnexal torsion (ovarian cyst accidents, pedunculated fibroid)	**Gastrointestinal** • Gastric/duodenal ulcer • Acute appendicitis • Acute pancreatitis • Acute gastroenteritis • Liver disease, including hepatitis, hepatic rupture • Intestinal obstruction or perforation • Strangulated hernia • Inflammatory bowel disease including toxic megacolon • Pancreatic pseudocyst • Splenic infarction or rupture **Urinary tract disorders** • Bladder/ureteral or renal stones • Rupture of renal pelvis • Ureteral obstruction with acute hydronephrosis **Vascular disorders** • Abdominal aortic dissection • Superior mesenteric artery syndrome • Ruptured aneurysm (e.g. mesenteric artery) **Rare (but, potentially life-threatening) incidental causes** • Intestinal volvulus • Abdominal trauma with intraperitoneal haemorrhage • Diabetic ketoacidosis • Acute intermittent porphyria • Meckel's diverticulitis

Table 23.3 Topographical guide to abdominal pain in pregnancy.

Abdominal region where pain is experienced	Organs to consider	Causes to be excluded
Supra-pubic	Bladder, uterus	Cystitis, placental abruption, uterine scar rupture
Left iliac	Sigmoid colon, left Fallopian tube and ovary	Inflammatory bowel disease, ectopic pregnancy, tubo-ovarian abscess, ruptured ovarian cyst, ovarian torsion
Right iliac	Appendix, caecum, right Fallopian tube and ovary	Appendicitis, caecal diverticulitis, ectopic pregnancy, tubo-ovarian abscess, ruptured ovarian cyst, ovarian torsion
Left hypochondrial	Spleen, pancreas, splenic flexure of colon	Splenic infarction, rupture or haemorrhage, colitis
Epigastric	Stomach, pancreas, aorta, heart	Gastritis, acute pancreatitis, aortic dissection/rupture, myocarditis, infarction
Right hypochondrial	Liver, kidney, hepatic flexure of colon, gallbladder	Hepatitis, cholecystitis, hepatic rupture or haemorrhage, acute fatty liver of pregnancy, HELLP syndrome, imminent preeclampsia
Right lumbar	Right kidney, ascending colon	Pyelonephritis, renal/ureteric calculi, inflammatory bowel disease
Umbilical	Transverse colon, appendix (early 'visceral pain'), uterus	Appendicitis (early), gastroenteritis, mesenteric lymphadenitis, acute pancreatitis, placental abruption, uterine scar dehiscence or rupture
Left lumbar	Left kidney, descending colon	Pyelonephritis, renal/ureteric calculi, inflammatory bowel disease

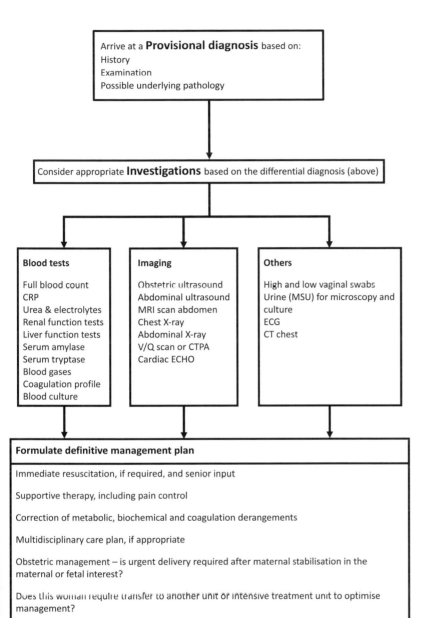

Figure 23.3 Suggested algorithm for management of abdominal pain during pregnancy.

- Understanding the topographical location of internal organs and their pathways for referred pain may help improve the diagnosis (Table 23.3).
- Rare causes such as secondary abdominal pregnancy, placenta percreta, acute pancreatitis and hepatic or splenic rupture should also be considered, especially if there is a diagnostic dilemma.

- Use of a management algorithm (Figure 23.3) may help clinicians to optimise management.

References

1. American College of Obstetricians and Gynecologists. *Guidelines for Diagnostic Imaging during Pregnancy*. ACOG Committee Opinion 158. Washington, DC: ACOG, 1995.

2. Royal College of Obstetricians and Gynaecologists. *Management of Early Pregnancy Loss.* Green-top Guideline No. 25. London: RCOG, 2006.

3. Schenker JG, Weinstein D. Ovarian hyperstimulation syndrome: a current survey. *Fertil Steril* 1978; 30: 255–268.

4. Golan A, Ron-El R, Herman A *et al.* Ovarian hyperstimulation syndrome: an update review. *Obstet Gynecol Surv* 1989; 44: 430–440.

5. Devarajan S, Chandraharan E. Abdominal pain in pregnancy: a rational approach to management. *Obstet Gynaecol Reprod Med* 2011; 21 (7): 198–206.

6. Centre for Maternal and Child Enquiries (CMACE). *Saving Mothers' Lives: Reviewing Maternal Deaths to make Motherhood Safer – 2006–2008. The Eighth Report on Confidential Enquiries into Maternal Deaths in the United Kingdom. Br J Obstet Gynaecol* 2011; 118 (Suppl. 1): 1–208.

7. Chandraharan E, Arulkumaran S. Acute abdomen and abdominal pain in pregnancy. *Obstet Gynaecol Reprod Med* 2008; 18 (8): 205–212.

8. Dellinger RP, Carlet JM, Masur H *et al.* Surviving Sepsis Campaign guidelines for management of severe sepsis and septic shock. *Crit Care Med* 2004; 32: 858–873.

9. Chandraharan E, Arulkumaran S. *Painful uterine contractions.* In Arulkumaran S (Ed.), *Emergencies in Obstetrics and Gynaecology.* Oxford: Oxford University Press, 2006.

10. Pedrosa I, Levine D, Eyvazzadeh AD *et al.* MR imaging evaluation of acute appendicitis in pregnancy. *Radiology* 2006; 238 (3): 891–899.

Chapter

24

Blurring of vision and sudden loss of vision in pregnancy

Anomi Panditharatne and Edwin Chandraharan

Key facts

Pregnancy is associated with anatomical, physiological, biochemical and functional changes in various organs and systems and the human eye is not an exception. Apart from capturing, processing and transmitting visual signals to the brain, the human eye acts as a 'window' and aids clinicians in diagnosing disorders of various systems, notably cardiovascular, neurological, endocrine and immunological.

Diseases that affect the eye in the non-pregnant population could also affect pregnant women for the first time or preexisting conditions may be modified by the physiological state of pregnancy. In addition, there are certain pregnancy-specific conditions such as preeclampsia that may present with visual symptoms and signs.

Ptosis or drooping of the eyelid may occur during or immediately after pregnancy. This is usually unilateral and is believed to be due to increased fluid within the levator aponeurosis associated with physiological oedema of pregnancy [1].

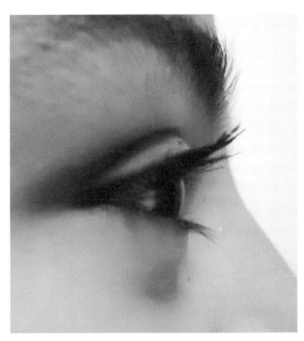

Figure 24.1 Physiological changes during pregnancy: drooping of eyelids (ptosis); changes in corneal surface; reduction in intra-ocular pressure; changes in tear film – increased dryness and irritation.

- Changes due to preexisting ocular disease or its altered course during pregnancy.

Key implications

The ocular conditions in pregnancy can be broadly subdivided into three main categories:

- Changes seen secondary to normal physiological changes observed during pregnancy.
- Changes due to pathological conditions – both pregnancy-specific and non-specific.

Visual symptoms due to physiological changes of pregnancy (Figure 24.1)

Tear film changes

The tear film consists of three layers, the outer lipid layer, the middle aqueous layer and the inner mucin layer. The stability of the tear film is dependent on

Obstetric and Intrapartum Emergencies, ed. Edwin Chandraharan and Sabaratnam Arulkumaran. Published by Cambridge University Press. © Cambridge University Press 2012.

all three layers functioning in an optimal, synergistic manner. The lipid layer is secreted by the Meibomian glands and the aqueous and the mucin layers by the lacrimal glands and goblet cells, respectively.

In pregnancy, the tear film becomes unstable and alters in composition, causing it to break up quickly resulting in irritation and discomfort to the patient. It is important to examine the eye under a slit lamp and exclude any other lid or corneal pathology, which could be contributing to these ocular symptoms.

Management

If no other disease process to explain ocular irritation is found, the patient can be reassured. Initially, simple steps can be tried such as ocular hygiene (use of cotton buds and warm water to clean the upper and lower eyelids to remove any dust) and creation of a more humid atmosphere at work or at home. The latter may include use of a humidifier and practical steps such as opening windows, having plants on the desk or around the home and keeping them watered. Smoke also irritates the eyes and patients should be advised to avoid smoking during pregnancy. When outdoors, 'wrap-around' sunglasses may help. Massaging the eyelids gently may encourage mucus to be pushed out of goblet cells.

Despite these measures, if the symptoms are troublesome and are affecting everyday activities, then preservative-free lubricants could be prescribed to alleviate discomfort and irritation.

Corneal changes

The cornea is the transparent structure located on the front of the eyeball that is important for clarity of vision. It consists of the following five layers:

- Stratified squamous non-keratinised epithelium.
- The Bowman's membrane, which is acellular.
- Stroma consisting of regularly arranged collagen fibres with a ground substance of proteoglycans.
- The Descemet's membrane of thin collagen fibres.
- Single-layered endothelium.

Thickness of the cornea changes during pregnancy and this could affect the clarity of vision. Changes in the shape and size of the eyeball secondary to physiological fluid retention and changes in blood pressure during pregnancy may result in minor changes in the refractive power of the eyes. In addition, contact lens wearers may feel they are intolerant of contact lenses during pregnancy and may find them 'ill-fitting'.

Management

It is important to exclude any other ocular pathology that may cause changes in vision by careful anterior and posterior segment examination. A refraction test may show slight changes in the power compared with the previous examination. If pathological causes have been excluded, explanation of the changes observed in vision should be explained to the patient and she should be reassured that these changes will subside following pregnancy and they need not change the prescription of their glasses or contact lenses [2]. However, contact lens wearers should be advised that if irritation and 'ill-fitting' contact lenses due to changes in the shape of the eyeball are a problem, changing to glasses during pregnancy may improve their symptoms.

Patients contemplating corneal surgery should be advised that the corneal thickness is variable during pregnancy and may affect the final outcome. Hence, corneal surgery should be recommended 3 months after birth.

Visual symptoms due to pathological conditions during pregnancy (Figure 24.2)

Blurring of vision and sudden loss of vision may occur due to pregnancy-specific pathological conditions as well as primary ocular or ocular manifestations of underlying systemic disorders that occur *de novo* during pregnancy.

Pregnancy-specific disorders: severe preeclampsia and eclampsia

Severe preeclampsia and eclampsia are potentially life-threatening conditions that are specific to the pregnant state. Although the exact aetiology is unknown, they are believed to be due to the widespread endothelial damage secondary to abnormal placentation and subsequent release of vasoactive factors. These result in systemic vasospasm, endothelial cellular damage (endotheliosis) and activation of the coagulation system resulting in disseminated intravascular coagulation. The diagnostic criteria for preeclampsia include blood pressure of over 140/90 mmHg in a pregnant woman after 20 weeks' gestation with proteinuria over 300 mg/24 hours. However, severe preeclampsia is diagnosed when the systolic blood pressure rises above

Figure 24.2 Management algorithm of blurring of vision or sudden loss of vision.

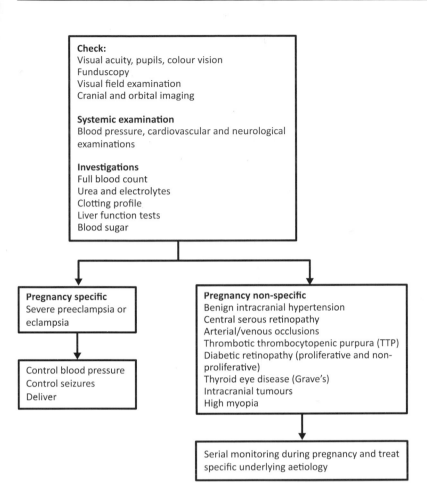

Check:
Visual acuity, pupils, colour vision
Funduscopy
Visual field examination
Cranial and orbital imaging

Systemic examination
Blood pressure, cardiovascular and neurological examinations

Investigations
Full blood count
Urea and electrolytes
Clotting profile
Liver function tests
Blood sugar

Pregnancy specific
Severe preeclampsia or eclampsia

Control blood pressure
Control seizures
Deliver

Pregnancy non-specific
Benign intracranial hypertension
Central serous retinopathy
Arterial/venous occlusions
Thrombotic thrombocytopenic purpura (TTP)
Diabetic retinopathy (proliferative and non-proliferative)
Thyroid eye disease (Grave's)
Intracranial tumours
High myopia

Serial monitoring during pregnancy and treat specific underlying aetiology

160 mmHg and/or the diastolic blood pressure rises above 110 mmHg with or without visual, hepatic or neurological symptoms. Onset of seizures is referred to as eclampsia.

Preeclampsia is common in primigravida and has an incidence of about 5%. Women with underlying chronic hypertension and renal disorders are at increased risk of developing 'super-imposed' preeclampsia during pregnancy. In addition, women with underlying immunological disorders (e.g. systemic lupus erythematosus (SLE)) and thrombophilia (congenital and acquired) are also at increased risk of developing preeclampsia.

Visual symptoms include blurred vision, double vision and photopsia, which are often associated with headaches and epigastric or right hypochondrial pain (hepatic involvement). Ocular manifestations of preeclampsia include features of optic neuropathy, which include papilloedema, optic neuropathy and optic atrophy.

On examination, visual acuity may be reduced depending on the severity and the location of the disease process within the eye. Retinopathy seen in preeclampsia is similar to hypertensive changes and is characterised by nerve fibre layer infarcts, hard exudates, flame-shaped haemorrhages, retinal oedema and narrowing of arterioles.

Swelling of the optic nerve head is a hallmark of malignant hypertension. Choroidal changes are less common in preeclampsia and would lead to Elschnig's spots which represent focal choroidal infarcts. There may also be bilateral exudative retinal detachments.

There is a correlation between the severity of preeclampsia and the extent of retinal involvement. Retinal changes are more marked in patients who have preexisting conditions such as renal disease and long-standing diabetes mellitus.

In preeclampsia, serous retinal detachments may also occur due to choroidal non-perfusion and sub-retinal leaks. These usually present as bilateral bullous detachments and resolve in the postpartum period.

Rarely, occipital infarcts and visual loss due possibly to cerebral oedema may occur in severe preeclampsia and these often resolve with the control of preeclampsia.

History of sudden onset of blurred vision should be taken very seriously and preeclampsia needs to be excluded in all pregnant women. Ocular symptoms improve with treatment of hypertension and usually resolve after birth. Excluding any other co-existing pathology is paramount.

Rarely, thrombotic thrombocytopenic purpura (TTP) may be confused with severe preeclampsia with HELLP (Haemolysis, Elevated Liver enzymes and Low Platelets) syndrome. Clinical presentation in TTP includes thrombosis of small vessels leading to thrombocytopenia, microangiopathic haemolytic anaemia associated with neurological and renal dysfunction. Patients are often febrile. Ocular manifestations in TTP occur due to narrowing of retinal artery, serous retinal detachment, retinal haemorrhage and oedema of optic disc. Rarely, patients may complain of homonymous hemianopia.

Pregnancy 'non-specific' disorders (primary ocular or systemic illnesses): benign intracranial hypertension

Benign intracranial hypertension refers to the presence of raised intracranial pressure in the absence of an intracranial mass or hydrocephalus. This condition is usually common in obese females in the third trimester but may occur throughout pregnancy.

Benign intracranial hypertension may cause sudden loss of vision and may occur due to papilloedema. Other associated symptoms include headaches, which are worse with postural changes and straining, transient visual obscuration lasting a few seconds and nausea and vomiting. Some patients may have drowsiness and horizontal diplopia.

On examination of the fundus, in the early stages, hyperaemia and mild disc swelling may be seen. Once papilloedema is established, visual acuity may be normal or reduced and the optic disc margins may appear indistinct. Appearance of venous engorgement, parapapillary flame-shaped haemorrhages and cotton wool spots as well as hard exudate around the macular forms, macular fan and the enlargement of the blind spot are the associated ocular signs.

Management

Regular ophthalmological examinations to observe optic nerve functions are essential. Serial visual field examinations are useful. Conservative measures include bed rest. Medications such as acetazolamide or steroids are best avoided in pregnancy in view of potential teratogenic effects. Intractable cases may benefit from lumbar puncture, optic nerve sheath decompression and lumbar peritoneal shunts to reduce the intracranial pressure.

Central serous retinopathy

Central serous retinopathy (CSR) is typically a sporadic self-limiting disease that affects the young, reproductive age group. It is characterised by unilateral localised detachment of the sensory retina at the macula with or without pigment epithelial detachment [3].

Aetiology

Central serous retinopathy is associated with hyperpermeability of the retinal pigment epithelium (RPE) or the choroidal vasculature.

Clinical features

Unilateral blurring of central vision with micropsia or metamorphopsia. Visual acuity 6/9–6/12. On ocular examination, round or oval detachments of the sensory retina at the posterior pole are observed and the fluid may be turbid or clear.

Management

Central serous retinopathy spontaneously resolves, usually in 1–6 months. Visual acuity returns to normal or near normal. Rarely, it may run a chronic course and persist for over 12 months with progressive changes at the macula. Argon laser treatment to the RPE leak or detachment may speed recovery but has no effect on the final visual outcome.

Aterio-venous occlusions causing sudden loss of vision

Pregnancy is associated with changes in the vessel walls and vascular endothelium as well as in the coagulation system. Incidence of optic or retinal arterial and venous occlusions may be increased in pregnancy, which may be due to the hyper-coagulable state that occurs due to changes in platelets, clotting factors and arterial–venous flow dynamics during pregnancy. Clinical features would depend on the location and severity of the occlusions and may range from sudden onset of loss or blurring of vision, usually in one eye but rarely both eyes may be affected.

On examination, the visual acuity would be reduced. Fundoscopic examination in arterial occlusions would confirm a pale retina and there would be arterial attenuations. In venous occlusions, the retina would appear haemorrhagic with venous dilation and tortuosity with haemorrhages and exudates in the involved areas of the retina. Other features include macular oedema and disc swellings.

In women with circulating anti-phospholipid antibodies, there may be features of vascular thrombosis of the retina with choroid, optic nerve and ocular motor involvement.

Management of vascular occlusions in pregnancy is similar to that in the non-pregnant state. Regular monitoring of visual acuity, intraocular pressure, optic nerve functions and retinal vascularity is essential. Complications such as macular oedema and retinal neovascularisation could occur and in this situation, laser treatment may be needed.

Preexisting systemic diseases with ocular manifestations in pregnancy: diabetic eye (retinopathy)

Diabetes mellitus is a complex condition associated with endocrine, metabolic, cardiovascular, renal and ophthalmological complications and is characterised by relative or absolute deficiency of insulin leading to sustained hyperglycaemia. There are two types of diabetes mellitus: Type I and Type II.

Diabetic retinopathy is a microangiopathy which affects arterioles, capillaries and post-capillary venules, although larger vessels may also be involved. Diabetic retinopathy does progress in pregnancy and such a progression depends on the extent of retinopathy prior to conception, duration and control of diabetes. Smoking, obesity, nephropathy and hyperlipidaemia are also associated risk factors for progression during pregnancy.

Non-proliferative diabetic retinopathy

This consists of background retinal changes that include microaneurysms, hard exudates, retinal oedema and haemorrhages. Fifty per cent of non-proliferative retinopathy may worsen in early and mid pregnancy, but usually improves by term and during the postpartum period. These patients should have an ophthalmological examination in each trimester.

Clinical features of pre-proliferative retinopathy

Cotton wool spots occur, which are focal infarcts of the retinal nerve fibre layer due to occlusion of the pre-capillary arterioles and the build-up of transported material within axons.

Intra-retinal micro-vascular abnormalities (IRMA) represent shunts that run from the arteriole to the venule bypassing the capillary bed. These are seen in areas of capillary closure. There is also venous dilation, arteriolar narrowing and silver wiring with blot haemorrhages.

Proliferative diabetic retinopathy

This is a more serious condition. Prior to frank proliferation there is pre-proliferation, which indicates progressive retinal ischaemia. The risk of pre-proliferation becoming proliferative retinopathy depends on the extent of ischaemia.

Clinical features of proliferative diabetic retinopathy

Proliferative retinopathy affects 5–10% of the diabetic population. Type I diabetics are at particular risk with an incidence of 60% in 10 years.

Neovascularisation is the hallmark of proliferative diabetic retinopathy. Neovascularisation can occur in the optic disc or elsewhere in the retina. It can lead to fibrosis that could lead to sight-threatening tractional retinal detachments.

Management

Pan retinal photocoagulation is the treatment of choice as this causes involution of new vessels and prevents visual loss from vitreous haemorrhage and retinal detachment. The extent of laser depends on the severity of the disease.

Regular follow-up of patients who have received laser therapy is mandatory to detect involution of new vessels. In advanced disease, early vitreous surgery may be necessary as there is a risk of vitreous haemorrhage and tractional retinal detachments. Approximately 45% to 50% progress during pregnancy and if severe retinopathy is detected, early laser treatment has been found to be beneficial. Monthly ocular assessments are indicated in those with more advanced disease. Macular oedema associated with diabetes also can be exacerbated in pregnancy and may present with visual symptoms. Visual acuity assessment with detailed dilated funduscopy would give the clinicians an indication of the level of diabetic control and also may help detect any ocular changes that may require treatment.

Intracerebral tumours

The common tumours that increase in size in pregnancy are pituitary adenomas and meningiomas. Pituitary adenomas cause visual field defects due the location of the optic nerve pathway and the pituitary gland. Non-secreting pituitary adenomas often present first to ophthalmologists whereas secreting adenomas may first present to endocrinologists.

Clinical features

Presenting symptoms include headaches, which are often non-specific. Visual symptoms are gradual in onset and examination of visual functions is useful. Visual field defects are another feature, especially bitemporal hemi-anopia due to compression of the optic chiasm by the enlarging pituitary adenoma. There may be evidence of colour desaturation across the vertical midline in early compressive lesions.

Optic atrophy is a late finding due to compression of the optic pathway. The optic disc would appear pale with clear margins and poor visual functions in the late stages. Examination of visual functions such as visual acuity, colour vision, pupil response, fundus examination as well as visual fields testing, would help clinch the diagnosis.

Brain imaging would indicate the relationship between the mass lesion and the optic chiasma and associated 'endocrine work-up' is also important.

During pregnancy, ocular examinations and visual field testing are done during every trimester and also at 6 weeks postpartum to detect any compressive signs. Pituitary adenomas tend to regress in size following pregnancy. If there are signs of compression of optic chiasma, medical treatment with bromocriptine or cabergoline for prolactinomas, steroids or transphenoidal surgery may be attempted. Radiotherapy is not recommended during pregnancy due to potential effects on the fetus, unless the tumour is rapidly enlarging and is life-threatening.

Pituitary apoplexy is a rare and sight-threatening condition due to sudden increase in the size of the gland secondary to haemorrhage [4]. Patients may complain of severe headaches, diplopia, visual loss and photophobia. Treatment with systemic steroids, and if unresponsive, urgent surgery may be needed to prevent blindness.

Meningiomas

Intracranial meningiomas typically affect middle-aged females but may also be seen during pregnancy. Visual field defects and clinical features depend on the location of the meningioma and its relationship to the intracranial centres. They commonly occur in the tuberculum sellae, sphenoidal ridge or in the olfactory groove. Meningiomas are generally slow-growing tumours and often regress following parturition. If there is compression on the optic nerve, surgical excision is the treatment of choice.

Thyroid (Graves') eye disease

This is an autoimmune disorder that usually presents in the third and fourth decade in females. The eye symptoms may increase in early pregnancy but usually settle down in the latter stages of pregnancy. Thyroid eye disease affects the soft tissue around the eye and causes globe protrusion. In addition it affects extra-ocular muscle movements and the eyelids as well as causing compressive optic neuropathy. Thyroid orbitopathy can be kept under observation by routine eye examination during pregnancy and by observing for signs of compressive optic neuropathy. Regular use of tear supplements can avoid corneal over-exposure and dryness.

High myopia

Myopia refers to short-sightedness and is associated with an increased size of the globe that results in distant images formed in front of the retina. It was thought earlier that patients who were 'high myopic' with or without previous retinal pathology or treatment would not be suitable to undergo spontaneous vaginal deliveries. This was because there was a concern that an increase in the intraocular pressure that occurs during spontaneous vaginal delivery would cause retinal tears or detachment. However, this has not been proved by scientific studies and recent evidence suggests that there may not be any significant increase in retinal detachment or tears in women with high myopia who attempt vaginal births.

In patients who have high myopia, clinical examination of the retina with dilation is useful to determine whether there are any untreated retinal lesions. If so they could be treated with laser and the patients could be reassured. Assisted vaginal birth should be considered to avoid a prolonged second stage of labour with active pushing.

References

1. Landau D, Seelenfreund MH, Tadmor O, Silverstone BZ, Diamant Y. The effect of normal childbirth on eyes with abnormalities predisposing to rhegmatogenous retinal detachment. *Graefes Arch Clin Exp Ophthalmol* 1995; 233 (9): 598–600.

2. Pizzarello LD. Refractive changes in pregnancy. *Graefes Arch Clin Exp Ophthalmol* 2003; 241 (6): 484–488. Epub 2003 May 8.

3. Kanski JJ (Ed.) *Clinical Ophthalmology: A Systematic Approach*. Fifth Edition. Boston: Butterworth Heinemann.

4. Chandraharan E, Arulkumaran S. Pituitary and adrenal disorders in pregnancy. *Curr Opin Obstet Gynecol* 2003, 15: 101–106.

Chapter

25

Psychiatric emergencies

Andrew Kent and Lorraine Cleghorn

Key facts

- Definition: serious disturbances of behaviour, cognition and emotion requiring immediate management to prevent a risk to self or others that are not attributable to an underlying medical illness or alcohol and substance misuse.

- Types:
  - Suicidal ideation – can present with any psychiatric disorder.
    - Deliberate self-harm – associated with depression, alcohol and substance misuse, and personality disorder; increased risk of suicide subsequently.
    - Severe anxiety – associated with significant subjective distress with retained insight; usually self-limiting in the short term.
    - Severe depression – associated with significant subjective distress, high suicide risk and self-neglect; usually not self-limiting.
    - Acute psychosis – associated with abnormal experiences and beliefs that may be florid and frightening and drive abnormal behaviour that can present a risk to self or others.

- Incidence:
  - Mild and transient psychiatric symptoms occur in up to 1 in 2 pregnancies.
    - Diagnosable psychiatric disorders are present in up to 1 in 5 pregnancies.
    - True psychiatric emergencies are relatively rare.

Key implications

- Maternal: Suicide is a preventable cause of maternal mortality. Misdiagnosis of medical illness as psychiatric disorder contributes to maternal morbidity and mortality.
- Fetal: Untreated psychiatric disorder is associated with a range of adverse fetal outcomes, including intra-uterine growth restriction and prematurity.

Key pointers

- Maternal distress.
- Concerned partner, relatives or friends.
- Already under the care of a specialist mental health service.
- Past history of emergency psychiatric presentations.

Key diagnostic signs

- No impairment of consciousness. This would imply delirium with an underlying medical cause.
- Subjective complaints of severe anxiety or depression.
- Acts or thoughts of deliberate self-harm, or suicidal thinking.
- Self-neglect, withdrawal or mutism.
- Marked emotional lability, euphoria, excitability, irritation or hostility [1].
- Delusional thinking: expressing rigid and unshakeable abnormal beliefs that are not understandable in the context of the patient's cultural, educational or social background; for example, the belief that staff are evil and trying to harm the unborn baby.

Obstetric and Intrapartum Emergencies, ed. Edwin Chandraharan and Sabaratnam Arulkumaran. Published by Cambridge University Press. © Cambridge University Press 2012.

- Hallucinations: perceptions in the absence of a stimulus; for example, hearing a voice commanding the patient to kill herself.

Key actions

Assess any immediate risks

The safety of the patient, other members of the public, including any accompanying children, and staff is the paramount consideration [2]. Whilst the very large majority of pregnant women presenting with a serious psychiatric problem are much more likely to be the victims of aggression and violence than they are to be the perpetrators, there are rare exceptions. If the possibility of any risk is anticipated then appropriate precautions should be taken. It is better to be over-prepared than caught off guard. Consider whether the patient presents any immediate risks to herself or others that will determine where and how the assessment should be conducted.

Indicators of potential risk include aggression, disinhibition, fearfulness, hyper-arousal, paranoia and sudden, unprovoked outbursts of anger. Recent alcohol or substance misuse may be a compounding factor as a result of their disinhibiting effects. Risk is increased if the patient is previously unknown and presenting in crisis in the maternity department for the first time.

If any risk is suspected, then assessment by more than one staff member in a safe and relatively quiet environment, such as a counselling room uncluttered by ultrasound machinery and other potentially hazardous clinical equipment, is preferred. If the assessment is being conducted by one staff member, then other staff should be aware of the situation and close at hand. The seating arrangements should allow patient and clinician to be at the same level, in the order of at least two arm lengths apart, and at an angle where eye contact can be made or avoided without discomfort. Both staff and patient should have easy access to the door. This is to avoid a frightened and paranoid patient feeling trapped and becoming more dangerous as a result.

If the assessment is taking place at the patient's home, then it is sensible to avoid assessing her in the kitchen or anywhere else where there are potential dangers should she become aroused and impulsive.

Obtain background information

It is rarely possible or necessary to conduct a full psychiatric assessment in an emergency 'triage' situation. Details of family and personal history, beyond the immediately relevant, such as family or personal history of any psychiatric disorder, can usually wait. Unless she is presenting for the first time, however, a large amount of background information will already be available in the woman's maternity record.

If the patient is already under the care of specialist psychiatric services, then she is likely to have a care plan that includes a risk assessment and a risk and contingency management plan. This can be an invaluable guide to any emergency obstetric mental health assessment. Midwives and obstetricians booking women for maternity care who are under the care of specialist mental health services should have sought these plans in advance so that they can be available in the maternity record [3].

If the patient is under the care of specialist mental health services she is likely to have a mental health care coordinator, for example a community psychiatric nurse, and it should be possible to contact him or her by telephone during normal working hours in an emergency situation in order to obtain any missing information on risk assessment and risk and contingency management plan [4]. Once again, contact details for the care coordinator should ideally have been recorded at booking and feature prominently in the list of key emergency contacts in the maternity record.

If a midwife specialising in mental health and/or a perinatal psychiatrist was involved at any previous stage of the pregnancy, then they may have provided further information in relation to perinatal risk and risk management.

Obtain collateral information

Depending on the circumstances, including the ability of the patient to provide clear information herself, information should be obtained from any accompanying partner, relative or friend. This may be during the assessment of the patient herself if she chooses to remain accompanied throughout, but if she is assessed on her own in the first instance it is important to ask anyone accompanying her to wait so that they can be interviewed subsequently.

Obtain history

If a patient is well enough to communicate without major difficulty, and not too distressed, then it is helpful to begin the assessment interview with one or two open questions. This has the advantage of putting the patient at her ease and emphasising that she is being listened to and that her concerns are being taken seriously. If she has any insight into the nature of her distress she may be very embarrassed and a calm, gentle and non-judgemental approach that allows her to explain her fears or concerns can be very therapeutic in itself. Many patients who go on to have specialist psychiatric assessment speak very positively about the experience of talking to a midwife or obstetrician who paid attention to their problems when they presented in crisis.

Identification of the presenting complaint or concern will guide subsequent enquiry.

If the patient complains of low mood or depression then further questions about the impact of depression on functional ability, feelings of hopelessness and despair, energy levels, ability to experience enjoyment or interest, sleep, appetite and weight disturbance, will all be helpful and positive answers confirmatory.

If the patient complains of fearfulness or severe anxiety, then further questions about potential antecedents (A) or triggers that might have precipitated the fear, a recent investigation for example that might have triggered fears that the unborn baby is at risk, any behaviour (B) evoked by the fear such as excessive reassurance seeking or escaping from a fear-inducing situation, and any consequences (C) of the fear, for example avoidance of any further investigations or fear-inducing situations, might give a clue as to the nature of the problem.

Sometimes fear is free-floating without any obvious cognitive association, as might occur in a patient experiencing her first panic attack for example, but asking the patient what thoughts were going through her mind when she was frightened will often elicit a cognitive component. It is also helpful to ask about specific physical concomitants of fear, including markers of autonomic arousal such as racing heart rate, hyperventilation and sweating.

If the patient presents as confused or perplexed, or if she describes abnormal beliefs or experiences, then it will be important to establish whether she is experiencing a psychotic illness such as schizophrenia. Delirium often has a very similar presentation and it is particularly important to consider the possibility in cases of suspected psychosis.

If the patient presents as aroused, emotionally labile, excitable and uncharacteristically irritable and argumentative, then hypomania or mania may be a possibility. Once again, the possibility of delirium needs to be carefully considered.

The presence of any suicidal ideation or intent should be sensitively explored in all patients presenting with a psychiatric problem in an emergency, and not just in patients with depression. It is also important to sensitively explore the possibility of any recent alcohol or substance misuse in all patients.

Patients from minority groups who do not speak the same language as the assessing clinician are particularly vulnerable, and should be assessed with the assistance of an interpreter whenever possible [5]. The use of a partner or relative is not an adequate substitute, although in an emergency situation with no access to an interpreter this may be necessary.

Mental state examination

A mental state examination, even if relatively brief, is a core component of any assessment of a psychiatric emergency. When the patient is uncooperative or uncommunicative, it will assume even more importance.

The process of mental state examination is very simple and largely accomplished 'automatically' during the assessment interview itself. Key points follow:

Appearance and behaviour: Any abnormalities of appearance or behaviour should be noted as they might give important clues about the underlying problem. These might include evidence of distractibility, fearfulness, perplexity or pre-occupation in a patient with a psychotic illness; over-excitability and over-activity in a patient with mania; agitation, withdrawal or neglect in a patient with a depressive illness; tremulousness, restlessness or reassurance seeking in a patient with an anxiety disorder.

Speech: Speech can be abnormal in flow, tempo, tone or volume. Subtle abnormalities can be difficult to spot, but in an emergency triage situation obvious problems such as loud verbosity, possibly suggesting mania; disorganised or muddled speech, possibly suggesting delirium or schizophrenia; and poverty of speech, possibly suggesting depression, should be noted.

Mood: The presence of any subjective and objective anxiety, depression, or perplexity should be recorded. If she has not been asked already, the patient should be asked if she is experiencing any active suicidal ideation.

Beliefs and experiences: If psychosis is suspected, it is appropriate to ask whether the patient has experienced any ideas that others have considered unusual or paranoid, and specifically whether she has worried that something strange has been going on, like people spying on her or wishing her harm. 'Normalisation' is a very useful technique when trying to elicit any abnormal beliefs or experiences. For example, questions can be phrased in the following way: 'Lots of people who have been under the kind of stress that you have been get so stressed out that they experience odd things, like paranoia or hearing voices when there is no one there. Has anything like that happened to you?'

Cognitive function: Any impairment of consciousness or disorientation should suggest delirium and an underlying medical cause requiring further investigation. Most people who are alert and orientated should be able to identify the time of day to the nearest half hour, and the day of the week and month, if not the exact date. In broad terms disorientation in time is the most sensitive marker of disorientation, followed by place and then person. Although there are specific tests for attention, concentration, immediate recall and recent memory, the patient's performance at interview will give a lot of information in the first instance. Additional tests of attention and concentration, like naming the days of the week backwards, or recalling three items in 1 minute, can be used to confirm initial impressions.

Insight: The degree of insight lies on a continuum. At one extreme a patient expressing floridly abnormal belief and behaving bizarrely may believe she is completely well. This would imply psychosis and the potential use of legal measures to enforce a safe assessment and subsequent treatment in hospital should the patient be a risk to herself or others. At the other end of the continuum a very distressed patient may recognise that she is unwell and in need of immediate help.

Next steps

Severe anxiety and panic attacks can usually be managed in the maternity department without recourse to specialist psychiatric intervention. Reassurance and explanation, particularly in relation to the benign nature of any physical symptoms of anxiety that the patient might have misinterpreted as signs of an imminent life-threatening problem, such as racing heart beat or hyperventilation, may be all that is required.

The hyperventilating patient should be instructed to take slow, even breaths. If she is experiencing physical symptoms of high pO_2, such as peri-oral tingling, she can be instructed to re-breath from a paper bag.

All of the other psychiatric emergencies described imply high risk and the need for an urgent specialist psychiatric assessment. If admission is required, and the patient is more than 32 weeks pregnant, then this should ideally be to a specialist psychiatric mother and baby unit.

Specific techniques

Risk assessment

Suicide risk is by far the more likely risk in a psychiatric emergency presenting in pregnancy. Psychiatric textbooks rightly emphasise the importance of actuarial risk factors in any assessment of suicide risk, but in an emergency triage setting it is much more vital to elicit whether the patient has any active thoughts of harming or killing herself. Active thoughts indicate high risk and the need for specialist psychiatric assessment. Associated factors indicating heightened risk include hopelessness, pessimism about the future, which may have particular connotations in the context of pregnancy, social isolation and lack of support.

Patients presenting with severe depression, mania or psychosis may be vulnerable to self-neglect, harm as a consequence of their abnormal beliefs and behaviours, and exploitation by others. The possibility of domestic violence should always be considered in vulnerable women in pregnancy, and discreetly and sensitively enquired about.

Any serious psychiatric illness presenting late in pregnancy has potential implications for the safety of the unborn baby following delivery, depending on the patient's circumstances and supports. Harm might arise as a result of neglect, emotional harm or the direct consequence of any abnormal beliefs or behaviours. If there is a risk, then consultation with the relevant social care agency responsible for child safeguarding is indicated.

De-escalation

If the patient should become very angry and aroused but she does not present an immediate danger, de-escalation may be attempted. The assessing clinician(s) should remain outwardly calm and helpful, and talk quietly and reassuringly. Reassurance may need to be repeated more than once if a preoccupied and distractible patient does not take it on board the first time. Staff should remain seated if it remains safe to do so as this will appear less threatening. Eye contact should neither be sustained nor avoided altogether as this can also appear threatening. Intermittent eye contact is usually perceived as more reassuring. Provocative, confrontational and threatening comments should be avoided and staff should never become visibly angry. It can be appropriate, however, to set clear boundaries and tell patients when their behaviour is intimidating or frightening.

De-escalation does not always work and departmental operational policies should include a protocol for the management of the very disturbed patient who becomes rapidly aggressive, identifying clear procedures for the rapid involvement of liaison psychiatry services and hospital security if required.

Restraint and rapid tranquillisation

It is very rarely necessary to attempt restraint or rapid tranquillisation in the maternity department, and the need to do so should be avoided. In all but the least well-resourced settings specialist psychiatric advice can be quickly sought and the patient transferred to a psychiatric ward or facility where there is on-site nursing expertise in control and restraint techniques.

The key principle of emergency restraint that applies to the pregnant patient is the avoidance of vena cava syndrome. She should not be restrained on her back or her right side, but to her left, ideally with the use of bean bags or similar for comfort and support. All hospitals should have rapid tranquillisation protocols that include consideration of the needs of a pregnant patient, and staff should be familiar with these [6]. The emergency use of a short-acting benzodiazepine, such as intramuscular lorazepam, is not contraindicated in a pregnant woman who requires rapid tranquillisation for her own safety and the safety of others.

Key pitfalls

- Failure to identify delirium.
- Failure to identify suicide risk.
- Failure to use an interpreter for a patient who does not speak the clinician's language.
- Failure to consider the safeguarding of needs of any children at home.

Key pearls

- Psychiatric assessment is very straightforward if a few key principles are observed.
- Whilst psychiatric disorders are common in pregnancy, true psychiatric emergencies are relatively rare and caused by a small number of conditions.
- Maternity units should have a midwife specialising in mental health and access to a specialist perinatal psychiatry service.
- Lessons learnt from adverse incidents due to psychiatric emergencies should be disseminated through the 'maternity dashboards' and clinical governance seminars.

Management in low-resource settings

In the absence of a specialist perinatal psychiatry service or hospital-based psychiatric liaison service the management of psychiatric emergencies is more complicated. All of the high-risk situations described in this chapter, with the exception of severe anxiety, imply the potential need for admission to a psychiatric hospital if the patient cannot be managed at home by a well-resourced, specialist psychiatric home treatment team. In such circumstances consideration should be given to admitting the patient to the maternity ward until a full psychiatric assessment can take place or transfer to a specialist psychiatric hospital arranged.

If psychiatric medication has to be used before specialist psychiatric advice can be obtained, for example if a patient is manic or psychotic and difficult to manage safely on the maternity ward, then advice should be sought from a pharmacist. Opinions on the safety of medications in pregnancy are subject to change, although at the time of writing haloperidol and olanzapine are considered reasonably safe antipsychotic medications in pregnancy, depending on the balance of risks, if used at appropriate dosages.

References

1. Glick RL, Berlin JS, Fishkind AB, Zeller SL. *Emergency Psychiatry. Principles and Practice.* Philadelphia, PA: Lippincott Williams & Wilkins, 2008.

2. Puri BK, Treasaden IH. *Emergencies in Psychiatry.* Oxford: Oxford University Press, 2008.

3. NICE. *Antenatal and Postnatal Mental Health. NICE Clinical Guideline 45.* London: National Institute for Health and Clinical Excellence, 2007.

4. Kent A. Psychiatric disorders in pregnancy. *Obstet Gynaecol Reprod Med* 2009; 19: 37–41.

5. Centre for Maternal and Child Enquiries (CMACE). *Saving Mothers' Lives: Reviewing Maternal Deaths to make Motherhood Safer – 2006–2008. The Eighth Report on Confidential Enquiries into Maternal Deaths in the United Kingdom. Br J Obstet Gynaecol* 2011; 118 (Suppl. 1): 1–208.

6. American College of Obstetricians and Gynecologists. Use of psychiatric medications during pregnancy and lactation. *ACOG Practice Bulletin No.* 92. *Obstet Gynecol* 2008; 111: 1001–1020.

Chapter

26

Drug overdose in pregnancy

Lakshman Karalliedde and Inidika Gawarammana

Key facts

- Intentional overdoses (suicide rates) are low and generally result in low toxicity to the mother.
- Risk of overdose is highest during the first few weeks of pregnancy and the first pregnancy, low socioeconomic status and in those who abuse ethanol.
- Antipyretics, analgesics and anti-rheumatics are the commonest drugs ingested.
- Adverse birth outcomes such as preterm labour and low birth weight have been reported in a very small number of patients.
- Most drug overdoses require only supportive care. However, a few drugs which may cause severe overdose are discussed in this chapter.
- Treat the poison if an antidote is available as the 'poison' is bound to be more toxic than the antidote to the fetus.
- Physiological changes in pregnancy may be associated with changes in pharmacokinetics and toxicokinetics following overdose. The delay in gastric emptying time of up to 50% would result in lower peak plasma concentrations. Similarly, the increase in plasma volume during pregnancy and the associated increase in the volume of distribution would also result in reduced peak plasma concentrations of the drug.
- Most drugs cross the placenta.

Key implications

- Maternal: some pharmaceutical agents may induce renal, liver and cardiac malfunction.
- Fetal: effects on the fetus following overdose of the mother are sparse or non-existent at present. Often effects on the fetus are considered to be directly related to maternal outcome.
- Some drugs are known to be mutagenic and/or teratogenic. Others have the potential to be carcinogenic.

Key diagnostic signs

These depend on the class of drug/s ingested. Always suspect poisoning when the presenting physical signs are not commonly associated with known disease states.

Some examples:

- Anticholinergic signs: dilated pupils, sweating, warm and red peripheries – e.g. tricyclic antidepressant or belladona alkaloid self-poisoning.
- Sympathomimetic signs: tachycardia, high blood pressure, sweating, dilated pupils – overdose of sympathomimetics e.g. amphetamines.
- Increased respiratory rate, sweating and tinnitus – salicylate self-poisoning.
- Bradycardia and hypotension – calcium channel blocker or beta-blocker self-poisoning.
- Depressed respiration, consciousness and small pupils – opioids (pinpoint pupils) or benzodiazepines self-poisoning.

Obstetric and Intrapartum Emergencies, ed. Edwin Chandraharan and Sabaratnam Arulkumaran. Published by Cambridge University Press. © Cambridge University Press 2012.

- Hyperthermia and rigidity – selective serotonin re-uptake inhibitors (SSRIs).
- Hypoglycaemia – self-poisoning with anti-diabetic medications.

Key actions

Assess and stabilise the patient

Drug overdose should be treated as a medical emergency. Attend to the patient immediately and stabilise (maintain vital physiological parameters, e.g. oxygen saturation, blood pressure) the patient as a priority (Table 26.1).

Use standard advanced cardiac life support

- Assess airway, breathing and circulation – use standard guidelines.
- Assess airway – talk to the patient. If she responds, the airway is patent. If there is no response, carry out airway opening manoeuvres (head tilt and jaw thrust).
- Assess breathing – look, feel and count respiratory rate – feel for air on palm. Cyanosis?
- Assess circulation – presence of pulse, measure blood pressure.
- Assess neurological disability – note score on Glasgow Coma Scale (GCS).
- Connect the patient to an ECG monitor and pulse oximeter. Measure blood sugar and serum electrolytes.

All patients who present with a 'threatened airway' (i.e. at risk of aspiration into the lungs) and low GCS should have endotracheal intubation.

Assess risk

- Ask for the name of the drug/s.
- Number of tablets, strength and preparation (ordinary release or slow release).
- Decide if the ingested dose is likely to cause toxicity. Examine to detect the presence of signs of toxicity.
- In the absence of signs of toxicity, assess probability of subsequent development of toxicity.

Decontaminate

- Decontamination may be effective for longer periods than the usually recommended 1-hour post-ingestion.
- Gastric lavage is not routinely recommended for a pregnant patient with drug overdose. Use activated charcoal.

For ordinary-release medications in overdose:

- Administer activated charcoal 1 g/kg (50 g) if the patient presents within 1 hour post-ingestion. Patient should have a protected airway and consent.
- Multiple doses of activated charcoal may be given in some cases of overdose with drugs such as carbamazepine and salicylates [1].
- Whole bowel irrigation should be carried out following overdose with drugs such as slow-release calcium channel blockers, lithium and iron.
- Method: Administer 1 litre of oral polyethylene glycol hourly until rectal effluent is clear.

Confirmation of poisoning

Serum drug assays – limited use but a necessity in some instances e.g. overdose with paracetamol, iron, salicylates, digoxin or lithium.

Other indicators of toxicity, for example:

- ECG: widened QRS (100 ms) complex in tricyclic antidepressant poisoning. Bradycardia and heart blocks in calcium channel blocker and beta-blocker poisoning.
- Tachyarrhythmias in tricyclic antidepressants (TCA), digoxin poisoning.
- Prolonged QT interval – beta-blockers poisoning.
- Metabolic acidosis – metformin poisoning (lactic acidosis), salicylate and iron poisoning.

Give antidotes

Some drug overdoses should be treated using specific antidotes.

Paracetamol

Mechanisms of toxicity

Paracetamol is largely metabolised in the liver to non-toxic glucuronide (~60%) and sulphate (~30%) conjugates, which are subsequently excreted in the urine.

177

Table 26.1 Clinical signs and management summary of some commonly ingested pharmaceutical agents.

Drug class	Clinical effects	Toxic dose	Action	Comments
ACE inhibitors	Hypotension and tachycardia. Hyperkalaemia	Variable	Supportive care. Intravenous fluids	
Amiadarone	Non-specific ECG changes, hypotension and bradycardia	Variable	AC and supportive care	
Antihistamines	Nausea, vomiting, retention of urine, tachycardia	Cyclizine 5 mg/kg, Dyphenhydramine > 300 mg	Aactivated charcoal (AC) and supportive care	
Antibiotics	Mainly gastrointestinal – variable signs depending on the agent		AC and supportive care	Some are teratogenic
Anticoagulants (warfarin)	Bleeding tendency and prolonged international normalised ratio (INR)	Variable	AC and vitamin K for up to 10 days	If mother is on long-term warfarin, correction should be gradual to prevent thrombosis
Barbiturates	Nystagmus, ataxia, small pupils, respiratory depression and coma		Manage airway. AC	
Benzodiazepines	CNS and respiratory depression	Variable	Manage airway. AC	Do not give flumazanil
Bromocriptine	Nausea, vomiting and hypotension. Psychosis and hallucinations	50–75 mg	AC. IV fluids and supportive care	
Clonidine	Drowsiness, coma, bradycardia and hypotension. Hypertension	Variable	AC. Supportive care, IV fluids	
Ergotamines	Cold cyanotic peripheries, abdominal pain	Variable	AC, glyceryl trinitrate, nitroprusside and nifedepine	Increases uterine tone, fetal hypoxia
Lithium (acute ingestions)	Nausea, vomiting, ataxia, myoclonic twitches, confusion and coma		Whole bowel irrigation if > 4 g of sustained release is ingested. Do lithium levels at 6 hours post ingestion. Observe for up to 24 hours. Manage airway and fluid balance	May induce congenital malformations. Haemodialysis if coma, convulsions and respiratory failure or levels > 7.5 mmol/l
MAOI	Drowsiness, confusion, agitation, coma, hypertension, hyperthermia		Airway management, diazepam, fluids	Symptoms may occur 24 hours post-ingestion
Opioids	Drowsiness, respiratory depression, hypotension, pinpoint pupils, coma		AC, naloxone (0.4 mg IV, increased every 2–3 minutes to a maximum bolus dose of 2 mg – use 2/3 the dose required as a maintenance each hour), airway management	Observe for minimum of 6 hours. In addicted patients, naloxone may precipitate withdrawal
Non-steroidal anti-inflammatory drugs	Variable – no symptoms to CNS depression and acidosis in massive doses	Variable	AC, supportive care	
SSRI	Nausea and vomiting. Drowsiness and serotonin syndrome (hyperthermia, rigidity, rhabdomyolysis)		AC. In serotonin syndrome – cooling, IV fluids, sedate with diazepam and cyproheptadine	
Theophylline	Nausea, vomiting, tachycardia, convulsions, hypokalaemia	1 g	Multiple dose AC	Observe 4 hours or up to 24 hours if sustained-release drug is ingested

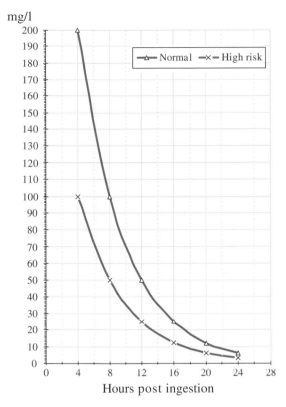

Figure 26.1 Paracetamol normogram.

A small fraction is also converted (by cytochrome P450-dependent mixed function oxidase enzymes) to the toxic metabolite, N-acetyl-p-benzoquinonimine (NAPQI). The toxic metabolite is inactivated by conjugation with hepatic glutathione and eventually excreted as cysteine and mercapturic acid conjugates. In overdose, there is accumulation of this toxic metabolite.

In healthy women, a dose greater than 200 mg/kg or 10 g in total (whichever is less) may be hepatotoxic. In those considered as high-risk, i.e. malnourished patients, patients on enzyme-inducing drugs (e.g. carbamazepine, phenytoin, rifampicin) or patients suffering from HIV, liver toxicity may occur at lower doses. The risk of liver damage is assessed using the paracetamol normogram (Figure 26.1) which plots the plasma paracetamol concentration in relation to the time of ingestion.

Those on or above the treatment line will require treatment with N acetylcysteine (NAC), without which severe liver damage could be expected in approximately 60% of patients. Where paracetamol has been taken chronically or in a staggered manner (e.g. > 2 hours between doses), or where the time of ingestion is unknown, the plasma paracetamol concentration cannot accurately be interpreted using the normogram. If the total dose in 24 hours exceeds 200 mg/kg or 10 g, whichever is the smaller (> 100 mg/kg in high-risk patients), NAC should be administered.

Investigations

Measure plasma paracetamol level 4 hours after ingestion. Obtain baseline values for INR, serum creatinine, aspartate transaminase (AST) and alanine transaminase (ALT).

A specialist liver centre should be contacted if:

- the INR is > 2 at 24 hours; > 4 at 48 hours; > 6 at 72 hours post-ingestion

    OR

- the PT in seconds is greater than the number of hours since overdose

    OR

- if the patient has any of the following:
- an elevated plasma creatinine (> 200 μmol/l).
- Hypoglycaemia.
- Acidosis.
- Hypotension (mean arterial pressure less than 60 mmHg) following accepted methods of resuscitation.
- Encephalopathy.

Treatment

It is important to treat within 8 hours post-ingestion as the recovery is almost 100%. If a plasma paracetamol level could be obtained within 8 hours, start treatment after the plasma paracetamol level is available. If the level is unlikely to be available within 8 hours of ingestion, start treatment when the ingested dose is considered potentially toxic. Continue/discontinue treatment after receiving the plasma paracetamol level.

NAC is the antidote and it should be administered as follows:

- 150 mg/kg body weight in 200 ml 5% dextrose by slow IV infusion over 15 minutes, followed by
- 50 mg/kg by IV infusion in 500 ml of 5% dextrose over 4 hours and 100 mg/kg in 1 litre of 5% dextrose over the next 16 hours.

Two hours after completion of the infusion, repeat measurements of INR, serum creatinine and AST. If the INR is stable or declining, there is no need for further treatment with NAC. If the patient is symptomatic and has an elevated INR, the patient is likely to require further doses of NAC.

Sulphonylureas and other blood sugar lowering agents

Clinical features are due to the hypoglycaemic effect. Patients may be asymptomatic or present with low GCS, nausea, vomiting, sweating, convulsions or even hemiparesis. Activated charcoal should be administered to all patients who present within 1 hour of ingestion of tablets.

Measure blood glucose 6-hourly. Monitor serum potassium levels as administration of dextrose may cause hypokalaemia. Occurrence of hypoglycaemia may be delayed if prophylactic dextrose has been given to patients with normal blood glucose levels or if the patient has had a recent meal. Hypoglycaemia may persist for days. Care must be taken to monitor for recurrent hypoglycaemia. Rebound hypoglycaemia may develop following cessation of dextrose therapy as dextrose could cause increased and persistent release of insulin.

Management of hypoglycaemia

Dextrose: Avoid intravenous administration of dextrose solutions prophylactically to patients with no clinical or laboratory evidence of hypoglycaemia, such therapy may delay the onset of hypoglycaemia. Oral glucose supplementation may be used as and when necessary.

In symptomatic patients and patients with significant hypoglycaemia (blood glucose < 4 mmol/l) 50 ml of 50% dextrose should be administered intravenously as a bolus followed by an infusion of 10% dextrose at a rate titrated to maintain blood sugar levels above 6 mmol/l. Patients with mild to moderate hypoglycaemia (blood glucose 4–6 mmol/l) could be managed using a 10% dextrose infusion titrated to maintain blood sugar level over 6 mmol/l.

For patients with severe hypoglycaemia who require large doses of 10% dextrose, 20% dextrose should be administered using a central line.

Glucagon: In severely poisoned patients with no IV access, 1 mg of glucagon could be administered intramuscularly. As glucagon causes release of endogenous insulin, continue administering dextrose with concurrent blood sugar measurements.

Aspirin

Self-poisoning with aspirin may be a challenging problem as it may on occasion cause serious complications. In overdose, salicylate stimulates the respiratory centre which results in a respiratory alkalosis. The body compensates by excreting bicarbonate, sodium and potassium ions and water in urine, resulting in electrolyte imbalance, dehydration and a decrease in the buffering capacity of the body. This allows the development of a high-anion gap metabolic acidosis, which enhances transfer of salicylate ion across the blood–brain barrier to produce effects on the central nervous system such as coma.

Salicylate uncouples oxidative phosphorylation resulting in a decrease in ATP production and oxygen consumption. Subsequently, the patient produces more lactic acid that contributes to the metabolic acidosis. These patients are generally fluid depleted, as there is associated vomiting and a decreased fluid intake.

Risk assessment

Ingestion of doses of 150 mg/kg, 250 mg/kg and 500 mg/kg lead to mild, moderate and severe salicylate toxicity respectively.

Peak plasma concentrations are generally reached by 2–3 hours post-ingestion. Patients who have taken significant overdoses should be symptomatic within a few hours post-ingestion. Presence of coma and convulsions indicates severe toxicity.

Plasma salicylate level provides a guide on the toxicity and the required level of care to such patients. As these patients may develop hypoglycaemia and electrolyte disturbances, frequent blood sugar and electrolyte measurements are a necessity.

Treatment

Administer a dose of activated charcoal. This dose should be repeated every 4 hours (about 4 doses) until salicylate level has reached a peak. Salicylates form pharmacobezoars which delay their absorption. Adequate fluid replacement is necessary to maintain hydration [2].

Urinary alkalinisation is the treatment of choice. In alkaline urine (urine pH 5–8), salicylate excretion is increased to 15–20 times the normal. Patients with salicylate levels above 500 mg/l require urinary alkalinisation. This is carried out by administering

1.26% sodium bicarbonate with 40 mmol/l of potassium intravenously over 4 hours.

Haemodialysis is recommended for severe salicylate intoxication. This includes any patient with coma, convulsions, severe metabolic acidosis who does not respond to fluids, or when mild CNS effects do not respond to the correction of acidosis. Other indications include congestive heart failure and noncardiogenic pulmonary oedema. If acid–base or electrolyte imbalances remain resistant to correction or if the salicylate concentration is persistently high despite an alkaline urine, haemodialysis should be started immediately.

Tricylic antidepressants (TCA)

Self poisoning with tricyclic antidepressants may be harmful to both the mother and the fetus.

Peak plasma concentrations and therefore signs and symptoms of toxicity should occur within about 6–8 hours. However, as TCA could cause a delay in gastric emptying, toxicity may develop later in some instances. The complications most often associated with a fatal outcome are severe hypotension and cardiac arrhythmias.

Clinical features

Initial clinical features are due to their anticholinergic effects: dilated pupils, hallucinations, dry mouth, tachycardia and urinary retention. Severe poisoning may result in deep coma, convulsions, hypotension, cardiac arrhythmias, respiratory depression and pulmonary oedema.

ECG changes

Prolongation of the QRS interval is the most distinctive feature of severe tricyclic poisoning. A QRS complex on ECG of duration greater than 100 ms is associated with a higher risk of convulsions. Cardiac arrhythmias such as ventricular arrhythmias are associated with QRS prolongations exceeding 160 ms. Continuous monitoring for at least 6–8 hours post-ingestion is necessary. If signs persist, continued monitoring is essential.

Specific treatment: gastric decontamination

Gastric lavage may be considered if patients present within 1 hour post-ingestion. This should be followed by a dose of activated charcoal. Because of delayed gastric emptying, a second dose of activated charcoal may be administered 2–4 hours after the initial dose.

Measure serum electrolytes and pH and normalise whilst maintaining adequate ventilation and oxygenation. Intravenous fluids should be used to maintain the blood pressure when required. Once oxygenation has been maintained, diazepam followed by sodium bicarbonate (see below) is the treatment of choice for convulsions.

If the patient is acidotic, showing definite signs of toxicity, has cardiovascular instability or a wide QRS complex on the ECG, sodium bicarbonate should be administered. The initial dose is 1–2 mmol/kg (1–2 ml/kg of 8.4% given IV) over approximately 15 minutes. A continuous IV infusion of 500–1000 ml of 1.26% may be administered when indicated. The arterial blood pH must be closely monitored and maintained between 7.45 and 7.55 with boluses of sodium bicarbonate.

Digoxin poisoning

Digoxin has a very narrow therapeutic index and a dose over 10 mg is considered toxic. It acts by altering the sodium/potassium ATPase transport system resulting in an increase in the availability of calcium ions to produce an increase in the force of contraction of the heart muscle. Digoxin toxicity affects the conduction system and the myocardium in overdose. In digoxin poisoning, extracellular potassium increases due to a defective Na^+/K^+-pump affecting the exchange of these two ions. The therapeutic plasma concentration is 0.5–2.0 ng/ml (0.64–2.56 nmol/l). Levels > 2 ng/ml (2.56 nmol/l) are associated with a higher risk of toxicity but toxicity is not always related to plasma level. Patients with healthy hearts are likely to tolerate large doses up to 5 mg. Overdose usually leads to onset of symptoms within 6 hours. The early symptoms are mainly associated with the gastrointestinal system: anorexia, nausea and vomiting being the commonest. CNS manifestations include headache, fatigue, lethargy, depression, confusion and hallucinations. Reversible visual disturbances, such as blurred vision, photophobia and alteration of colour perception, may also be observed.

Biochemically, hyperkalaemia may be a prominent feature in acute toxicity.

Different cardiac effects may be seen and occur within 6 hours.

- Bradyarrhythmias such as AV conduction disturbances (first-degree heart block, second-degree heart block and complete heart block).
- Tachyarrhythmias are common. Ventricular tachycardia and fibrillation indicate severe toxicity.
- Hypotension and cardiac arrest may also occur.

Treatment

Gastric decontamination with activated charcoal should be carried out when a patient presents within 1 hour of ingestion. Observe the patient on a cardiac monitor for at least 6 hours following ingestion. If the patient develops signs of toxicity, continue observations until signs of toxicity abate.

Hyperkalaemia should be treated aggressively with insulin/dextrose. Sodium bicarbonate or calcium resonium exchange resin may be used as alternatives if required. Calcium gluconate is contraindicated as VF may follow its administration.

Bradycardias may respond transiently to intravenous boluses of atropine.

Digibind is the antidote of choice and is indicated in the presence of any of the following:

- Hyperkalaemia > 5.5 mmol/l, or resistant to correction.
- Bradyarrhythmias (e.g. high-grade AV block) unresponsive to atropine or associated with hypotension.
- Tachyarrhythmias, especially if associated with hypotension.

One of the following methods may be used to calculate the required dose of digibind.

(a) Number of vials = $\dfrac{\text{amount of digoxin ingested (mg)} \times 0.8}{0.5}$

(b) Number of vials = $\dfrac{\text{serum digoxin concentration in ng/ml} \times \text{weight in kg}}{100}$

If dose ingested or serum concentration is not known 20 vials of digibind could be administered as a single dose. Alternatively, 10 vials may be administered initially and the remainder later if indicated.

Calcium channel blocker overdose

The calcium channel blockers are used in the treatment of hypertension, angina and arrhythmias. There are three groups of calcium channel blockers: the dihydropyridines (e.g. nifedipine), benzothiazepine (diltiazem) and a phenylalkylamine (verapamil). All three groups do produce serious toxicity in overdose. In overdose, these drugs produce profound hypotension while some agents may cause bradyarrhythmias whilst others may cause tachyarrhythmias.

Most of these agents are also available as sustained release (SR) preparations. Following ingestion of SR preparations, signs and symptoms may occur as late as 18 hours afterwards and therefore it is important to confirm whether the patient had ingested a SR preparation. Consequently all individuals who have ingested SR preparations should be observed for at least 18 hours from the time of ingestion. As deterioration may occur suddenly, close monitoring is a necessity.

Clinical features

Hypotension is the commonest feature to all the agents in this class of drugs. Some agents (verapamil and diltiazem) may produce varying degrees of conduction blocks including complete heart block. Nifedepine may cause a tachycardia.

Treatment

These patients need close observation. Following ingestion of SR preparations, cardiac monitoring should be continued for at least 18 hours. Gastric decontamination may be attempted within 1 hour post ingestion. In very severe overdoses, whole bowel irrigation can be attempted. All symptomatic patients should be managed in a facility for cardiac monitoring.

Hypotension should initially be treated with intravenous fluids. If there is no response, intravenous calcium gluconate should be administered (3 g in a 10% solution, i.e. 30 ml repeated every 10–20 minutes for 3–4 doses). Severe overdoses may not respond to this therapy. In the absence of a response to fluids and calcium gluconate, patients should be treated with insulin and dextrose. Usually high doses of insulin are administered – initially 1–2 units/kg of soluble insulin as a bolus. Thereafter, an infusion of 0.5–1 unit/kg per hour in 10% dextrose should be administered. Measure blood sugar and serum potassium levels every 1–2 hours.

Beta-blockers

Beta-blockers are widely used antihypertensive and anti-angina agents. Poisoning with these drugs is not uncommon. They act by blocking the beta-adrenergic receptors. Consequently beta$_1$ receptors regulate heart rate and blood pressure. Some beta-blockers e.g. atenolol and bisoprolol are more 'cardio-selective' than others, i.e. they selectively block the beta$_1$ receptors more than the beta$_2$ receptors at therapeutic doses, resulting in fewer side effects. Some beta-blockers block fast sodium channels and thus cause myocardial depression whilst others are lipid soluble and hence cross the blood–brain barrier causing central nervous system effects following an overdose.

After ingestion, most patients develop symptoms within 2–4 hours. Hypotension is common and is mostly due to the negative inotropic effect on the heart. Bradycardia may also occur but this is less common with cardio-selective beta-blockers.

ECG changes may include prolonged PR interval, first-degree AV block and bundle branch block. Severe toxicity may result in disappearance of P waves, total AV block, asystole and intraventricular conduction defects. Agents with membrane-stabilising activity may prolong the QRS interval. Cardiogenic shock and pulmonary oedema are possibilities especially in patients with preexisting cardiac disease.

CNS effects such as drowsiness are more commonly seen in overdose with beta-blockers with membrane-stabilising activity.

Treatment

Gastric decontamination with activated charcoal to patients presenting within 1 hour of ingestion. All patients require cardiac monitoring for at least 6 hours post-ingestion. If patients have ingested slow-release preparations observe patients for at least 12 hours.

Hypotension should initially be treated with IV fluids; this should be done cautiously in patients with pre-existing cardiac disease or in those at risk of serious poisoning. In such cases CVP (central venous pressure) monitoring is advisable.

Glucagon is the drug of choice for patients who are haemodynamically unstable.

An average patient should receive a 10 mg IV bolus of glucagon and repeated as required or a 1–10 mg/hour IV infusion, depending on the response. Vomiting is a useful indicator that an adequate dose has been given.

Iron overdose

Iron tablets are easily accessible to pregnant mothers. Iron poisoning is dangerous to the mother. It causes mitochondrial damage, interfering with cellular respiration and resulting in cellular dysfunction, metabolic acidosis and, ultimately, cell death, particularly in the liver.

Toxic doses of elemental iron are:

< 30 mg/kg – mild toxicity.
> 30 mg/kg – moderate toxicity.
> 60 mg/kg – severe toxicity.
> 150 mg/kg could be lethal.

The clinical course of iron poisoning may be divided into four phases; the time scale is variable. What is presented below is only a guide.

- Phase 1: Predominantly vomiting, diarrhoea, abdominal pain occurring 30 minutes to 6 hours post-ingestion. The vomitus and stools may be dark or bloodstained and may have a metallic smell. Leukocytosis and hyperglycaemia may occur. In severe cases, drowsiness, lethargy, coma, convulsions, metabolic acidosis, shock and gastrointestinal haemorrhage may occur.
- Phase 2: Apparently asymptomatic phase occurring 6–24 hours post-ingestion. Some patients would not proceed beyond this phase.
- Phase 3: At about 12–48 hours post-ingestion relapse may occur with severe lethargy, coma, convulsions, gastrointestinal haemorrhage, shock, cardiovascular collapse, metabolic acidosis, liver failure with hypoglycaemia, coagulopathy, pulmonary oedema and renal failure.
- Phase 4: At 2–5 weeks stricture formation, pyloric stenosis and small bowel obstruction.

Treatment

Patients who ingest > 30 mg/kg body weight elemental iron require assessment and treatment.

Radiological assessment and gut decontamination

An abdominal X-ray should be performed following ingestion of a potentially toxic dose to determine the need for gut decontamination [3]. As there are potential fetal risks, this examination should be done after discussion with the patient. Iron tablets are radio-opaque and they may be visualised on X-ray. If tablets are visible in the stomach, gastric lavage may be performed. If they are detected further down the gastrointestinal tract, whole bowel irrigation should be carried out. Some tablets may not be seen on an X-ray.

Measure serum iron level 4 hours after ingestion. Patients with serum iron levels between 55 and 90 μmol/l require only observation and intravenous fluids. A concentration over 90 μmol/l indicates severe toxicity and warrants treatment with desferrioxamine. A dose of 15 mg/kg per hour as a continuous infusion (in 0.9% saline or 5% dextrose) should be administered. The dose should be reduced as soon as the clinical situation permits, usually after 4–6 hours, to prevent exceeding a dose of 80 mg/kg in any 24-hour period. Chelation therapy should be continued until there are no radiological abnormalities and all symptoms have resolved.

Extracorporeal drug removal

Some drugs may be effectively removed by haemodialysis. It is not contraindicated in pregnancy and should be offered to all mothers when indicated.

Supportive care

Most drug overdoses require only supportive care. This includes management of the airway in drug overdoses that may lead to reduced consciousness. Antiepileptics and sedatives are the commonest drugs in this group. Some drugs may cause stimulation of the sympathetic nervous system. Salbutamol and theophylline are known examples. These patients present with an elevated blood pressure and tachycardia. Fluid replacement and sedatives such as benzodiazepines should be administered to such patients. Some drugs may induce a serotonin syndrome (e.g. selective serotonin reuptake inhibitors). These patients develop high temperatures and muscle rigidity. Such patients require active cooling measures and liberal IV fluids.

Most overdoses with ordinary-release drugs require monitoring for at least 6–8 hours. Signs and symptoms should appear by this time lag. However, sustained-release drugs may produce symptoms as late as 18–24 hours post-ingestion.

References

1. McClure CK, Patrick TE, Katz KD, Kelsey SF, Weiss HB. Birth outcomes following self-inflicted poisoning during pregnancy, California, 2000 to 2004. *J Obstet Gynecol Neonatal Nurs* 2011; 40 (3): 292–301.

2. Czeizel AE. Attempted suicide and pregnancy. *J Inj Violence Res* 2011; 3 (1): 45–54.

3. Dart RC (Ed.) *Medical Toxicology*. Third Edition. Philadelphia, PA: Lippincott Williams and Wilkins, 2003.

Chapter

27

Diabetic ketoacidosis in pregnancy

Ingrid Watt-Coote and Julia Kopeika

Key facts

- Definition: Diabetic ketoacidosis (DKA) is an acute medical emergency characterised by dehydration, acidosis, hyperglycaemia and ketonuria. This is a complex metabolic disorder. It increases the morbidity and mortality for both mother and fetus.
- Commonly seen in patients with Type I diabetes but can occur in the presence of Type II and gestational diabetes [1].
- Pregnancy is a state of insulin resistance which increases as gestation advances.
- DKA in pregnant diabetics may occur at lower blood glucose levels than in the non-pregnant state.
- Incidence: In pregnancy this is about 2% (range 1–3%) [2, 3]. Most presentations occur in the second and third trimesters. The incidence in developing countries is unknown but anticipated to be higher [4–6].

Key implications

- Maternal: Significant morbidity and mortality. The mortality rate is less than 1% with prompt diagnosis and management.
  - There were no deaths from DKA in the latest UK Confidential Enquiry into Maternal deaths [2]. The mortality rate is higher in developing countries [7].

- Fetal: Hypoxia and metabolic acidosis increase the risk of fetal death. The fetal mortality is about 9%. Perinatal mortality has been reported as 30% in poorly managed patients and as high as 60% if there is coma [1].

Key pointers

- Predisposing factors; nausea and vomiting, infections especially of the urinary tract, poor or non-compliance, poor management.
- Corticosteriods (betamethasone, dexamethasone) for preterm labour can precipitate hyperglycaemia for up to 48 hours following the last dose.
- Prednisolone for asthma can precipitate hyperglycaemia.
- Consider sliding scale insulin if capillary blood glucose is greater than 8 mmol/l during steroid therapy.

Key diagnostic signs

Presentation will be as in the non-pregnant patient. These patients may present to the accident and emergency department or directly to the maternity unit. They may sometimes present to their local general practitioner.

All healthcare professionals working in these areas and the community must therefore have a high index of suspicion of the diagnosis of DKA when caring for a pregnant diabetic.

Diabetic ketoacidosis can develop very rapidly in insulin-dependent diabetics who omit their injections or have inter-current illnesses.

Diabetic ketoacidosis must always be considered when a diabetic pregnant patient is admitted to hospital [8] especially if they are in the second or third trimester.

Obstetric and Intrapartum Emergencies, ed. Edwin Chandraharan and Sabaratnam Arulkumaran. Published by Cambridge University Press. © Cambridge University Press 2012.

This may be the first presentation for an undiagnosed diabetic.

Acute confusion is a **late** indicator of physical ill health or deterioration. This requires immediate admission to an intensive care facility.

Symptoms are attributed to three main features +/− possible signs of infection:

- Hyperglycaemia.

  · Polyuria (at initial stage).
  · Polydipsia.

- Acidosis.

  · Vomiting.
  · Abdominal pain, generalised malaise.
  · Hyperventilation.
  · Tachypnoea.

- Dehydration (consequence of hyperosmolarity and polyuria).

  · Oliguria.
  · Tachycardia.
  · Drop of blood pressure.
  · Lethargy, coma (cerebral dehydration and possible hypoxia).

- +/− Infection.

  · Cough, if chest infection.
  · Dysuria and/or loin pain if urinary tract infection/pyelonephritis.

Findings:

- Maternal: Anxiety, confusion, dehydration, smell of ketones on the breath, hyperventilation, hypotension, tachypnoea, tachycardia, hypoxia.

Investigations:

- Venous blood: acidosis pH < 7.3 [9]

  · Bicarbonate (HCO_3) < 15 mmol/l.
  · Capillary ketone > 3 mmol/l.
  · Glucose > 11 mmol/l.

- Urinanalysis: Ketonuria $> 2+$

The presentation varies from mild to severe DKA. Only one of these abnormal results may be present.

Remember pregnancy is a state of relative alkalosis with bicarbonate level of 18–20 mmol/l.

- Hyperglycaemia 11–13 mmol/l (note much lower levels than in the non-pregnant state) [1].
- Fetal: Electronic fetal heart rate monitor may reveal evidence of fetal compromise or absent fetal heart rate.

Key actions (Management algorithm)

This is a medical emergency and the woman must be admitted to the high dependency unit (HDU) or intensive care facility. Both the senior obstetrician and diabetologist must be involved in the immediate care as the first 24 hours following admission are crucial. The major risk to the pregnant woman is delay in recognition of severe illness, poor management at admission and failure to involve senior doctors [2].

- Delay in diagnosis and appropriate treatment increases both maternal and fetal morbidity and mortality.
- Thus, a rapid clinical assessment must be performed to assess severity.
- If the woman presents in a coma then she must be admitted directly to the intensive therapy unit (ITU) without any delay except for life-saving interventions.

Resuscitation

Airway, **B**reathing and **C**irculation (ABC) including oxygen saturation.

- AVPU (Alert, Voice, Pain and Unconsciousness) assessment tool can be used.
- Glasgow Coma Score (GCS) system is more sensitive to assess neurological status.
- 'Back to Basics' and the use of the Modified Early Obstetric Warning System (MEOWS) [2] (Table 27.1).
- Remember the left lateral tilt for pregnancies beyond 20 weeks.

Immediate (within the first hour):

- Summon senior assistance (obstetrician, anaesthetist, diabetic team).
- Secure intravenous access with two large-bore cannulae e.g. size 16G.
- Clinical assessment of blood pressure, heart rate (peripheral pulse), temperature, respiratory rate.
- Bloods: Urea and electrolytes, capillary and venous glucose, full blood count (FBC), blood cultures.

Table 27.1 Modified Early Obstetric Warning System (MEOWS) score.

Observation	2	1	0	1	2
Pulse	< 40	41–50	51–100	101–120	> 120
Systolic BP	< 80	80–99	100–150	151–170	> 170
Diastolic BP	< 40	–	40–90	91–110	> 110
Resp rate	≤ 8	–	9–20	21–26	> 26
O$_2$ Sats	< 94	–	94–100		
Oxygen delivery				≥ 8 litres or 40%	
Temp	< 35.0	35.0–36.0	36.1–38.0	–	> 38.0
Conscious level	Respond to pain only	Drowsy, respond to voice only	Alert	Acute confusion or agitation	
	Score	If MEOWS 2–3 medical review			
	Score	If MEOWS 4–5 medical review – urgently			
	Score	If MEOWS > 6 call senior obstetrician and critical care team			

- Venous blood gas [9].
- Measure capillary blood glucose using a Ward glucose meter.
- Septic screen (blood and urine cultures), swabs as indicated.
- ECG and pulse oximetry (continuous).
- Request chest X-ray.
- Urinalysis for ketones.
- Catheterisation and connect to an urometer for hourly urine if no urine passed in 3 hours.

A Ward glucose meter will be accurate up to 30 mmol/l but if the values are above 25 mmol/l it is important to obtain a value from the laboratory as soon as possible.

Fetal assessment

- Cardiotocograph if gestation > 28 weeks otherwise intermittent auscultation. The role of the cardiotocograph in extreme prematurity (24–28 weeks) is controversial.
- Will not change management during the acute resuscitation phase as maternal care takes priority. **Do not waste time to do this**.
- The timing of delivery can be decided once the mother is fully resuscitated and this usually refers to gestations beyond 34 weeks.
- **Do not** deliver for acute fetal compromise unless there is complete resolution of maternal condition.

Fluid resuscitation

Vital to reverse the acute acidosis state and correct the intravascular depletion.

This is a rapid process which can potentially cause complications in pregnancy mainly of pulmonary oedema and less so of cerebral oedema. Thus, involvement of the anaesthetist is vital because of the possibility of the need for central venous pressure (CVP) monitoring.

- Start 0.9% sodium chloride solution. Crystalloid solution of choice administered via an infusion pump.
- 1000 ml in 60 min (first hour).
- 500 ml/hour for next 4 hours.
- 250 ml/hour for next 8 hours.
- 125 ml/hour for next 12 hours.
- **Potassium chloride (KCl)** 40 mmol/l **must** be added to each litre of fluid to maintain serum potassium between 3.5 and 5.5 mmol/l (available premixed with sodium chloride solution).

A faster infusion rate can take place in the first hour if the blood pressure is < 90/65 mmHg.

- Start 10% dextrose solution at 125 ml/hour if glucose < 14 mmol/l.
  - Administered simultaneously with sodium chloride infusion.

This is vital to avoid hypoglycaemia and associated complications.

Insulin

- Start intravenous short-acting soluble insulin (Actrapid®, Humulin S®) at a fixed rate of 0.1 unit/kg per hour [5, 10].

- Standard variable rate can cause premature reduction of insulin dosage.
- Booking weight may be used if current weight is not available.

- 50 units soluble insulin (50 units/ml) added to 49 ml sodium chloride 0.9% solution to give a mixture of 50 units in 50 ml or 1 unit/ml.

  - Bolus insulin is not needed but if there is a delay with the insulin infusion then give this intramuscularly (IM) at 0.1 units/kg.

Do not discontinue long-acting or basal insulin (e.g. Levemir®, Lantus® and Insulatard®). Continue this at the current dosing regime and route [4].

Electrolyte replacement

This applies mainly to serum potassium as both hyperkalaemia and hypokalaemia are dangerous since they can precipitate cardiac arrhythmia thus increasing the maternal morbidity and mortality risk. Continuous ECG monitoring is essential.

- Aim for potassium level 3.5–5.5 mmol/l. Add KCl 40 mmol to each litre of 0.9% sodium chloride solution.
- If potassium > 5.5 mmol/l **do not** add potassium.
- If potassium < 3.5 mmol/l, additional potassium replacement is needed therefore liaise with senior intensivist/physician.
- Bicarbonate will correct itself with the aggressive fluid resuscitation [11].
- No need to give sodium bicarbonate.
- Phosphate measurement and replacement is not necessary [3, 12].

Reassess, Reassess, Reassess

- Patient's mental state using AVPU or GCS.
- To ensure acidosis is corrected.

  - Venous blood gas hourly for 2 hours then 2-hourly. If still **hypoxic** perform arterial blood gas (ABG).
  - Potassium and bicarbonate level from blood gas report.

- To ensure ketonemia is reversing.

  - This has been reported as the best indicator of resolution of diabetic ketoacidosis [13].
  - Bedside ketone meter if available.

Table 27.2 Thromboprophylaxis in pregnancy recommended by the RCOG [14].

Weight (kg)	Suggested thromboprophylactic dose of Enoxaparin
< 50	20 mg daily
50 to 90	40 mg daily
91 to 130	60 mg daily
131–170	80 mg daily
> 170 kg	0.6 mg/kg/day
High prophylactic dose (for 50 to 90 kg)	40 mg twice daily

- **Do not use ketonuria to assess resolution because this will be the last parameter to disappear**.

- To ensure hyperglycaemia is reversing.

  - Capillary glucose hourly using a Ward glucose meter (send sample to the laboratory for venous glucose if level > 20 mmol/l).

- To ensure rehydration.

  - Fluid balance chart showing input and output.
  - Monitor urine output and aim for 0.5 ml/kg/hour; 30 ml/hour or average 100 ml/4 hours.
  - Monitor heart rate and blood pressure.

- To ensure electrolyte imbalance is reversed.
- Continue infusion of sodium chloride solution.
- Start thromboprophylaxis – give pregnancy regime/doses (Table 27.2).

  - Venous thromboembolism is increased in pregnancy.
  - The risk is further increased with hospital admission, diabetes, dehydration and the acute illness [14].

- Fetal heart

  - CTG may show evidence of reversal of fetal compromise as maternal condition improves. (Remember the risk of fetal intra-uterine demise is more likely the more severe the DKA.)
  - Neonatologist review if viable gestation.

Table 27.3 Suggested variable rate insulin infusion with Actrapid® or Humulin S®.

Blood glucose (mmol/l)	Insulin rate (ml/hour)	Dextrose rate (ml/hour)
0–2.9	0.1	80
3–3.9	0.5	63
4–4.9	1.5	63
5–5.9	2.0	63
6.0–6.9	2.5	63
7.0–7.9	3.0	63
8–8.9	4.0	63
9–9.9	5.0	63
10+	6.0	30

50 units Actrapid (50 units/ml) added to 49 ml 0.9% NaCl solution to give a solution of 50 units/50 ml or 1 unit/ml or 1 unit = 1 ml.

Resolution

Resolution is occurring if:

- Bicarbonate is increasing at a rate of 3 mmol/l/hour OR
- Glucose is reducing by 3 mmol/l/hour OR
- Ketonemia is reducing at a rate of 0.5 mmol/l/hour.

If resolution is not taking place at the rates indicated above then increase the insulin infusion at **1 unit/hour** increments [10].

For example: if current rate is 70 units/hour then increase this to 71 units/hour then 72 units/hour and continue with monitoring aiming for at least one of the changes above.

Caution in pregnancy as glucose levels are normally lower therefore venous gas PH is important to confirm resolution of acidosis.

Post-resolution

- Introduce food.
- May change to variable rate insulin if there is no ketonaemia (Table 27.3).
- Reintroduce subcuticular insulin if eating normally, biochemically stable and asymptomatic.
- Fetal medicine ultrasound scan if fetus alive.
- Continue with diabetic team review.

Key pitfalls

- Not getting senior help quick enough.
- Not starting 10% dextrose solution.

- Stopping basal insulin. If occurred, do not discontinue insulin infusion until the basal or long-acting insulin is restarted for 12–24 hours.
- Remember there is a risk of error and hence danger if KCl is added because pre-prepared solution of sodium chloride with KCl is not available or a higher concentration of KCl is needed. Be cautious and double check.
- Insulin measurement 50 units/ml. Do not add more than 49 ml of sodium chloride to 1 ml of soluble insulin to achieve a mixture of 1 unit/ml.
- Assumption of resolution of acidosis if glucose is in the normal range. Ensure venous gas pH is in the normal range to confirm resolution.

Key pearls

- Prime the infusion tubing prior to infusion of intravenous insulin to prevent insulin sticking to the walls.
- Always start 10% dextrose solution infusion in pregnancy simultaneously with other fluids as the glucose level at which DKA occurs in pregnancy is usually 11–13 mmol/l.

  - Generally, start 10% dextrose if glucose < 14 mmol/l.

- Remember discharge from hospital must not take place until there has been a diabetic consultation and patient education about risk and factors to avoid preventing recurrence of DKA.
- Ensure patient has enough supply of insulin, testing sticks including ketostix and a workable machine.

  - Advise if unwell, do regular ketostix testing at home and if positive to attend hospital.

- For patients on continuous insulin pump therapy, re-education on the use of the pump.
- Outpatient appointment to be seen by the diabetic team in 48 hours.
- An outpatient appointment must be arranged for review in the combined obstetric and diabetic antenatal clinic in a week.
- Arrange a fetal medicine ultrasound scan.
- Ensure all causes were addressed.

  - If there was a confirmed urinary tract infection consider prophylactic antibiotic for the duration of the pregnancy especially if there have been previous confirmed laboratory reports.

Management in low-resource settings

- Lack of infusion pumps for both insulin and rehydration fluids.

  - Therefore give insulin intramuscularly (IM) and be extremely cautious with intravenous fluid as iatrogenic fluid overload can precipitate respiratory distress secondary to pulmonary oedema. Likewise the development of cerebral oedema. Strict fluid balance.

- If bedside ketone meter is not available then use bicarbonate levels to assess response to treatment (remember this is less reliable after 6 hours) [10]. Less reliable after 6 hours as glucose normalised especially in pregnancy where glucose level is usually < 14 mmol/l. Remember 10% dextrose infusion.
- If there is no 'y' connector for infusion of both insulin and sodium chloride then two separate intravenous lines can be used.
- Ideally 0.9% sodium chloride solution is best, however Ringer's lactate (Hartmann's solution) may be used.
- Intermittent fetal auscultation with a sonicaid or Pinard stethoscope listening for a minimum 60 seconds hourly for a viable fetus. For a non-viable fetus this can be less frequent (remember this is not a priority as maternal resuscitation is more important).
- May not be able to provide neonatal care for gestation < 24 weeks or < 500 g therefore manage as facilities available. Discuss with local neonatal team.
- Dextrose 5% solution may be used.

References

1. Kamalakannan D, Baskar V, Barton DM, Abdu TA. Diabetic ketoacidosis in pregnancy. *Postgrad Med J* 2003; 79 (934): 454–457.
2. Centre for Maternal and Child Enquiries (CMACE). *Saving Mothers' Lives: Reviewing Maternal Deaths to make Motherhood Safer – 2006–2008. The Eighth Report on Confidential Enquiries into Maternal Deaths in the United Kingdom. Br J Obstet Gynaecol* 2011; 118 (Suppl. 1): 1–208.
3. Hawthorne G (Ed.) Diabetic ketoacidosis in pregnancy. In *Maternal Complications in Diabetic Pregnancy*. London: Elsevier, 2011.
4. Zargar AH, Wani AI, Masoodi SR *et al.* Causes of mortality in diabetes mellitus: data from a tertiary teaching hospital in India. *Postgrad Med J* 2009; 85 (1003): 227–232.
5. Gokel Y, Paydas S, Koseoglu Z, Alparslan N, Seydaoglu G. Comparison of blood gas and acid-base measurements in arterial and venous blood samples in patients with uremic acidosis and diabetic ketoacidosis in the emergency room. *Am J Nephrol* 2000; 20 (4): 319–323.
6. Raghavan VA. Diabetic ketoacidosis. http://emedicine.medscape.com/article/118361-overview
7. Otieno CF, Kayima JK, Omonge EO, Oyoo GO. Diabetic ketoacidosis: risk factors, mechanisms and management strategies in Sub-Saharan Africa. *East African Med J* 2005; 82: S197–203.
8. National Institute of Health and Clinical Excellence. *Diabetes in Pregnancy*. London: NICE, 2008.
9. Kelly AM. The case for venous rather than arterial blood gases in diabetic ketoacidosis. *Emerg Med Australas* 2006; 18 (1): 64–67.
10. Joint British Diabetes Societies Inpatient Care Group. *The Management of Diabetic Ketoacidosis in Adults*. London: NHS, 2010.
11. Glaser N, Barnett P, McCaslin I *et al.*; Pediatric Emergency Medicine Collaborative Research Committee of the American Academy of Pediatrics. Risk factors for cerebral edema in children with diabetic ketoacidosis. *N Engl J Med* 2001; 344 (4): 264–269.
12. Liu PY, Jeng CY. Severe hypophosphatemia in a patient with diabetic ketoacidosis and acute respiratory failure. *J Chin Med Assoc* 2004; 67 (7): 355–359.
13. Sheikh-Ali M, Karon BS, Basu A *et al.* Can serum beta-hydroxybutyrate be used to diagnose diabetic ketoacidosis? *Diabetes Care* 2008; 31 (4): 643–647. Epub 2008 Jan 9.
14. Royal College of Obstetricians and Gynaecologists. *Reducing the Risk of Thrombosis and Embolism during Pregnancy and the Pueperium*. Green-top Guideline No. 37a. London: RCOG, 2009.

Convulsions and epilepsy

Julia Kopeika and Ingrid Watt-Coote

- Definition: Epilepsy is a neurological condition characterised by recurrent epileptic seizures unprovoked by any immediately identifiable cause. An epileptic seizure is the clinical manifestation of an abnormal and excessive discharge of a set of neurons in the brain [1].
- Incidence: Approximately 40–70 new cases per 100 000 per year in high-income countries and 100–190 per 100 000 per year in low-income countries.
- Prevalence: Varies between 3 and 40 per 1000 worldwide. Epilepsy affects 0.5–1% of pregnant women; 3.5% of epileptic women will have a seizure in labour [2] and 1–2% of epileptics will develop status epilepticus.

Types of seizure [3]

Focal seizures

Focal indicates that the seizures originate primarily within networks limited to one cerebral hemisphere.

These include simple and complex. Such seizures can present as a twitching of one limb or part of a limb, an unusual smell or taste, a strange feeling such as a 'rising' sensation in the stomach or 'pins and needles' in part of the body or a sudden intense feeling of fear or joy. Sometimes patients can start wandering around or behaving strangely and they may not know what they are doing. They may pick objects up for no reason, fiddle with their clothes or make chewing movements with their mouth.

Generalised

Generalised epileptic seizures originate within, and rapidly engage, bilaterally distributed networks. The person becomes unconscious, and afterwards will not remember what happened during the seizure.

- Myoclonic seizures: Involve the jerking of a limb or part of a limb, and often happen shortly after waking up from sleep.
- Clonic seizures: During the seizure the person usually falls to the ground and shakes or makes jerking movements (convulses).
- Tonic seizures: The person's muscles suddenly become stiff. If they are standing they often fall backwards and may injure the back of their head.
- Tonic–clonic seizures: During a tonic–clonic seizure the person goes stiff, usually falls to the ground and shakes or makes jerking movements (convulses). Their breathing can be affected and they may go pale or blue, particularly around their mouth. They may also bite their tongue.
- Atonic seizures: In an atonic seizure (sometimes called a 'drop attack') the person's muscles suddenly relax, and they become floppy. If they are standing they often fall forwards and may injure their face or head.

Absence seizures

- During an absence a person becomes unconscious for a short amount of time, usually a few seconds. They may look blank and not respond to what is happening around them.

Obstetric and Intrapartum Emergencies, ed. Edwin Chandraharan and Sabaratnam Arulkumaran. Published by Cambridge University Press. © Cambridge University Press 2012.

Key implications

- Maternal: increase of seizure frequency in 10–30% during pregnancy; deterioration of disease in those with poorly controlled epilepsy before pregnancy; modest increase in preeclampsia and caesarean section [4]; premature labour (especially if woman is a smoker) [5]; placental abruption; trauma; indirect cause of maternal death; sudden unexpected death in epilepsy.
- Fetal: Increased risk of congenital abnormalities due to antiepileptic drugs (higher with polytherapy); risk of epilepsy in child; risk of fetal hypoxia if prolonged convulsive seizures or status epilepticus develop; possible neurocognitive effects [4].

Key pointers

Risk factors for seizures in pregnancy/labour

- Decreased compliance to take medication due to concern about teratogenicity.
- Decreased drug absorption because of nausea and vomiting.
- Decreased drug levels due to increased volume of distribution in pregnancy, increased drug metabolism and renal elimination.
- Impaired sleep/rest, hyperventilation.

Key diagnostic signs

Epilepsy is, in most cases, diagnosed before pregnancy, however it may occasionally present for the first time during pregnancy. Seizure that occurred in pregnancy/labour needs to be differentiated from syncope.

The following questions could be used to help differentiation [1].

Questions used that, if positive, support a diagnosis of epileptic seizure:

- At times do you wake up with a cut tongue after your spells?
- At times do you have a sense of *déjà vu* or *jamais vu* before your spells?
- At times is emotional stress associated with losing consciousness?
- Has anyone noticed your head turning during a spell?
- Has anyone ever noted that you are unresponsive, have unusual posturing or have jerking limbs during your spells or have no memory of your spells afterwards?
- Has anyone noticed that you are confused after a spell?

Questions used that, if positive, support a diagnosis of syncope:

- Have you ever had light-headed spells?
- At times do you sweat before your spells?
- Is prolonged sitting or standing associated with your spells?

Differential diagnosis for convulsions in pregnancy should include the following:

- Eclampsia.

  Associated with proteinuria, raised blood pressure.

- Epilepsy.

  Usually previous history.

- Cerebral venous thrombosis.

  Associated with headache, vomiting, photophobia, focal neurological signs.

- Thrombotic thrombocytopenic purpura.

  Associated with headache, drowsiness, fever, renal impairment with haemolytic anaemia; hypertension is not common.

- Stroke (ischaemic/haemorrhagic).

  Associated with headache and raised blood pressure, often secondary to preeclampsia or ruptured arterio-venous malformations.

- Encephalitis/meningitis.

  Associated with headache, neck stiffness signs or psychiatric features, meningism, focal central nervous system signs.

- Cerebral tumours.

  Might be preceded by symptoms associated with space-occupying lesion in the head.

- Cerebral trauma.

  Signs of trauma, history from friends, relatives, witnesses.

- Drug withdrawal

  History from friends and relatives.

- Toxicity.

  Epidural, overdose of tricyclic antidepressants.

- Metabolic disturbances (hypoglycaemia, hypocalcaemia, hyponatraemia).

  Associated with tremor, hunger prior to attack, paraesthesia, carpo-pedal spasm.

- Postdural puncture.

  Preceded by postdural headache that is relieved by lying down, associated neck stiffness, tinnitus, visual symptoms.

- Amniotic fluid embolism.

  Presence of predisposing factors (age, induction of labour, hyperstimulation, uterine trauma), respiratory distress, cyanosis, shock with further vaginal bleeding.

- Cardiogenic (Stokes–Adams attacks, arrhythmias).

  Associated with palpitation, chest pain or shortness of breath, during the attack pallor and pulse is slow or absent.

- Infection.

  · Neurocysticercosis (history of eating uncooked pork or drinking contaminated water).
  · Cerebral malaria (living or visiting endemic area, recent high fever with rigors, sometimes jaundice).
  · Tetanus (recent 'unclean' delivery, unsafe abortion, trismus, arched back, board-like abdomen).
  · Septicaemia (high fever, abdominal pain, purulent discharge, very ill patient with delirium, signs of septic shock).

Evaluation of a pregnant woman who has had a seizure

- Obtain as much history as possible from patient and witnesses.
- Try to establish associated symptoms (headache, visual disturbances, epigastric pain, neck stiffness, tinnitus, palpitation, shortness of breath, chest pain).
- Check urine for proteins.
- Check blood pressure, pulse, oxygen saturation, temperature and respiratory rate.

- Send blood for FBC, U & E, LFTs, urea, Ca^{2+}, PO_4^{3-}, glucose, international normalized ratio (INR)/partial thromboplastin time (PTT), blood film, serum and urine toxic screen, thrombophilia screen.
- Imaging: CT, MRI or magnetic resonance angiography (MRA) (if seizure occurs for the first time in pregnancy).
- ECG, 24-hour ECG, EEG.

Key actions (management algorithm)

Immediate management of short-lasting self-limiting convulsions in pregnancy

During the seizure

- Summon senior staff, call for help, but try not to leave the patient on her own. You would need the most senior obstetricians, anaesthetist, midwife, other nursing and ancillary staff. Specify that it is maternal seizure.
- Note the time the seizure starts – note the exact time when seizure was witnessed to be started. Allocate one of the staff to record the events and watch the time. Also ask to inform you if seizure lasts more than 4–5 minutes. Most tonic–clonic seizures last less than 2 minutes [6].
- Prevent injury. Most of the seizures are self-limiting. Do not try to restrict the convulsions. Only move the patient if she is in a dangerous place, e.g. on the edge of a staircase. Preferably try to ease the patient down onto the floor if she was sitting down before. Try to put padding on the side rails of the bed, move objects away if they might hurt the patient.
- Semi-prone position if possible. Place wedge under right hip or nurse in left lateral position. After the convulsion subsides put patient in recovery position.
- Secure airway and administer high-flow oxygen. Do not try to open the mouth and introduce anything solid in the mouth during the fit. After the convulsive movements subside check the airway is not obstructed.

Immediately after the seizure

- Monitor vital signs including blood pressure, pulse, ECG, respiration rate, temperature, saturated O_2 and fetal heart rate. It will not be possible to obtain accurate readings for some of the vitals, such as blood pressure for example, during tonic–clonic phase. However, it should be done immediately after seizure. Ensure there is no apnoea and pulse is maintained.

- Secure intravenous access and draw blood for FBC, U&Es, LFTs, clotting screen, cross match.
- Administer anticonvulsant drugs – see below. Short-lasting tonic–clonic seizures do not require emergency drug treatment [7] during the convulsion, however you may consider administration of the drug to prevent recurrence.
- Commence CTG following the seizure. It could show reduced variability up to 1 hour following administration of diazepam.
- Catheterise bladder, monitor urine output and test urine for protein after resolution of the seizure.
- Document the events with clear description of the type of the seizure and length of time.
- Debrief patient and relatives when fully recovered and conscious.
- Time of delivery. Self-limiting epileptic seizure is not an indication for immediate delivery. However, if the nature of the seizure is not known further history and investigation should be undertaken as soon as possible. If the seizure is attributed to eclampsia in this case the delivery should be considered after appropriate stabilisation of the mother.

Drug treatment

An individual who has a prolonged convulsion (lasting 5 minutes or more) or serial seizures (three or more seizures in an hour) or lasting longer than usual should receive medical treatment. Otherwise, the medical treatment could be administered after self-limiting seizure to prevent recurrence (Table 28.1).

Treatment of status epilepticus

Convulsive status epilepticus is defined as a generalised convulsion lasting 30 minutes or longer or repeated tonic–clonic convulsions occurring over a 30-minute period without recovery of consciousness between each convulsion. This definition is specific to convulsive status epilepticus, but there are other types, for example non-convulsive status epilepticus [1].

- Summon senior staff.
- Note the time the seizure starts.

- Secure airway and administer high flow oxygen 100%.
- Assess cardiac and respiratory function.
- Gain IV access = 2 large-bore cannulas.
- Obtain blood and send urgent arterial/venous gases, FBC, U & E, LFTs, coagulation, glucose, calcium, AED levels.
- Administer:
  - IV bolus lorazepam 4 mg.
  - IV fluid (correct hypotension).
  - 50 ml of 50% glucose if hypoglycaemia.
- Start IV infusion:
  - IV phenytoin 15 mg/kg at a rate of < 50 mg/min.
  - Or diazepam infusion 100 mg in 500 ml of 5% dextrose: infuse at 40 ml/hour.
- Intubate if not intubated already, sedation.
- Monitor ECG and blood pressure.
- General anaesthesia phase.
- Transfer to intensive treatment unit.

Intrapartum care for women with known epilepsy

- Continue to take regular anti-epileptic drugs.
- Keep hydrated.
- Maternal exhaustion and hyperventilation should be avoided.
- Secured intravenous access could be recommended.
- Labour should take place in obstetric-led units.
- Labour in the pool should be avoided.
- Do not leave woman unattended.
- If seizure occurs see Figure 28.1 for protocol.

Key pitfalls

- Failure to record/note the time the convulsion started.
- Do not restrain the patient, allow the seizure to happen.
- Do not try to move patient during the seizure, unless there is an imminent danger of trauma.
- Do not put anything in their mouth.
- Do not assume it is epileptic seizure in pregnant patients with no known history (think eclampsia until proven otherwise!).

Table 28.1 Emergency anticonvulsant drugs that can be used in pregnancy.

Name of drug	Dose	Route of administration	Cautions
Diazepam	10–20 mg 10–20 mg	IV bolus (rate not more than 2–5 mg/min), per rectum	Carries risk of respiratory depression, hypotension and cardiovascular collapse Pulse, BP, RR, saturated O_2 should be monitored after administration of the drug CTG should be commenced Reduced variability could be observed up to 1 hour
Lorazepam	4 mg	IV bolus	Longer lasting than diazepam, less lipid soluble so can be given faster Monitoring of cardio-respiratory function is essential
Midazolam	10 mg	Buccal (medication is drawn up into syringe and administered in mouth through the catheter)	Has equal efficacy and as rapid in action as rectal diazepam More convenient and faster to administer, less stigmatising, more socially accepted [5] Beware of effects on cardiovascular system
Magnesium sulphate[1]	4 g (20 ml of 20% magnesium sulphate) – loading dose 1 g/hour – maintenance dose	IV over 20 minutes IV 50 ml magnesium sulphate 20%; for 24 hours	Respiratory depression, loss of patellar reflexes, drowsiness, slurring of speech, muscle weakness

[1] In a pregnant patient with uterus above umbilicus (> 20 weeks) and no previous history available, the clinician should have a high suspicion of eclampsia. These patients should be treated as if they are eclamptic until further history and observations are available.

- Do not focus on fetal distress before having mother stabilised. (Mother is always the highest priority: always follow ABC algorithm for mother even if there is evidence of fetal distress.)
- Delay anticonvulsant treatment in prolonged seizure if no IV access gained.
- Do not leave patient unattended following the resolution of the seizure especially if benzodiazepines were given.

Key pearls

- Remember to summon senior help.
- Anticipate and prevent (keep a woman with known epilepsy well hydrated, have adequate pain relief, remember to give antiepileptic drugs regularly, do not leave a woman on her own in labour and after delivery).
- Remember that the dose of antiepileptic drugs needs to be adjusted in pregnancy.
- Regular drills and skills for staff.
- If eclampsia suspected magnesium sulphate should be first line of treatment, since it has better outcome for mother and baby in comparison with diazepam [8].

- Remember the immediate postnatal period is a high risk for seizure (do not leave woman on her own).
- Counsel woman with epilepsy about the risk of drowning, recommend to use shower, rather than bath.
- Remember that there are multiple causes of seizures apart from eclampsia and epilepsy.
- Refer to a specialist with experience of managing epilepsy or status epilepticus.
- In the management of seizure in a pregnant woman follow the main principles [9]:
  - Speed (timely help is crucial).
  - Skills (summon help of people with right skills (obstetricians, anaesthetists, medics, ITU specialists, neurologists).
  - Priority (prevent the injury, secure airways, provide oxygen, secure IV access, control blood pressure, administer anticonvulsant drugs).

Management in low-resource settings

It is believed that the incidence of epilepsy in low-income countries is much higher (100–190 per 100 000 people) than in the high-income world (40–70 per 100 000) [10]. The management of epilepsy in

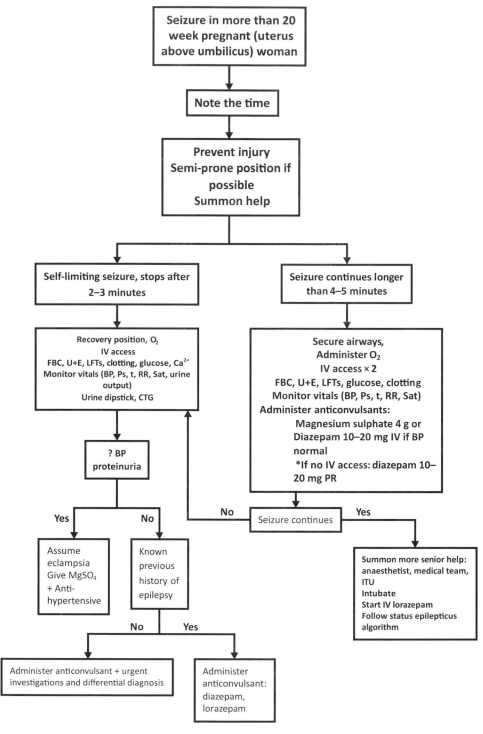

Figure 28.1 Algorithm for management of seizure in pregnant woman.

low-resource settings should start with proper recognition of the problem. Recent data show that more than 50% of people with epilepsy are not properly treated due to poor recognition of the symptoms [11]. The next barrier is a widespread stigmatisation and misperception about epilepsy that causes under-reporting of symptoms by women with epilepsy.

There is also a wide disparity in the availability of treatment through the world. Nonetheless, phenobarbital carries the lowest cost among the anti-epileptic drugs and can be accessed in most of the countries [12].

Seizure in pregnant woman is an emergency that requires immediate actions that do not require any high-tech facilities or drugs. The management of seizure in a pregnant patient described above can be applied in any setting. In resource-poor settings, where most obstetrical care occurs later in pregnancy and home births are the norm, women with epilepsy, especially those with poorly controlled seizures, should be encouraged to deliver at the hospital [13].

References

1. Stokes T, Shaw EJ, Juarez-Garcia A, Camosso-Stefinovic J, Baker R. *Clinical Guidelines and Evidence Review for the Epilepsies: Diagnosis and Management in Adults and Children in Primary and Secondary Care.* London: Royal College of General Practitioners/NICE, 2004. http://www.nice.org.uk/nicemedia/live/10954/29533/29533.pdf

2. *The EURAP Study Group.* Seizure control and treatment in pregnancy. *Neurology* 2006; 66: 354–360.

3. Berg AT, Berkovic SF, Brodie MJ et al. *Revised Terminology and Concepts for Organization of the Epilepsies: Report of the Commission on Classification and Terminology.* International League Against Epilepsy, 2009. http://www.ilae-epilepsy.org/Visitors/Documents/ClassificationSummaryReportweb Aug2009.pdf

4. Walker SP, Permezel M, Berkovic SF. The management of epilepsy in pregnancy. *Br J Obstet Gynaecol* 2009; 116 (6): 758–767.

5. Harden CL, Hopp J, Ting TY et al. Practice parameter update: management issues for women with epilepsy – focus on pregnancy (an evidence-based review): obstetrical complications and change in seizure frequency. Report of the Quality Standards Subcommittee and Therapeutics and Technology Assessment Subcommittee of the American Academy of Neurology and American Epilepsy Society. *Neurology* 2009; 73 (2): 126–132.

6. Scottish Intercollegiate Guidelines Network (81). *Diagnosis and Management of Epilepsies in Children and Young People.* 2005. http://www.sign.ac.uk/pdf/sign81.pdf

7. Shorvon S. *Handbook of Epilepsy Treatment.* Third edition. Oxford: Wiley-Blackwell, 2010.

8. Duley L, Henderson-Smart DJ, Walker GJ, Chou D. Magnesium sulphate versus diazepam for eclampsia. *Cochrane Database Syst Rev* 2010; 12: CD000127.

9. World Health Organization. *Managing Eclampsia. Education Materials for Teachers of Midwifery. Midwifery Education Modules.* Second edition. Geneva: Department of Making Pregnancy Safer, Family and Community Health, World Health Organization, 2006.

10. World Health Organization, International Bureau for Epilepsy, International League against Epilepsy. *Global Campaign against Epilepsy out of the Shadow.* The Netherlands, 2003.

11. Meinardi H, Scott RA, Reis R, Sander JW; ILAE Commission on the Developing World. The treatment gap in epilepsy. *Epilepsia* 2001; 42: 136–149.

12. World Health Organization. *Epilepsy: The Services. Epilepsy Atlas.* Geneva: WHO, 2005. http://www.who.int/mental_health/neurology/Epilepsy_atlas_r1.pdf

13. Birbeck GL. Epilepsy care in developing countries. Part II of II. *Epilepsy Curr* 2010; 10 (5): 105–110.

Chapter

29

Musculoskeletal considerations in pregnancy

Hiran Amarasekera

Key facts

Pregnancy causes several changes to the musculoskeletal system that should be remembered when treating injuries during pregnancy. The main changes are shift in centre of gravity (Figure 29.4), increase in body weight and increase in ligament laxity mainly caused by increased relaxin release during pregnancy.

As a result of these changes in pregnancy women are more prone to certain musculoskeletal conditions (Table 29.1). Some of the common conditions are [1]:

- Low back pain.
- Hip problems, e.g. transient osteoporosis, AVN (avascular necrosis of hip) leading to hip pain and even femoral neck fractures.
- Compression neuropathies and tendonopathies e.g. carpal tunnel syndrome, De Quervain's tenosynovitis.
- Leg cramps/deep vein thrombosis (DVT).
- Tinel's test: Light tapping of the median nerve over carpal tunnel causes pain and tingling sensation radiating to lateral $3\frac{1}{2}$ fingers.
- Phalen's test: Hyperflexion of the wrist and holding for about 30 seconds causes numbness over the medial nerve distribution (lateral $3\frac{1}{2}$ fingers)
- Finkelstein's test: Flex the thumb and grasp inside a closed fist, and ulna deviate the hand. This stretches the extensor pollicis brevis and abductor pollicis longus tendons causing sharp pain along the radial side.

- Faber/Patrick's test: The affected side knee is flexed to 90 degrees and the foot is rested on the opposite knee. Pelvis is firmly held against the table and the affected side knee is pushed towards the examination table. If this causes pain it's more likely to originate from the sacroiliac joint [2].

Cauda equina syndrome

Key facts

- Rare complication seen in 1/10 000 pregnancies [3].
- When diagnosed it is an emergency that requires an acute surgical intervention.
- This is caused by lumbar disc herniation compressing the cauda equina.

Key implications

- It is important to differentiate normal back pain from cauda equina syndrome.
- If not treated early could result in permanent neurological deficit such as incontinence, foot drop.

Key pointers (Predisposing factors)

- Preexisting lumbar disc disease.
- Pregnancy-related changes (see above).
- Increase in maternal age [4].

Obstetric and Intrapartum Emergencies, ed. Edwin Chandraharan and Sabaratnam Arulkumaran. Published by Cambridge University Press. © Cambridge University Press 2012.

Table 29.1 Musculoskeletal conditions in pregnancy.

	Key implications	Key pointers	Key diagnostic signs	Key actions	Key pearls	Key management options
Low back pain	Caused by lumbar lordosis Shift in centre of gravity and ligament laxity	Previous low back pain Previous pregnancy Conditions causing large abdomen	Low posterior pelvic pain, relieved by lying or sitting	Early education Early training	If pain originates from sacroiliac joint, direct compression over joint causes pain Faber test is positive	Activity modification/ physiotherapy, mild NSAIDs Pelvic support Steroid injections Epidural analgesia Pregnancy is a relative contraindication for any surgery except in caudal equina syndrome
Transient osteoporosis (TO) and avascular necrosis of the hip (AVN)	Rare conditions Aetiology unknown	Hip pain At rest Pain on movement Pain on weight-bearing Sometimes night pain	Limited movement of hip MRI, pelvic ultrasound X-rays	TO – No action required, self limiting AVN – need early orthopaedic referral	Remember to rule out more sinister conditions such as fractured neck of femur	Treatment is similar to non-pregnant symptomatic patients Needs referral to an orthopaedics unit Initial management is non-surgical (conservative) Surgical intervention is reserved for failed cases
Compression neuro/ tendinopathies 1. Carpal tunnel syndrome (CTS) 2. Dequavain's Tenosynovitis (DT)	Both caused by increased fluid retention	CTS – Pain, numbness tingling over lateral 3½ fingers DT – pain radial side of hand	CTS – Tinel's test, Phalen's test Ultrasound DT – Tenderness near radial styloid Finkelstein's test	Mild conditions do not require any intervention Identifying the condition, observing the progression and reassurance are important initially	Both: Avoid surgery when possible. 95% resolve after delivery	CTS – Conservative: Night splints (80%) respond to this Surgery: Carpal tunnel decompression for severe cases DT – Conservative Splints Steroid injections Surgery if conservative measures fail

Key diagnostic signs

- Acute onset or progressively increasing back ache.
- Pain spreading down the legs.
- Motor involvement, muscle weakness mainly L4, L5, S1 roots.
- Lower limb motor weakness (L4, L5, S1).
- Foot drop.
- Bladder sphincter involvement either causing urinary retention or incontinence.
- Bowel involvement mainly loss of the anal sphincter tone.
- Saddle anaesthesia around the peri-anal area.

Key actions

- If cauda equina is suspected it should be referred to the spinal team urgently (orthopaedic or neurosurgery depending on the hospital) as early surgery gives best results.

- In pregnancy clinical features can be easily missed therefore a high index of suspicion is needed to make a diagnosis.
- Early diagnosis.
- Early referral.

Management in a low-resource setting

MRI scans are often not required as the diagnosis is mainly clinical. However, when surgery is indicated an MRI scan is taken as it allows localisation of the lesion and acts as a road map for the surgeon. If MRI is not available a CT scan is an option. However it is worth noting that CT exposes the patient to radiation and has a limited value in showing soft tissues.

Key actions/management

Lower back pain and lumbar disc herniation does not need an acute surgical intervention as it is self-limiting and likely to resolve after delivery.

Indications for surgical intervention

- Cauda equina syndrome (bowel bladder involvement).
- Motor deficit such as acute foot drop.
- Progressive neurological deficit.

Surgical options

- Open surgery: laminectomy, partial hemi-laminectomy [4].
- Micro-discectomy.

Symphysis pubis diastasis (SPD)

Key facts

- Pubic symphysis separation is a recognised complication of pregnancy with incidence estimates ranging from 1 : 600 to 1 : 3400 among obstetric patients [5].
- Most cases are self-limiting and spontaneously resolve during the postpartum period and do not require any acute intervention.
- Most respond to conservative management. However, severe disruptions, persistent symptoms and unstable SPD will require surgical intervention.

Key implications

Symphysis pubis diastasis, in most cases, is self-limiting. Most cases do not require any surgical intervention because full recovery is seen with conservative management, in the majority of patients. However it is important to identify the patients who may need surgery (Figure 29.1).

Patients may have skeletal or soft-tissue injuries:

- Skeletal: associated damage to sacroiliac joints.
- Soft tissue:

    Bladder injuries, bladder herniation [6].
    Vaginal injuries (rare).
    Rectal injuries (rare).

Key pointers

- Interventions such as forceps delivery.
- Large head.
- Forceful separation of legs (forced flexion abduction).
- Prolonged labour and/or rapid descent during second stage [7].
- This is an under-diagnosed, under-reported condition, which can be easily missed if a high index of suspicion is not exercised [7].

Key diagnostic signs

- Intrapartum care (difficult labour, instrumentation).
- Postpartum pain around pubis symphysis.
- Urinary incontinence with change of position.
- Pain when walking.
- Gait changes.
- On examination palpable gap within the symphysis.

Key actions

- Initial bed rest.
- Check soft-tissue injuries.
- X-ray will confirm diagnosis; if X-rays are contraindicated ultrasound scan can be used.

Key pitfalls

- Failure to diagnose.
- Failure to assess severity.

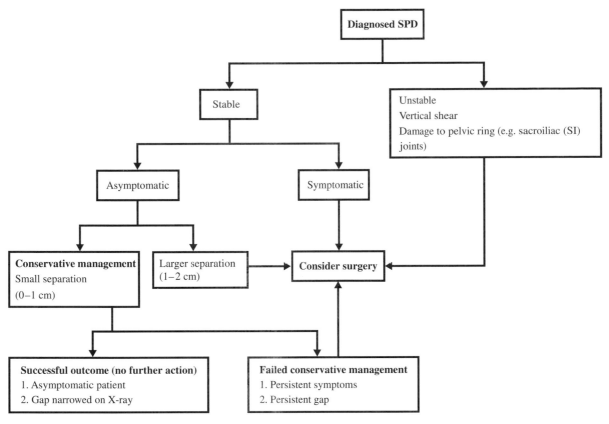

Figure 29.1 Symphysis pubis diastasis (SPD) management algorithm.

- Failure to follow up mainly when patient is asymptomatic following delivery 3–6 months postpartum.

Key pearls

- High index of suspicion is the utmost important aspect in the diagnosis [8].
- When a diagnosis of SPD is made, exclude associated soft-tissue injuries such as bladder injuries or herniation.

Management in low-resource setting

Commercially made pelvic binders (Figure 29.2) may not be available in every setting.

Therefore it is important to note that the compression can be achieved by using a sheet that can be wrapped around the pelvis and both hips and tied tightly so that it brings compression from sides towards the pubic symphysis (Figure 29.3a, b). This

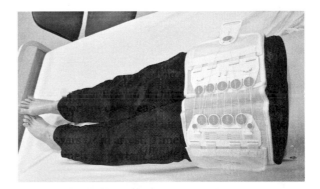

Figure 29.2 Supporting the pelvic girdle in pregnancy.

will bring the two halves of the symphysis together. This was extensively used previously before stabilisers were commercially marketed. Nevertheless the principle remains the same and this is an ideal option in a low-resource setting.

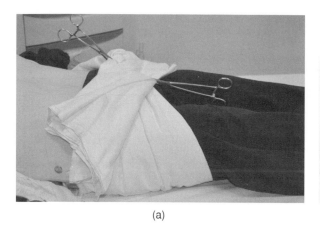

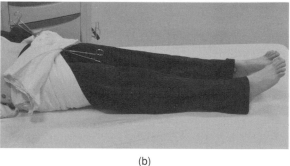

(a)

(b)

Figure 29.3 Supporting the pelvic girdle in a low-resource setting.

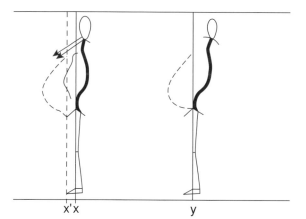

Figure 29.4 A line diagram showing the shifting of centre of gravity anteriorly during pregnancy (from X to X¹) The body compensates by hyperlordosis to correct the shift (y).

Key management options

- Pelvic ring includes pubic symphysis, superior rami of pubis iliac bones, sacroiliac (SI) joints and the sacrum.
- Degree of separation, stability of the pelvic ring, pain, patient's symptoms, as well as associated damage to soft tissues should be considered in managing the patient.

Conservative management includes the following options:

- Physiotherapy.
- Occupational therapy.
- Pelvic floor muscle-strengthening exercises.
- Bed rest.

- Pain control.
  - Mild analgesics
  - Transcutaneous Electrical Nerve Stimulation (TENS)
  - Alternative therapies e.g. acupuncture, cryoanalgesia [9].

- Use of pelvic stabilisation devices such as pelvic binders and slings.

Pelvic stabilisation devices can be used initially to achieve reduction in large SPD. However there is little evidence to support long-term use [10]. As soon as the patient is comfortable physiotherapy and muscle-strengthening exercises should be started.

Surgical options include [11]:

- External fixation devices [12, 13].
- Internal fixation

  Screws.
  Plates and screws [14].
  Wiring.

Fractures during pregnancy

It is worth noting that some fractures such as femoral neck, lower limb, and pelvic fractures can occur during pregnancy.

Pregnancy may contribute indirectly as the gait changes, transient osteoporosis, AVN and weight gain all may be risk factors.

Pregnant women are also exposed to general risk factors for fractures such as major trauma, falls and other impact injuries.

It is worth noting that pregnancy does not affect the principles of most fracture management as standard fractures are managed in the same way as in a non-pregnant woman. It is important to obtain early orthopaedic advice when a fracture is noted.

Final management should involve multidisciplinary input from the orthopaedic, trauma, obstetric, anaesthetic and radiology teams.

Major trauma is another area where the principle of 'Mother's life comes first' should be applied.

References

1. Ritchie JR. Orthopedic considerations during pregnancy. *Clin Obstet Gynecol* 2003; 46: 456–466.

2. Doro CJ, Forward DP, Kim H *et al*. Does 2.5 cm of symphyseal widening differentiate anteroposterior compression I from anteroposterior compression II pelvic ring injuries? *J Orthop Trauma* 2010; 24: 610–15.

3. LaBan MM, Perrin JC, Latimer FR. Pregnancy and the herniated lumbar disc. *Arch Phys Med Rehabil* 1983; 64: 319–321.

4. Brown MD, Levi AD. Surgery for lumbar disc herniation during pregnancy. *Spine (Phila Pa 1976)* 2001; 26: 440–443.

5. Senechal PK. Symphysis pubis separation during childbirth. *J Am Board Fam Pract* 1994; 7: 141–144.

6. Fuhs SE, Herndon JH, Gould FR. Herniation of the bladder. An unusual complication of traumatic diastasis of the pubis. *J Bone Joint Surg Am* 1978; 60: 704–707.

7. Taylor RN, Sonson RD. Separation of the pubic symphysis. An underrecognized peripartum complication. *J Reprod Med* 1986; 31: 203–206.

8. McIntosh JM. Diastasis of the pubic symphysis. *Br J Gen Pract* 1994; 44: 386–428.

9. Glynn CJ, Carrie LE. Cryoanalgesia to relieve pain in diastasis of the symphysis pubis during pregnancy. *Br Med J (Clin Res Ed)* 1985; 290: 1946–1947.

10. Depledge J, McNair PJ, Keal-Smith C, Williams M. Management of symphysis pubis dysfunction during pregnancy using exercise and pelvic support belts. *Phys Ther* 2005; 85: 1290–1300.

11. Lange RH, Hansen ST, Jr. Pelvic ring disruptions with symphysis pubis diastasis. Indications, technique, and limitations of anterior internal fixation. *Clin Orthop Relat Res* 1985; 201: 130–137.

12. Chang JL, Wu V. External fixation of pubic symphysis diastasis from postpartum trauma. *Orthopedics* 2008; 31: 493.

13. Dunivan GC, Hickman AM, Connolly A. Severe separation of the pubic symphysis and prompt orthopedic surgical intervention. *Obstet Gynecol* 2009; 114: 473–475.

14. Webb LX, Gristina AG, Wilson JR *et al*. Two-hole plate fixation for traumatic symphysis pubis diastasis. *J Trauma* 1988; 28: 813–817.

Chapter

30

Endocrine emergencies in pregnancy

Manilka Sumanatilleke

Introduction

Pregnancy is a state where a woman's hormonal milieu changes in a manner which is unrivalled by any other period in life. Effect of placental hormones, changes in the level of hormone-binding proteins, changes in plasma volume, physiological hypertrophy of many glands etc. can have myriad effects on the endocrine system. A number of endocrine diseases and emergencies can have unique characteristics in pregnancy and many early symptoms of common endocrine conditions may be difficult to differentiate from common symptoms experienced during a normal pregnant state.

Furthermore, pregnancy itself may alter the course of underlying endocrine conditions such as autoimmune disorders and pituitary disease. Graves' disease usually improves during pregnancy but occasionally may flare up. Development of lymphocytic hypophysitis and enlargement of existing pituitary adenomas – especially prolactinomas, which may result in apoplexy – are a few good examples of this phenomenon.

Hence, careful analysis of symptoms and investigations, early recognition of warning signs and instituting a management plan keeping in mind the complexities of the maternal–fetal unit can be both very challenging and extremely rewarding.

Thyroid

Thyroid disease is a very common endocrine disease affecting women of reproductive age and thyrotoxicosis causing a thyroid storm is comparatively much more common than hypothyroidism causing myxoedema coma.

Thyroid storm

Key facts

- Thyroid storm is a clinical and biochemical state resulting in acute, severe over-production of and exposure to thyroid hormones.
- Incidence: 1–2% of women with hyperthyroidism receiving thionamide treatment [1].
- Overt hyperthyroidism complicates approximately 2 in 1000 pregnancies and maternal mortality with a thyroid storm is approximately 3%.
- Graves' disease is responsible for approximately 90% of cases. Toxic multinodular goitre, solitary toxic adenoma, exogenous thyroid hormones and rare causes such as struma ovarii, HCG-producing trophoblastic tumour and excessive exogenous iodine will contribute to the rest of the cases.

Key implications

Maternal

- Severe hypertension.
- Congestive cardiac failure.
- Coma or seizures, confusing with eclampsia.
- Miscarriage/placental abruption/preterm labour.

Fetal

- Stillbirth.
- Neonatal hyperthyroidism.
- Prematurity.
- Central hypothyroidism.

Obstetric and Intrapartum Emergencies, ed. Edwin Chandraharan and Sabaratnam Arulkumaran. Published by Cambridge University Press. © Cambridge University Press 2012.

Diagnostic approach

Clinical

- Symptoms of mild hyperthyroidism may mimic symptoms of normal pregnancy:
  - Fatigue.
  - Palpitations.
  - Tachycardia.
  - Vomiting.
  - Increased appetite.
  - Heat intolerance.
  - Increased urinary frequency.
  - Insomnia.
  - Emotional lability.

- More specific symptoms and signs described below should increase the suspicion of thyrotoxicosis which warrants close clinical evaluation and biochemical testing:
  - Tremor.
  - Nervousness.
  - Frequent passage of stools – formed or loose.
  - Muscle weakness – especially proximal muscle weakness.
  - Brisk reflexes.
  - Excessive sweating.
  - Weight loss.
  - Hypertension.
  - Goitre (normal pregnancy can cause up to 15% increase in size of thyroid gland).
  - Bruit over the thyroid.

- Diagnostic signs:
  - Graves' ophthalmopathy – exophthalmos, ophthalmoplegia, changes in visual acuity and colour vision.
  - Thyroid acropachy (clubbing).
  - Dermopathy (pretibial myxoedema).

Diagnosis of a thyroid storm

This is essentially a clinical diagnosis and encompasses hypermetabolic complications of severe thyrotoxicosis including hyperpyrexia, cardiovascular compromise, gastrointestinal symptoms and changes in the central nervous system. As treatment should be initiated even before confirmatory biochemical test results are available the diagnostic criteria [2] given in Table 30.1 are a very useful guidance and should **not** be a substitute for good clinical judgement on an individual basis.

Table 30.1 Diagnosis of a thyroid storm.

Diagnostic parameters	Scoring points
Thermoregulatory dysfunction	
Temperature F (C)	
99–99.9 (37.2–37.7)	5
100–100.9 (37.8–38.2)	10
101–101.9 (38.3–38.8)	15
102–102.9 (38.9–39.4)	20
103–103.9 (39.5–39.9)	25
≥ 104.0 (40)	30
Central nervous system effects	
Absent	0
Mild (agitation)	10
Moderate (delirium, psychosis, extreme lethargy)	20
Severe (seizures, coma)	30
Gastrointestinal–hepatic dysfunction	
Absent	0
Moderate (diarrhoea, nausea/vomiting, abdominal pain)	10
Severe (unexplained jaundice)	20
Cardiovascular dysfunction	
Tachycardia (beats/minute)	
90–109	5
110–119	10
120–129	15
≥ 140	25
Congestive heart failure	
Absent	0
Mild (pedal oedema)	5
Moderate (bibasilar rales)	10
Severe (pulmonary oedema)	15
Atrial fibrillation	
Absent	0
Present	10
Precipitating event	
Absent	0
Present	10

Scoring system: A score of 45 or greater is highly suggestive of thyroid storm; A score of 25–44 is suggestive of impending storm; A score below 25 is unlikely to represent thyroid storm.
Adapted from Burch HB, Wartofsky L. Life-threatening thyrotoxicosis. Thyroid storm. *Endocrinol Metab Clin North Am* 1993; 22 (2): 263–277.

Precipitating factors

- Poorly controlled hyperthyroidism/poor compliance with medication.
- Infection.
- Surgery.
- Thromboembolism.

- Preeclampsia.
- Parturition.

Biochemistry

Impact of pregnancy on the thyroid:

- Alpha subunit of TSH molecule is common to those found on LH and hCG and high levels of these hormones will stimulate the TSH receptors in the thyroid gland to produce thyroid hormones.
- Gestational transient thyrotoxicosis is typically associated with hyperemesis gravidarum and molar pregnancies.
- By 20 weeks' gestation plasma thyroxine binding globulin (TBG) levels increase 2.5-fold due to reduced hepatic clearance and oestrogen-induced change in the structure of TBG prolonging its half-life [3].
- 25–40% increase in serum total T4 (TT4) and 30% rise in total T3 in the first trimester and 50–60% rise later [4].
- Monitoring free T4 and TSH is recommended and close liaison with the laboratory is essential to obtain the trimester-specific values for the type of assay used.

Laboratory tests

- High free T4 and suppressed TSH.
- Leukocytosis.
- Occasionally elevated liver enzymes.
- Mild hypercalcaemia.
- Routine biochemistry for any acutely ill patient should be done.

Management

Principles of management:

- Reduce the synthesis and release of thyroid hormones.
- Block the peripheral actions of thyroid hormones/decrease sympathetic outflow.
- Block the peripheral conversion of T4 to more active T3.
- Identify and treat any precipitating factors such as infection.
- Identify and treat complications.
- Supportive care.

Supportive care:

- Patient best managed in an obstetric intensive care unit (ICU) or an ICU where continuous fetal monitoring and an emergency delivery could be handled.
- IV fluids and correct electrolyte imbalances.
- Cardiac monitoring and consider central haemodynamic monitoring to guide beta-blocker therapy if there is cardiac failure due to hyperdynamic circulation.
- Cooling measures to control the hyperpyrexia.

  - Sponge bath.
  - Acetaminophen (avoid aspirin).
  - Chlorpromazine 50–100 mg IM (inhibits central thermoregulation, useful in severe agitation).

- Oxygen therapy.
- Nasogastric tube if indicated (useful to administer medication especially propylthiouracil which is not available in IV form).

Medication

- Propylthiouracil orally or via nasogastric tube, 300–800 mg loading dose followed by 150–300 mg 6-hourly.

  - Inhibits iodination of tyrosine and thyroid hormone production.
  - Blocks peripheral conversion of T4 to T3.
  - Lower incidence of aplasia cutis in newborns compared with carbimazole.

- Iodides: Inhibit proteolysis of thyroglobulin and block the release of stored thyroid hormones. Ideally started at least 1 hour after the loading dose of propylthiouracil but should not be delayed if it is the only preparation available immediately.

  - Potassium iodide 60 mg oral/NG tube 6-hourly.
  - Lugol's iodine 6–8 drops 6-hourly.

- Beta-blockers: Control of autonomic symptoms especially tachycardia. Some inhibition of peripheral conversion of T4 to T3. Propranolol, labetalol and esmolol have been used in pregnancy [5].

  - Propranolol 160–480 mg per day in divided doses(4–6 hourly) or an infusion at a rate of 2–5 mg/hour with an aim to reduce the heart rate to < 90/minutes.

- Esmolol: 250–500 μg /kg of body weight loading dose followed by an infusion of 50–100 μg/kg per minute.

- High-dose glucocorticoids: Blocks peripheral conversion of T4 to T3 and release of stored thyroid hormones. Will supplement adrenal function and prevents adrenal insufficiency.

  · Hydrocortisone – 100 mg IM 6-hourly.
  · Prednisolone – 60 mg PO daily.
  · Dexamethasone – 8 mg PO daily.

Glucocorticoids and iodides can be discontinued after initial clinical management and when the clinical status is stable. Safer to continue for at least 24–48 hours.

Therapeutic options in special situations

- Calcium channel blockers can be used when beta-blockers are contraindicated.
- Lithium carbonate can be substituted for iodides in patients allergic to iodine.
- Plasmapheresis and peritoneal dialysis may be effective in patients resistant to usual pharmacological measures.
- Colestyramine (3 g tds) improves thyrotoxicosis by reducing the enterohepatic circulation of thyroid hormones.
- Near-total thyroidectomy (in second trimester) if conventional therapy fails.
- Radioactive iodine – postpartum.

Key pitfalls

- Failure to consider the diagnosis in an acutely ill patient with a history of thyroid illness and overlooking highly suspicious or diagnostic symptoms and signs.
- Delaying treatment awaiting thyroid function tests in a person with a history of thyroid disease.
- Failure to look for treatable aggravating factors such as infection.
- Failure to recognise common complications such as heart failure and continuation of high-dose beta-blockers without central haemodynamic monitoring.

Key pearls

- Diagnosis is essentially clinical and presence of hyperpyrexia (> 41 °C) and neuropsychiatric

symptoms with a history of weight loss in pregnancy will be highly suspicious.
- Laboratory tests cannot confirm the diagnosis and serum thyroid hormone levels can be similar to levels seen in uncomplicated hyperthyroidism.
- Symptoms of sympathetic over-activity will be prominent as thyroid hormones sensitise the peripheral tissues to the action of catecholamines.
- Start propylthiouracil at least 1 hour before the iodides as the iodine load in them can initially increase the production of thyroid hormones, but if there is a delay in obtaining propylthiouracil, iodides should be given without any delay.

Myxoedema coma

Key facts

- Vanishingly rare in pregnancy (usually seen during winter in the elderly with self-neglect).
- End stage of long-term untreated or insufficiently treated hypothyroidism.
- Severe hypothyroidism usually causes anovulation and infertility.
- Suspect in a woman with a history of thyroid disease – thyroid surgery, radioiodine therapy, poor compliance with medication.
- Can occur in a woman with previously undiagnosed mild to moderate hypothyroidism progressing rapidly due to a precipitating factor.

Key implications

- Cretinism and congenital anomalies in the newborn if severely hypothyroid in first trimester.
- Higher incidence of miscarriage, stillbirth, prematurity, placental abruption, postpartum haemorrhage, anaemia and cardiac dysfunction.

Diagnosis

History of progressively worsening typical hypothyroid symptoms:

- Lethargy.
- Increased sleepiness.
- Cold intolerance.
- Constipation.
- Hoarseness of voice.

Development of hypothermia, severe bradycardia, slow relaxing or diminished reflexes and confusion will herald the onset of myxoedema coma.

- May be complicated by pleural, pericardial effusions and ascites.
- Common precipitating factors:
  - Cold exposure.
  - Infections – pneumonia, upper respiratory tract.
  - Administration of sedatives, opioids and diuretics.
  - Cardiovascular event.
  - Surgery.

Laboratory tests

- Severe hyponatraemia due to poor water excretion is common and adds to the severity of the symptoms.
- Low free T4 and markedly raised TSH would be the hallmark.
- If the TSH is not raised with a low free T4 suspect pituitary disease.
- Blood sample for random cortisol.
- Routine investigations including renal, liver functions and muscle enzymes should be done.

Management

- Supportive care including cardiac monitoring and oximetry – may need ICU care if comatose.
- Identify and treat any precipitating factors.
- Passive external re-warming if hypothermic – aim for a rise of 0.5 °C/hour.
- Mild fluid restriction (1–1.5 l/day) if hyponatraemic.
- Levothyroxine 300–500 µg IV or by nasogastric tube stat and 100 µg daily until oral medication can be taken.
- If no improvement in 24–48 hours T3 10 µg tds could be added.
- Hydrocortisone 50–100 mg IM 6-hourly if cortisol deficiency is suspected.

Key pitfalls

- Failure to detect hypothermia in a comatose patient (low-reading thermometer may be needed).

- Failure to detect complications such as hyponatraemia, pleural and pericardial effusions which may complicate the clinical picture.

Key pearls

- Suspect in any confused person with hypothermia, hyponatraemia and diminished or absent reflexes.
- Always obtain personal and family history of thyroid disease.
- Intravenous T4 and T3 are hard to find and if there is any practical difficulty of having a nasogastric tube in place treatment can be given per rectal using a higher dose than usual.
- Monitor with core body (rectal) temperature.

Adrenals

Among the emergencies involving the adrenals, hypocortisolism would be the commonest but the much rarer phaechromocytoma crisis would be a diagnostic challenge while causing a high percentage of maternal and fetal mortality.

Acute adrenal insufficiency

Although many hormones are produced by the adrenal cortex and the medulla this term is usually used to denote the deficiency of cortisol, which is essential for life.

Key facts

- It can be due to a disease process in the adrenal cortex (primary) or due to pituitary or hypothalamic disease (secondary).
- Usually no fetal morbidity unless placental circulation is affected by prolonged low maternal blood pressure. Fetus produces and regulates its own adrenal steroids and maternal cortisol is inactivated by the placenta.
- It is commonly associated with diagnosed or undiagnosed preexisting primary or secondary disease aggravated by a stressful situation such as an infection, surgery or labour.
- Acute onset in pregnancy, although rare, can be due to adrenal haemorrhage or pituitary apoplexy.

Common causes

- Primary (Addison's disease).
  - Autoimmune destruction of adrenal cortex.

- Tuberculosis of adrenals.
- Infarction due to thrombosis in antiphospholipid syndrome.
- Acute haemorrhage due to disseminated intravascular coagulation (DIC), anticoagulants or Waterhouse–Friderichsen syndrome (in meningococcal septicaemia).
- Congenital adrenal hyperplasia.

- Secondary.

  - Suppression of hypothalamo-pituitary-adrenal axis by administration of exogenous glucocorticoids.
  - Lesions of the pituitary and hypothalamus.
    - Tumours such as adenomas and craniopharyngiomas.
    - Infections such as tuberculosis.
    - Inflammation due to sarcoidosis, histiocytosis X, haemochromatosis, lymphocytic hypophysitis.
    - Previous surgery, radiotherapy and trauma.
    - Acute onset in pituitary apoplexy.

Diagnosis

Symptoms of early disease can be difficult to distinguish from those of pregnancy but persisting symptoms should heighten the suspicion: as will the presence of vitiligo or other endocrinopathy (type 1 diabetes, thyroid disease).

- Nausea, vomiting and abdominal pain.
- Lethargy, tiredness.
- Hyperpigmentation – especially involving the mucosae, palmar creases, under bras and belts and recent scars.
- Postural dizziness/postural hypotension.
- Pyrexia of unknown origin.
- Symptomatic hypoglycaemia.

Laboratory investigations

- Hyponatraemia.
- Hyperkalaemia.
- Eosinophilia.
- Raised blood urea.
- Marginally raised serum calcium.

Unique features of secondary causes

- Absence of pigmentation (due to decreased ACTH).

- Features of pituitary and hypothalamic disease – other endocrine deficiencies, visual field defects, cranial diabetes insipidus.
- Electrolyte imbalances less common and absence of mineralocorticoid deficiency (aldosterone synthesis usually independent of ACTH control).

Biochemical confirmation

- This would be a challenge in pregnancy and careful analysis by an expert with collaboration with a biochemist and laboratory would be helpful.
- Maternal cortisol levels rise 2–3-fold during pregnancy.
- Effect of oestrogen causes the rise of corticosteroid binding globulin (CBG) resulting in raised total cortisol and impaired clearance of cortisol from the kidneys.
- Non-pregnant 'normal' levels can be too low during pregnancy.
- No consensus on normal levels of ACTH and interpretation of short synacthen test.

Suggested values

- In the first and early second trimester a 09.00 h cortisol level of 3 µg/dl (83 nmol/l) is suggestive of deficiency and a level more than 19 µg/dl (525 nmol/l) in a clinically stable patient could safely exclude the diagnosis.
- A 09.00 h ACTH level of > 100 pg/ml (22 pmol/l) is suggestive of primary adrenal insufficiency.
- Short synathen test (250 µg IM) in normal pregnant women in the second and third trimester showed responses 60–80% more than in non-pregnant women.

Diagnosis and treatment should not be delayed awaiting laboratory confirmation.

Suggestive symptoms and signs with supportive non-hormonal biochemistry should be sufficient to initiate emergency management which will be life-saving and a sample should always be taken for cortisol and ACTH (Table 30.2). Expert advice should be sought for interpretation of the results.

Management

- Hydrocortisone would be the cornerstone of management.

  - Hydrocortisone 200 mg IV stat.

Table 30.2 Normal plasma total and urinary free cortisol and ACTH levels in normal pregnancy.

	Non-pregnant	Third trimester
Total cortisol 09.00 h 24.00 h	11.34 ± 3.5 µg/ml 324 ± 100 nmol/l 3.6 ± 2.6 µg/ml 103 ± 76 nmol/l	36.0 ±7 µg/ml 1029 ± 200 nmol/l 23.5 ± 4.34 µg/ml 470 ± 124 nmol/l
Urinary free cortisol	4.7–9.5 µg/day 13–256 nmol/day	82.4–244.8 µg/day 229–680 nmol/day
Plasma ACTH	15–70 pg/ml 3.3–15.4 pmol/l	20–120 pg/ml 4.4–26.4 pmol/l

· Hydrocortisone 100 mg IM 6-hourly until oral therapy can be taken.

· Double the standard replacement dose of oral hydrocortisone until well – 20 mg/10 mg/10 mg (on waking/midday/evening).

· In primary adrenal insufficiency fludrocortisone 100 µg daily can be added when dose of hydrocortisone is reduced to normal replacement dose. (High-dose glucocorticoids have sufficient mineralocorticoid activity.)

- Fluids.

  · Intravenous 0.9% saline will be needed to correct the volume depletion and the hyponatraemia during the first 24–48 hours.
  · If hyponatraemia has been chronic, correction should not exceed more than 10–12 mmol/l in the first 24 hours.
  · Glucose supplementation.
  · Close monitoring of blood sugar and replacement as required.
  · Monitor treatment with electrolytes, urea and glucose.
  · Investigate and treat any underlying or precipitating condition.

Key pitfalls

- Delaying treatment pending confirmation of diagnosis.
- Failure to look for associated electrolyte and metabolic abnormalities.
- Overzealous correction of hyponatraemia may cause central pontine myelinosis.

Key pearls

- Consider in any emergency when suspicious features, suggestive basic biochemistry and hypotension not responding to inotropes.
- Unexplained fever, abdominal pain and hypoglycaemia will help to clinch the diagnosis with confidence.
- Have a low threshold to treat with hydrocortisone when above features are present.

Phaeochromocytoma crisis

Key facts

- Very rare but potentially lethal condition with a maternal mortality of around 17% and a fetal mortality of around 30% if not treated.
- Highest risk of hypertensive crisis and death during labour.
- Rarely may present as 'flash pulmonary oedema'.

Diagnosis

- Suspect in a woman with:

  · Persistent or intermittent hypertension associated with paroxysms of headache, palpitations and sweating.
  · Hypertension developing early in pregnancy (< 20 weeks).
  · Hypertension in the absence of proteinuria and oedema.
  · Hypertension associated with diabetes or persistent glycosuria.
  · Family history of MEN-2 or von Hippel–Lindau syndrome.

- Biochemical diagnosis by two 24-hour urine catecholamine and metanephrine collections and plasma catecholamines, ideally at a time of a paroxysm or elevated blood pressure.
- MRI of adrenals if diagnosis is confirmed by biochemistry.

Management

- Alpha blockade with phenoxybenzamine intravenous or oral according to the clinical status.

  · 0.5 mg/kg in 500 ml 0.9% saline or 5% dextrose over 4 hours IV.

> 10 mg 12-hourly (oral) building up gradually to a maximum of 20 mg 8-hourly.

- Beta blockade with propranolol only after adequate alpha blockade and tachycardia persists or develops – 40 mg 8-hourly (oral).
- Monitor with postural blood pressure, haemoglobin, packed cell volume (PCV) and filling up with IV fluids as required and supportive therapy.
- Surgery.

  > Can be considered before 24 weeks but controversial – depends on severity and response to medical management.
  > After 24 weeks delay until fetal maturity and consider combined caesarean section and tumour removal (should be pretreated with IV phenoxybenzamine for at least 3 days).

Pituitary

The pituitary gland enlarges during pregnancy mainly due to oestrogen-stimulated hypertrophy and hyperplasia of the lactotrophs and may appear hyperintense on MRI. The size of the gland usually reaches its maximum size around the third day postpartum and may measure up to 12 mm on MRI.

The hormonal milieu of pregnancy will stimulate the growth of pituitary adenomas, especially prolactinomas.

Acute hypopituitarism

Three common causes in pregnancy are given below. The terminology used can sometimes be confusing.

Sheehan's syndrome is a unique situation seen in pregnancy characterised by acute pituitary necrosis occurring immediately postpartum commonly due to ischaemia caused by hypotension subsequent to an obstetric haemorrhage.

Pituitary apoplexy (stroke) encompasses a broader spectrum of acute pituitary injury which can result from either haemorrhage or infarction, most commonly of an existing pituitary adenoma which can occur during any stage of pregnancy.

Lymphocytic hypophysitis is an autoimmune, infiltrative condition which is more common during pregnancy.

Pre-existing hypopituitarism with inadequate replacement can precipitate an acute insufficiency state with advancing gestation, labour, infection or surgery.

All these conditions will cause varying degrees of hypopituitarism, and when severe will present as an emergency in the form of secondary adrenal failure and hypopituitarism, but they have their own unique features which will be explained below.

Sheehan's syndrome

Key facts

- Physiologically enlarged pituitary gland in pregnancy is susceptible for any compromise to its blood supply.
- Postpartum haemorrhage, sickle cell disease are common risk factors while amniotic fluid embolism and disseminated intravascular coagulation can be rare associations.
- Involvement of the anterior pituitary, which derives its vascular supply from a low-pressure portal system, is more common than the more resilient posterior pituitary which has its own arterial supply.

Common clinical presentation

- Failure of lactation and involution of breasts.
- Dizziness, lethargy.
- Prolonged amenorrhoea.
- Loss of axillary and pubic hair.
- Features of acute adrenal insufficiency without the effects of mineralocorticoid deficiency as described earlier.
- Symptoms of hypothyroidism.

Pituitary apoplexy

Key facts

- Catastrophic event with consequences which can be life or sight threatening.
- Occurrence is more common with known or unknown pituitary disease/adenomas.
- Prolactinomas show the greatest propensity to rapidly enlarge in size during pregnancy.
- Can occur in the physiologically enlarged gland during pregnancy.
- Head injury or anticoagulation therapy can be rare causative factors.

Common clinical presentation

- Sudden onset of symptoms.
- Severe headache, nausea and vomiting.
- Bitemporal hemianopia or other visual field defects.
- Reduced visual acuity, colour vision if optic nerve is compressed.
- Cranial nerve palsies – commonly 3rd, 4th and 6th if severe.
- Meningeal symptoms especially after a haemorrhage.
- Hypotension and other features of acute secondary adrenal insufficiency.

Lymphocytic hypophysitis

Key facts

- Rare inflammatory condition of the pituitary gland thought to be autoimmune in nature occurring more commonly in females, usually presenting in late pregnancy or postpartum.
- 20–25% associated with other autoimmune disorders; majority being Hashimoto's thyroiditis.
- Pituitary enlarges due to inflammatory infiltrate.

Common clinical presentation

- More sub-acute in presentation compared with apoplexy.
- Symptoms are mainly due to pressure effects – headaches, visual field defects.
- Hormonal deficiencies can occur and posterior pituitary involvement (diabetes insipidus) will be more common than in other acute pituitary diseases discussed.
- Course is variable and pituitary function can either continue to deteriorate or improve with time.
- Symptoms of acute secondary adrenal insufficiency or hypothyroidism will be more common than gonadotrophin or growth hormone deficiency.

Pre-existing hypopituitarism

Key facts

- Commonly due to previous surgery and/or radiotherapy and pituitary damage due to any other cause.

- Dose of hydrocortisone may need to be increased during pregnancy due to rising CBG levels reducing the bioavailability of hydrocortisone.
- Thyroxine requirement usually increases with advancing pregnancy.
- Vasopressinase synthesised by the placenta will break down vasopressin and those having untreated partial diabetes insipidus may manifest symptoms.
- Unlikely to have pressure or visual symptoms unless an untreated large non-functioning adenoma is present.

Diagnosis

- Essentially clinical as mentioned above.
- Non-contrast CT pituitary to rule out haemorrhage if clinically suspected as in apoplexy and MRI pituitary (diffusion-weighted imaging and special protocols may be able to pick up infarcts early).
- Lymphocytic hypophysitis shows diffuse homogeneous contrast enhancement, in contrast to apoplexy or Sheehan's which will be non-homogeneous, and may characteristically show enlargement of the pituitary stalk and sometimes the absence of the posterior pituitary bright spot when diabetes insipidus is present. Pituitary biopsy will be needed for a definitive diagnosis although not essential for treatment when all typical features are present.
- Hormonal measurement would be purely academic in the acute setting but low prolactin levels seen in association with disruption of other hormonal axes are characteristic of apoplexy and in lymphocytic hypophysitis it can be normal or marginally low and sometimes it can be raised.
- In a sub-acute setting serial hormonal measurements along with clinical assessment would be useful.

Management

- Whatever the underlying cause, acute secondary adrenal insufficiency should be managed immediately with hydrocortisone, fluids and correction of hypoglycaemia if present (as explained earlier in this chapter).
- Fludrocortisone replacement is not necessary as aldosterone production is mainly independent of ACTH control.

- Dexamethasone 4 mg tds (IV/oral) can be used instead of hydrocortisone in severe lymphocytic hypophysitis initially and to reduce the oedema in apoplexy when vision is affected or other cranial nerve involvement is present, although there is no strong evidence of superiority of one over the other.
- If pressure symptoms persist, early surgical decompression via the trans-sphenoidal route would be indicated.
- Deterioration in visual acuity would be an urgent indication.
- Replacement of other anterior pituitary hormones can be done if there is persistent clinical and biochemical evidence of deficiency once the patient has recovered from the initial insult.
- If there is polydipsia and polyuria with increased nocturnal urine volumes and rising plasma osmolality with relatively dilute urine, subcutaneous or oral desmopressin can be given. Strict fluid balance should be maintained and the dose of desmopressin should be adjusted according to the serum electrolytes, plasma and urine osmolalities.

Key pearls

- Never give thyroxine in the acute setting or prior to a few days of proper replacement of hydrocortisone.
- Replacing hydrocortisone may 'unmask' an undiagnosed partial diabetes insipidus.
- Apoplexy always does not need surgery but careful monitoring of visual acuity and other upper cranial nerves is essential.

References

1. Molitch ME. Endocrine emergencies in pregnancy. *Baillières Clin Endocrinol Metab* 1992; 6 (1): 167–191.

2. Momotani N, Nob J, Oyanagi H *et al.* (1986) Antithyroid drug therapy for Graves' disease during pregnancy. *New Engl J Med* 1986; 315: 24–28.

3. Van der Spuy ZM, Jacobs HS. Management of endocrine disorders in pregnancy. Part 1 – thyroid and parathyroid disease. *Postgrad Med J* 1984; 60: 245–252.

4. Schenker JG, Granat M. Phaeochromocytoma and pregnancy – an updated appraisal. *Austral N Z J Obstet Gynaecol* 1982; 22: 1–10.

5. Chandraharan E, Arulkumaran S. Endocrine disorders of pregnancy. *Int J Gynecol Obstet India* 2002; 5: 68–85.

Chapter

31

General anaesthesia and failed intubation

Sarah Hammond and Christina Wood

Key facts

- Definition: Failed intubation is the inability to successfully intubate the trachea after two attempts despite optimal positioning and the use of adjunctive techniques.
- Incidence: 1 in 300. Almost 10 times higher in the obstetric population than in the general surgical population.
- There were no reported deaths from failed intubation in the Confidential Enquiry into Maternal Deaths (CEMACH) 2003–2005 [1]. In the more recent Confidential Enquiry (CMACE 2006–2008) two deaths occurred after airway problems: one after persistent attempts to intubate following the placement of an intubating laryngeal mask; and one after the misplacement of a tracheostomy tube on an intensive care unit [2].
- The incidence of general anaesthesia continues to decline as regional techniques are now performed for complex obstetric indications such as placenta praevia and maternal cardiac conditions that were previously indications for general anaesthesia.
- General anaesthesia may be indicated in cases of urgency, maternal refusal of regional technique, inadequate regional or when regional technique is contraindicated such as in cases of coagulopathy or the use of anticoagulants.
- The Royal College of Anaesthetists' standard for best practice states less than 5% of elective and less than 15% of non-elective

caesarean sections should be under general anaesthetic [3].
- According to NICE, 41% of category 1 caesarean sections were under general anaesthesia in the UK in 2004.

Key implications

Maternal

- Major complications of general anaesthesia include failed intubation, aspiration of gastric contents, increased blood loss and awareness.

  - Anatomical changes in pregnancy such as increased adipose tissue, pharyngeal and laryngeal oedema, large tongue and enlarged breasts result in decreased Mallampati scores and contribute to the likelihood of difficult laryngoscopy. Mallampati scores have also been shown to deteriorate during labour [4, 5].
  - In pregnancy there is an increase in volume and acidity of gastric contents, a reduction in lower oesophageal sphincter tone and raised intra-abdominal pressure due to the gravid uterus. The incidence of acid aspiration in caesarean section under general anaesthesia is 1 in 400–600 [6]. Morbidity is reduced by the use of antacids, prokinetics, head-up tilt and a rapid sequence induction.
  - The average blood loss for caesarean section under general anaesthesia is estimated to be 100–200 ml greater than under regional techniques [7].

Obstetric and Intrapartum Emergencies, ed. Edwin Chandraharan and Sabaratnam Arulkumaran. Published by Cambridge University Press. © Cambridge University Press 2012.

- In the past The Royal College of Anaesthetists has estimated the incidence of awareness to be 1 in 250 during general anaesthesia for caesarean section. This has been attributed to a fear of volatile agents causing over-sedation of the fetus and reduced contractility of the uterus, resulting in the administration of lower doses of anaesthetic drugs.

Neonatal

- Placental transfer of general anaesthetic drugs has been implicated in causing lower 1 minute Apgar scores in neonates [8]. More recently there has been shown to be an increased requirement for resuscitation and intubation in neonates born by caesarean section under general anaesthesia. This was more likely in cases of fetal distress where the fetus may already be compromised to some extent [9].
- Opioids are not used routinely as part of the anaesthetic induction but in cases of maternal cardiac disease or hypertensive disorders of pregnancy opioids may be given in order to attenuate the hypertensive response to laryngoscopy and intubation. These drugs often result in neonatal respiratory depression and the neonatal team must be made aware of their use so that appropriate support may be given.
- Periods of prolonged maternal hypoxia that can occur during a failed intubation may adversely affect neonatal neurological outcome.

Key pointers

- General anaesthesia is often administered in emergency situations and out of hours by trainees whose experience may be limited. It is more commonly required in category 1 caesarean sections when there is a considerable amount of pressure on the anaesthetist to act quickly. The recent reduction in hours worked by junior doctors in the UK due to the European Working Time Directive has compounded this situation.
- Physiological and anatomical changes of pregnancy result in reduced functional residual capacity that is worsened by the supine position. In addition, oxygen requirements and cardiac output are increased resulting in a tendency to rapid oxygen desaturation during periods of apnoea.

Key diagnostic signs for general anaesthesia

- Consent for general anaesthesia is difficult as it is frequently administered in emergency situations. High-risk patients should be identified on the delivery suite allowing earlier identification of problems.
- A full pre-operative assessment including evaluation of the airway must be performed prior to administering general anaesthesia, especially as the obstetric population is becoming more medically complex. Even in the category 1 emergency caesarean section there is time to ascertain a succinct medical and drug history and examine the airway.
- Cardiovascular history is particularly relevant as cardiac disease is the commonest cause of indirect maternal death in the UK.
- Current haemoglobin and confirmation that a valid group and save sample has been processed are equally important.
- Obesity poses specific challenges for general anaesthesia. Regional anaesthetic techniques are preferable but technically more difficult [10, 11]. These patients also have a higher incidence of surgical delivery [12]. Anaesthetic problems relating to obesity include:

  - Increased likelihood of difficult airway management.
  - Reduced chest wall compliance results in high inflation pressures required for ventilation.
  - Anatomical and physiological changes which predispose to oxygen desaturation are exaggerated in the obese parturient.

- A pertinent obstetric history should be elicited to ascertain specific anaesthetic concerns such as: risk of postpartum haemorrhage (PPH), evidence of preeclampsia, multiple surgical deliveries and fetal condition.
- An anaesthetic history is required to identify issues with previous general anaesthetics or a family history of problems. There are two specific conditions of note:

  - Plasma cholinesterase deficiency is an autosomal recessive inherited condition, which results in a reduced level of the enzyme that metabolises suxamethonium. This causes

215

prolonged muscle paralysis and the need for mechanical ventilation and sedation on an intensive care unit.

· Malignant hyperthermia is an autosomal dominant inherited condition. It is a life-threatening condition caused by abnormal skeletal muscle contraction and increased metabolism that results in severe metabolic acidosis, hyperkalaemia, severe pyrexia and rhabdomyolsis. It is triggered by suxamethonium and volatile inhalational anaesthetic agents; consequently these patients must receive total intravenous anaesthesia and the avoidance of suxamethonium.

• A thorough airway evaluation must be performed on all patients presenting for general anaesthesia to identify those with anticipated airway difficulties. The following are a selection of bedside tests which can be performed in less than a minute and can identify potential difficulties with intubation:

· Mouth opening; patient opens mouth as wide as possible. Distance of less than 3 finger breadths between incisors predicts reduced airway access.
· Mallampati assessment; ability to visualise different structures within the oropharynx (Figure 31.1). Grades III and IV are predictors of difficulty.
· Range of neck movement, reduced flexion significantly restricts views at laryngoscopy.
· Thyro-mental distance; distance between the chin and thyroid cartilage of less than 7 cm is a predictor of short neck and difficulty with intubation.
· Jaw protrusion; assesses temporo-mandibular joint movement. The patient attempts to bite their top lip with their lower teeth. Lower incisors should move further forward than the upper. The inability to perform this manoeuvre can also indicate difficulties.
· Prominent dentition; protruding incisors can cause difficulty with instrumenting the airway. Loose teeth pose an aspiration risk if dislodged into the airway.
· Facial trauma or tongue swelling.
· Hoarseness, stridor or change in voice character predict oedema of the larynx and

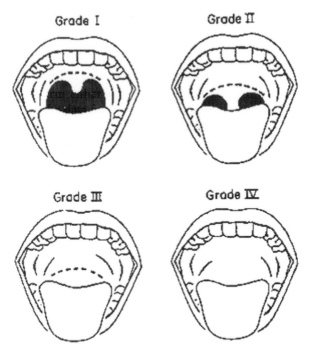

Figure 31.1 Mallampati assessment of airway.

may indicate the need for a smaller endotracheal tube.

General anaesthesia key actions

Equipment and preparation

• Most general anaesthetics are administered in emergency situations therefore drugs and equipment must be prepared in advance. Every 24 hours the anaesthetic machine and airway equipment must be checked and emergency drugs prepared ready for immediate use.
• A size 7 cuffed endotracheal tube is most commonly used, however smaller and bigger tubes must be present on the airway trolley. Different laryngoscopy blades, in addition to the standard Macintosh, are necessary; short handle, McCoy and Polio laryngoscopes can aid intubation in the patient with limited mouth opening and large breasts.
• The gum elastic bougie is a useful adjunct in difficult intubation and is easy and cheap to use. Rescue supra-glottic airway devices, most commonly a laryngeal mask airway, must be readily available on the airway trolley.

Starvation and antacid prophylaxis premedication

- For elective cases patients should be starved for 6 hours for solids and 2 hours for clear fluids. They should also receive pre-operative antacid prophylaxis and metoclopramide to increase gastric emptying. Sodium citrate antacid is also administered orally to all patients just prior to induction due to its short duration of action.
- Women in labour at high risk of surgical intervention should receive regular prophylactic antacid medication.
- All pregnant women beyond the first trimester presenting for general anaesthesia are at risk of aspiration and should receive a rapid sequence induction.

Rapid sequence induction

- The purpose of rapid sequence induction is to secure a definitive airway with a cuffed endotracheal tube as quickly as possible in patients at high risk of aspiration. A force of 30 Newtons of cricoid pressure is applied to the cricoid cartilage to occlude the oesophagus and prevent aspiration of gastric contents. This must be performed by a skilled operator familiar with the technique and can only be removed once tube position is confirmed and the cuff inflated.
- The patient must be appropriately positioned on the operating table to aid intubation, and lateral tilt applied until the baby is delivered to relieve aortocaval compression. Large-bore intravenous access must be secured with intravenous fluids attached and running at an appropriate rate. Mandatory standards of monitoring must be attached; non-invasive blood pressure, pulse oximetry, capnography and three-lead ECG should be in use until the patient is fully awake. Suction must be turned on and easily accessible in case of regurgitation at induction.
- Strict pre-oxygenation is fundamental to a safe rapid sequence induction. The purpose is to ensure an adequate oxygen reservoir to prevent the patient profoundly desaturating when apnoeic. The functional residual capacity is de-nitrogenised by administering 100% oxygen for 3 minutes, or if time is limited by asking the patient to take four vital capacity breaths. Ideally the expired oxygen should be greater than 90% and a capnography trace should be seen to ensure there is an adequate seal of the anaesthetic circuit. This is performed whilst the surgeon is scrubbing and prepping the patient.

- The patient must be reassured that surgery will not commence until anaesthesia has been induced but all preparations are made before starting, to minimise placental transfer to the fetus.
- Specific drugs are licensed for use in rapid sequence induction in obstetrics.

  - Thiopentone is a barbiturate used to induce anaesthesia. The dose is 3–5 mg/kg, it has a quick onset of action causing unconsciousness within one arm to brain circulation time, and the half-life is 3 minutes.
  - Suxamethonium is a depolarising muscle relaxant. The dose is 1–2 mg/kg, the time of onset is 30 seconds leading to widespread fasciculations followed by rapid paralysis that facilitates intubation; it has a half-life of 3 minutes.

- Commencement of surgery should only occur once intubation has been confirmed with capnography, bilateral chest movement and audible bilateral air entry. Clear communication with the obstetrician is essential.

Peri-operative care

- Anaesthesia is typically maintained by ventilation with 1% isoflurane, a volatile inhalational agent, in a mixture of 50% oxygen and 50% nitrous oxide until delivery. This can then be reduced to a 40 : 60 ratio. Nitrous oxide has anaesthetic and analgesic properties that allow a lower inspired fraction of volatile agent to be used. Volatile agents can contribute to uterine atony.
- Awareness, a state of muscle paralysis but without loss of consciousness, occurred in the past when very low doses of anaesthetic agent were used to minimise placental transfer to the fetus. The advent of inhalational agent monitoring through minimum alveolar concentration (MAC) has reduced the incidence of awareness. Additional muscle relaxation may be required to assist mechanical ventilation if surgery is prolonged. A non-depolarising agent is used with duration of action of 20 minutes.

- Following delivery of the baby 5 IU of syntocinon should be given by slow intravenous infusion to aid uterine contraction and placental delivery followed by an infusion of 40 IU over 4 hours in cases at high risk of PPH. A prophylactic dose of broad-spectrum antibiotic is also given.
- The patient must be extubated when fully awake in the left lateral position, after ensuring adequate protective airway reflexes have returned.
- Intra-operative analgesia without a preceding regional technique should be multimodal: intravenous paracetamol, non-steroidal anti-inflammatory drug such as diclofenac, if no contraindication, and morphine. Postoperative analgesia can be provided by intermittent oral morphine or intravenous morphine via a patient-controlled analgesia device. Alternative techniques include ultrasound-guided transversus abdominis plane (TAP) block with local anaesthetic.
- A neonatal resuscitation team must be in attendance for all deliveries requiring general anaesthesia. They must be informed of indications for caesarean section and if maternal opiates have been given.

Key diagnostic signs of failed intubation

- A thorough airway assessment, as detailed previously, is the best way of predicting difficulties with intubation. If difficulties are anticipated it is imperative to call for senior help early and reconsider the need for a general anaesthetic. This should be communicated to the obstetrician as maternal safety must be paramount. Cases of unanticipated failed intubation still occur despite a favourable airway assessment. Capnography is mandatory for all general anaesthesia cases to detect oesophageal intubation. A consistent endtidal CO_2 will only be seen if the endotracheal tube is positioned within the trachea or bronchus.
- In all general anaesthetic cases a rescue airway device must be ready for use prior to induction and strict pre-oxygenation for 3 minutes and endtidal oxygen of 90% achieved.
- The patient position should be optimised in the first instance. For an obese patient this requires ramping the head, neck and upper body with

pillows to ensure horizontal alignment between the sternal notch and external auditory meatus. Arms should be placed on arm boards to either side of patient.

- If difficulties are encountered with intubation:
  - Adjust head and/or neck position.
  - Adjust cricoid pressure which may have been incorrectly applied.
  - Use alternative laryngoscope, gum elastic bougie or smaller tube.
  - A second dose of suxamethonium is absolutely contraindicated.

Key actions

A failed intubation occurs following two unsuccessful attempts despite improving the patient position and conditions. The anaesthetist must declare a failed intubation out loud to the theatre team, ask for senior help and immediately proceed to the failed intubation algorithm. This should be practised regularly as part of an obstetric drill exercise. The management algorithm is outlined below.

- Ask for help: contact senior anaesthetist.
- Oxygenate the patient with 100% oxygen via face mask; an oropharyngeal airway may aid airway management.
- Cricoid pressure may need to be released to aid face mask ventilation.
- If no improvement in oxygen saturation, proceed to:
  - Insertion of LMA (classic, ILMA or proseal depending on familiarity of use).
- If still no improvement in oxygen saturation, proceed to:
  - Needle/surgical cricothyroidotomy.
- If clinical circumstances allow maintain the airway, abandon procedure and wake the mother. A regional technique or an awake fibreoptic intubation must be utilised next time.
- In cases of maternal cardiac arrest or massive haemorrhage maternal wake-up is not feasible. Airway must be maintained with 100% oxygen and manual ventilation must continue until spontaneous respiration returns.
- Needle or surgical cricothyroidotomy must be performed in cases of 'can't intubate can't

ventilate' (CIVCV) scenario as a last attempt to maintain maternal oxygenation.

Cricothryroidotomy

This is a life-saving rescue airway procedure performed in cases of severe hypoxia when all other airway manouvres have been unsuccessful. The cricothyroid membrane is avascular and has clear anatomical landmarks making it easy to identify and therefore ideal for emergency airway access. A cannula over needle technique should only be employed if a high-pressure jet ventilation system is available. Otherwise a small endotracheal tube (size 5) can be inserted through an incision in the membrane.

Key pitfalls

- Many general anaesthetics are given out of hours in emergency situations by a relatively junior anaesthetist.
- The urgency of the clinical situation often causes added anxiety for the clinical team.
- Inadequate pre-assessment and lack of recognition of the difficult airway.
- Inadequate checking of equipment and no immediate availability of rescue techniques such as LMA.
- Omission of antacid medication, especially sodium citrate, prior to induction of anaesthesia.
- Inadequate pre-oxygenation due to the urgency of the obstetric management.
- Failure to wait long enough for suxamethonium to work, or an inadequate dose causing difficulties with intubation.
- Inadequate positioning of patient for intubation.
- Incorrectly applied cricoid pressure can distort the view at laryngoscopy.
- Distorted situational awareness, especially the time taken to call for help.
- Failure to recognise oesophageal intubation with a lack of capnography trace.
- Remember – lack of oxygen kills, not lack of intubation.

Key pearls

- Thorough airway assessment of all women presenting to anaesthetist for interventions.
- Two anaesthetists present for emergency general anaesthesia for caesarean section.

- Mandatory capnography to confirm correct endotracheal tube placement.
- Difficult-airway trolley which is regularly checked and is familiar to all anaesthetists who use it.
- Regular rehearsal of a failed intubation drill with all team members including 'Can't intubate, can't ventilate' scenario.

Management in a low-resource setting

- Thorough airway assessment – to be forewarned is to be forearmed.
- The gum elastic bougie is a simple and cheap aid to difficult intubation.
- Good communication with all team members including midwives and obstetricians.
- Awareness of risks and management of failed intubation by the whole team.
- Rehearsal of drills and identification of role of each team member in emergency situations.

References

1. The Confidential Enquiry into Maternal and Child Health (CEMACH). *Saving Mothers' Lives': Reviewing Maternal Deaths to make Motherhood Safer – 2003–2005. The Seventh Report on Confidential Enquiries into Maternal Deaths in the United Kingdom.* London: CEMACH, 2007.

2. Centre for Maternal and Child Enquiries (CMACE). *Saving Mothers' Lives: Reviewing Maternal Deaths to make Motherhood Safer – 2006–2008. The Eighth Report on Confidential Enquiries into Maternal Deaths in the United Kingdom. Br J Obstet Gynaecol* 2011; 118 (Suppl. 1): 1–208.

3. http://www.rcoa.ac.uk/docs/arb-section8

4. Pilkington S, Carli F, Dakin MJ *et al.* Increase in Mallampati score in pregnancy. *Br J Anaesth* 1995; 74 (**6**): 638–642.

5. Boutonnet M, Faitot V, Katz A *et al.* Mallampati class changes during pregnancy, labour and after delivery: can these be predicted? *Br J Anaesth* 2010; 104 (1): 67–70.

6. Rawlinson E, Mincon A. Pulmonary aspiration. *Anaesth Intensive Care* 2007; 8: 365–367.

7. Afolabi BB, Lesi FE, Merah NA. Regional versus general anaesthesia for caesarean section. *Cochrane Database Syst Rev* 2006; 18 (4):CD004350.

8. Reynolds F, Seed PT. Anaesthesia for caesarean section and neonatal acid-base status analysis. *Anaesthesia* 2005; 60 (7): 636–653.

9. Algert CS, Bowen JR, Giles BW *et al*. Regional block versus general anaesthesia for caesarean section and neonatal outcomes: a population based study. *BMC Med* 2009; 7: 20.

10. Vricella LK, Louis JM, Mercer BM *et al*. Anaesthesia complications during scheduled caesearean delivery for morbidly obese women. *Am J Obstet Gynecol* 2010; 203 (3): 276. E1–5.

11. Hood DD, Dewan DM. Anaesthetic and obstetric outcome in morbidly obese parturients. *Anaesthesiology* 1993; 79 (6); 1210–1218.

12. Weiss JL, Malone FD, Emig D *et al*. Obesity, obstetric complications and caesarean delivery rate. A population-based screening study. *Am J Obstet Gynecol* 2004; 190: 1091–1097.

Chapter

32

Fluid overload and underload

Renate Wendler

Key facts

- Definitions:
  - Overload – Excessive accumulation of fluid in the body – intravascular, interstitial and/or intracellular.
  - Underload – Marked decrease in the amount of fluid in the body – intravascular, interstitial and/or intracellular.

- The maternal body accumulates water in pregnancy. Total body water can increase by up to 8 litres. Plasma osmolality decreases by about 10 milliosmol/kg below non-pregnant levels [1]. Oestrogens increase plasma renin activity with enhanced renal sodium absorption and water retention (renin–angiotensin–aldosterone system) [2]. These changes promote sufficient placental perfusion. Reduced maternal plasma volume is associated with abnormal pregnancy outcome [3].

- The normal human heart is able to tolerate recurrent episodes of pregnancy-related volume overload without compromising normal function [4].

- Disturbances in the cardiovascular system and the regulation of fluid balance can lead to changes in blood pressure and to hypotension or hypertension. Imbalance in salt and fluid regulation is common and can cause oedema in later stages of pregnancy. During labour, demands on the regulatory systems further increase.

- The re-absorptive capacity of renal tubules for sodium, chloride and water increases by as much as 50% due to increased production of steroid hormones by the placenta and adrenal cortex. Glomerular filtration rate can increase by up to 50% during pregnancy, with increase of water and electrolyte excretion in the urine [5].

- Whilst in the first and second trimester maternal fluid regulation appears normal, water load is not easily excreted in the last trimester. Fluid regulation is more vulnerable with the risk of overload and underload [1].

- In the postpartum period, mobilisation of fluids can lead to a drop in colloid osmotic pressure of up to 30%.

- All the outlined physiological changes to maternal fluid balance through the stages of pregnancy emphasise the need for careful fluid management, especially in patients with underlying medical disease or acute illness.

- Incidence of pulmonary oedema in pregnancy: approximately 0.08% [6].

Key implications

Fluid overload

- Pulmonary oedema, although uncommon in pregnancy, is associated with an increase in maternal and fetal morbidity and mortality.

Obstetric and Intrapartum Emergencies, ed. Edwin Chandraharan and Sabaratnam Arulkumaran. Published by Cambridge University Press. © Cambridge University Press 2012.

- In patients with preeclampsia, fluid overload can lead to cerebral oedema with high maternal mortality [7].
- If necessary, central venous access and non-invasive cardiac output monitoring should be established to guide fluid therapy in critically ill pregnant patients who present with signs of fluid overload.

Fluid Underload

- Inadequate plasma volume expansion in pregnancy is linked to poor fetal outcome.
- Patients with preeclampsia have decreased plasma volume and are at higher risk of fluid balance disturbance [7].
- Volume loss due to hyperemesis gravidarum or haemorrhage can lead to maternal hypotension, collapse and fetal distress due to poor placental perfusion.
- Severe hypovolaemia and hypovolaemic shock can lead to reduced organ perfusion and multi-organ failure including myocardial infarction and stroke.

Key pointers

Risk factors for fluid overload

- Use of tocolytic agents: Simultaneous use of (multiple) tocolytic agents, particularly ritodrine and terbutaline, is a relatively common cause of maternal pulmonary oedema. This may be explained by the prolonged catecholamine exposure with maternal myocardial dysfunction, changes in pulmonary capillary permeability and also iatrogenic volume overload due to maternal tachycardia and attempted fetal resuscitation.
- Maternal cardiac disease: Diminished myocardial function or cardiac outflow tract obstruction frequently deteriorates in pregnancy with a high risk of peripheral and/or pulmonary oedema and congestive cardiac failure. Patients with hypertension can develop diastolic cardiac dysfunction and left ventricular hypertrophy with reduced cardiac compliance to fluid challenges. The majority of cardiac deaths in pregnancy occur with no previous cardiac history, therefore it is important to pay attention to cardiac risk factors (maternal age, lifestyle, ethnicity, clinical history) when administering intravenous fluids.

- Severe infection: In patients with sepsis and generalised increase in capillary permeability, fluid resuscitation should be guided by invasive haemodynamic monitoring.
- Preeclampsia: Preeclampsia leads to endothelial damage with increased capillary permeability and decreased colloid osmotic pressure [6]. In addition, there is a frequent increase in peripheral vascular resistance with myocardial diastolic dysfunction. These patients are at a high risk of fluid overload and should be treated with fluid restriction and close monitoring of their fluid balance.
- Iatrogenic fluid overload: Common in patients with long, complicated labour and frequent episodes of fetal distress, when fluid boluses are given to restore normal maternal haemodynamic state. It is important to monitor the fluid intake of all patients in labour and postpartum carefully.

Risk factors for fluid underload

- Underlying medical disease: Diarrhoea and vomiting, hyperemesis gravidarum and/or endocrine disorders can lead to significant volume underload with hypotension or maternal collapse.
- Haemorrhage: This remains the leading cause of maternal mortality and morbidity worldwide. Young healthy pregnant women can lose up to 30% of their blood volume without significant haemodynamic disturbance. The blood pressure can remain normal for a while with anxiety or confusion, combined with tachycardia and oliguria, as the first signs of significant fluid underload. It is important to have a high index of suspicion especially in cases of concealed haemorrhage.

Key diagnostic signs

Fluid overload

- Peripheral oedema, dyspnoea, tachypnoea, inappropriate weight gain.
- Paroxysmal nocturnal dyspnoea, inability to lie flat.
- End-expiratory crackles on auscultation, pink frothy sputum.
- Hypoxia and radiological signs of pulmonary oedema in chest X-ray (Figure 32.1).

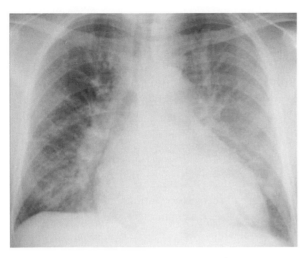

Figure 32.1 Chest X-ray showing pulmonary oedema.

Fluid underload

- Tachycardia, nausea and vomiting, light-headedness, confusion, collapse.
- Dry skin and mouth, skin flushing, dark-coloured (concentrated) urine.
- Hypotension and oliguria.

Key actions

Strict attention must be paid to fluid balance. This includes careful monitoring of fluid input and output on an early-warning or high-dependency chart in a dedicated high-dependency unit. A senior clinician should have the overall responsibility of the management. Consultant obstetric anaesthetists and/or intensivists should be involved early as part of a multidisciplinary approach. Always check for signs of fetal distress due to maternal compromise and consider early delivery to improve maternal outcome.

Fluid overload

If the patient is distressed with pulmonary oedema start treatment before investigations.

Principles of management

- Look for causes of volume overload, e.g. underlying cardiac disease, sepsis, tocolytic therapy or preeclampsia.
- Administer oxygen – position the patient upright. Check airway, breathing and circulation. Remember laryngeal swelling can make mask ventilation and/or intubation significantly more

difficult, therefore careful airway assessment is essential. Establish venous access – this may be difficult because of extensive peripheral oedema. Consider central venous access and/or invasive haemodynamic monitoring with arterial line.

- Urinary catheter with hourly fluid balance – aim for urine output > 0.5 ml/kg per hour [8]. Patients with preeclampsia will frequently have a brief period of oliguria up to 6 hours after delivery. This should be anticipated and not overcorrected [7].
- Fluid restriction – pay attention to intravenous drug therapy in addition to fluid maintenance. Overall fluid input should not exceed 85 ml/hour or 1 ml/kg per hour. It may often be necessary to double/triple concentrations of drugs to avoid infusion of excessive amounts of fluid. The choice between colloid or crystalloid solutions remains controversial. Crystalloid may reduce plasma colloid pressure even further. Colloid solutions may contribute to volume overload during postpartum fluid mobilisation [9]. Use colloid solutions if the colloid osmotic pressure is markedly decreased (< 12 mmHg).
- Take blood for renal and liver function (including albumin) tests and full blood count. Consider blood gas analysis, especially in cases where the cause of fluid overload is unclear.
- Arrange for a chest X-ray to identify pulmonary oedema but look for other underlying causes (pneumonia, cardiac disease).
- Consider central venous pressure (CVP) monitoring. Non-invasive cardiac output monitoring and echocardiography may be useful in patients with severe preeclampsia or underlying cardiac disease.
- Use diuretics in cases of acute pulmonary oedema with underlying cardiac disease or iatrogenic fluid overload. The use of diuretics in patients with preeclampsia is still controversial because of the hypovolaemic state of preeclamptic patients, despite the presence of peripheral oedema. The current opinion is to avoid diuretic therapy in these cases [7].

Fluid underload

Look for signs of hypovolaemic shock with cardiac, renal or other organ failure and call for help accordingly. Restoration of normovolaemia is the first priority. Remember that young pregnant patients may lose large volumes without obvious cardiovascular disturbance.

Principles of management

- Look for causes of volume depletion, especially haemorrhage and treat accordingly.
- Administer oxygen. Check airway, breathing and circulation. Establish venous access.
- Take blood for cross matching, full blood count (FBC), clotting and electrolytes.
- Replace circulating volume with crystalloid or colloid infusion. An initial fluid challenge of 1000 ml in 250 ml boluses is well tolerated by a young, fit pregnant woman (beware of underlying preeclampsia).
- Urinary catheter with hourly fluid balance. Aim for urine output > 0.5 ml/kg per hour.
- If bleeding is the underlying cause of hypovolaemia, give blood as soon as possible. Only use uncross-matched O negative blood in cases of massive haemorrhage (> 40% of circulating blood volume).
- Remember the risk of dilutional coagulopathy in cases of massive volume replacement. Always substitute fresh frozen plasma and platelets in cases of massive transfusion. Check FBC and clotting (including fibrinogen) regularly.
- Establish invasive haemodynamic monitoring (CVP and arterial line) in cases of ongoing volume loss [10].

Key pitfalls

- Failure to involve experienced clinicians early.
- Failure to call for help/communicate clearly in an emergency.
- Failure to use obstetric early-warning chart for maternal surveillance.

Volume overload

- Failure to anticipate risk factors for volume overload in pregnancy.
- Uncontrolled fluid challenges in patients with preeclampsia and/or impaired renal function.
- Use of multiple tocolytic agents simultaneously without attention to side effects.
- Failure to diagnose and treat pulmonary oedema promptly and adequately.

- Failure to recognise underlying cardiac disease in pregnancy.

Volume underload

- False reassurance from normal blood pressure readings in relation to degree of volume depletion. Young healthy patients can tolerate large volume loss without initial blood pressure changes.
- Failure to restore normovolaemia as a first priority to prevent organ damage.
- Failure to recognise dilutional coagulopathy in cases of severe haemorrhage and massive transfusion.
- Failure to keep patient warm.

Key pearls

- All staff providing intrapartum care should undergo regular skills and drills training on maternal early warning charts, management of the sick obstetric patient and massive obstetric haemorrhage.
- Lessons learned from confidential enquiries into maternal deaths and adverse incidents should be disseminated to the entire team.
- All staff should have regular updates on basic life-support skills.

Management in low-resource settings

Maternal fluid overload and underload can be life threatening for the mother and fetus and require immediate attention by a senior clinician, ideally in a multidisciplinary team. If facilities for high-dependency care and invasive haemodynamic monitoring are unavailable, it is important to concentrate efforts on strict control of fluid balance.

Fluid overload

Patients with clinical signs of fluid overload should be positioned upright and oxygen administered. Fluid input should be restricted and hourly urine output noted, as well as vital parameters recorded. In cases of respiratory compromise diuretics should be administered.

Fluid underload

Restoration of normovolaemia should be the first priority. Venous access should be established and an initial fluid challenge of 1000 ml crystalloid or colloid solution in 250 ml boluses administered. Further fluid boluses may be necessary in cases of continued volume loss to prevent hypovolaemic shock. In cases of haemorrhage the cause of bleeding should be established and treated immediately.

Case study

Your patient is a 39-year-old primigravida who develops preeclampsia at 36 weeks' gestation. Labour is induced at 37 weeks due to worsening of her preeclampsia. She has a prolonged first stage of labour with oxytocin augmentation, but unfortunately has to have an emergency caesarean section because of fetal distress at 8 cm dilation. She loses 800 ml of blood during surgery due to uterine atony and receives crystalloid and colloid infusions in theatre. She is now 3 hours post-surgery and is still on a postoperative oxytocin infusion. She has not received a blood transfusion. Her baby is doing well and stays with the mother.

Your patient is cared for on an obstetric high-dependency unit and monitored with an obstetric early-warning chart, and has so far showed no abnormalities apart from poor urine output (10–20 ml/hour), which is attributed to the oxytocin infusion. She is on fluid restriction of 85 ml/hour and currently kept nil by mouth.

At shift handover, the patient is found to be slightly breathless, with SpO_2% of 95% on air, respiratory rate 20/min, BP 102/82 mmHg and pulse 120/min. On auscultation of the chest, there are a few basal crackles. Her urine is very concentrated and she has passed 10 ml in the last hour. On examination her peripheries are cold with partially mottled skin. She does not complain of any pain, but seems slightly confused.

Differential diagnosis should include:

- *Sepsis with fluid underload*. Tachypnoea, poor oxygenation, tachycardia can be early signs of evolving maternal sepsis. Cold peripheries and mottled skin are classical signs for evolving septic shock. The history of prolonged first stage could also support the diagnosis. Clinical examination should focus on signs of infection (foul-smelling discharge) in search for a focus.

- *Cardiac failure with fluid overload*. Maternal age is a risk factor for cardiac problems in pregnancy. Especially in combination with preeclampsia, myocardial diastolic dysfunction can be expected, and this may lead to congestive cardiac failure with pulmonary oedema and oliguria. The blood pressure appears to be relatively normal, is however low for a preeclamptic patient and could suggest myocardial failure. Clinical examination should focus on signs of congestive cardiac failure (raised jugular venous pressure, peripheral oedema and third heart sound).

- *Hypovolaemia/haemorrhage with fluid underload.* The history of postpartum haemorrhage during the caesarean section with a blood loss of 800 ml should raise suspicion of further haemorrhage. Tachycardia and oliguria are typical signs of hypovolaemia. Blood pressure is probably low for a preeclamptic patient; however, hypotension is usually a late sign for fluid underload in pregnant patients. Clinical examination should focus on signs of haemorrhage (open or concealed).

It is important to establish a diagnosis quickly as this patient is already showing signs of haemodynamic compromise. Basic measures should include high-flow oxygen via face mask and adequate intravenous access. Observations including temperature should be checked regularly. Urgent blood samples should be sent for full blood count (FBC), clotting, electrolytes, renal function and sepsis parameters. It is important to note that initially normal haemoglobin may not reflect the extent of haemorrhage until fluid resuscitation occurs.

Outcome

A thorough clinical examination found a large uterus, tender on palpation. There were no signs of sepsis or cardiac failure. The patient was transferred to theatre with a diagnosis of concealed postpartum haemorrhage, which was confirmed by ultrasound. Intraoperative findings were 1.5 litres of blood clots in the uterine cavity, possibly due to an atonic uterus immediately after caesarean section.

A massive obstetric haemorrhage call was put out and blood products were administered accordingly. The patient was stabilised and had a full recovery with discharge 4 days postpartum.

References

1. Risberg A. Hormones and fluid balance during pregnancy, labor and post partum. *Digital Comprehensive Summaries of Uppsala Dissertations from the Faculty of Medicine* 2009; 478.

2. Wilson M, Morganti AA, Zervoudakis I *et al.* Blood pressure, the renin-aldosterone system and sex steroids throughout normal pregnancy. *Am J Med* 1980; 68: 97–104.

3. Bernstein IM, Ziegler W, Badger GJ. Plasma volume expansion in early pregnancy. *Obstet Gynecol* 2001; 97: 669–672.

4. Katz R, Karliner JS, Resnik R. Effects of a natural volume overload state (pregnancy) on left ventricular performance in normal human subjects. *Circulation* 1978; 58: 434–441.

5. Dunlop W. Serial changes in renal haemodynamics during normal human pregnancy. *Br J Obstet Gynaecol* 1981; 88: 1–9.

6. Sciscione A, Ivester T, Largoza M *et al.* Acute pulmonary oedema in pregnancy. *Obstet Gynecol* 2003; 101: 511–515.

7. Engelhardt T, MacLennan FM. Fluid management in pre-eclampsia. *Int J Obstet Anesth* 1999; 8: 253–259.

8. Mackenzie MJ, Woolnough MJ, Barrett N, Johnson MR, Yentis SM. Normal urine output after elective caesarean section: an observational study. *Int J Obstet Anesth* 2010; 19: 379–383.

9. Park GE, Hauch ME, Curlin F, Datta S, Bader AM. The effects of varying volumes of crystalloid administration before caesarean delivery on maternal haemodynamics and colloid oncotic pressure. *Anaesth Analg* 1996; 83: 299–303.

10. ASA Task Force on Obstetric Anesthesia. Practice guidelines for obstetric anesthesia: an updated report by the American Society of Anesthesiologists Task Force on Obstetric Anesthesia. *Anesthesiology* 2007; 106: 843–863.

Chapter

33

Transfusion, anaphylactic and drug reactions
Transfusion reactions

Rehana Iqbal and Cheron Bailey

Key facts

- Definition: An adverse effect that results from transfusion of blood or blood products.
- Serious or life-threatening reactions are rare but symptoms and signs must be taken seriously, as they may be early warnings of a serious reaction.

Acute complications

- Acute haemolytic reaction.
- Infusion of a blood pack contaminated by bacteria.
- Transfusion-related acute lung injury.
- Transfusion-associated circulatory overload.
- Allergic reactions.

  - Anaphylaxis.
  - Less severe allergic reactions.
  - Febrile non-haemolytic transfusion reactions.

Delayed complications [1]

- Delayed haemolytic transfusion reaction.
- Transfusion associated graft-versus-host disease.
- Post-transfusion purpura.
- Iron overload.

Infections

- Viral, bacterial and others.

Other

- Massive blood transfusion [2].

Immune reactions

- Immune haemolytic reactions are due to sensitisation of the recipient to donor red cells, white cells, platelets or plasma proteins.
- Immune non-haemolytic reactions are due to sensitisation of the recipient to donor white cells, platelets or plasma proteins.

Acute haemolytic reactions

- Most commonly due to ABO incompatibility and are reported with a frequency of about 1 : 250 000 transfusions. The risk of a fatal reaction is about 1 : 1 000 000 transfusions [3].

Delayed haemolytic reactions

- These are generally mild and usually caused by antibodies to non-D antigens of the Rh system and several other antibodies such as Kell and Duffy systems. Typically, these occur about 1–2 weeks after the transfusion. The incidence is about 1 : 1000 transfusions.

Non-haemolytic immune reactions

- Febrile reactions 1 : 200 transfusions. Most febrile reactions are due to the immune destruction of leukocytes or platelets.
- Urticarial reactions 1 : 200 transfusions. Cutaneous allergic reactions.
- Anaphylactic reactions 1 : 150 000. Individuals with antibodies against IgA molecules may develop these when exposed to plasma-containing components.

Obstetric and Intrapartum Emergencies, ed. Edwin Chandraharan and Sabaratnam Arulkumaran. Published by Cambridge University Press. © Cambridge University Press 2012.

- Post-transfusion purpura (PTP). This is a rare but potentially lethal complication of transfusion of red cells or platelets. It is more often seen in female patients. It is caused by platelet-specific alloantibodies. Typically 5 to 9 days after transfusion, the patient develops an extremely low platelet count with bleeding [4].
- Immunosuppression is more common especially with blood products containing leukocytes.

Infections

Viral infections such as hepatitis are especially due to hepatitis B and C viruses.

The incidence of hepatitis B is low because of better screening and most viral hepatitis is caused by hepatitis C. Although the signs and symptoms are mild, it can lead to chronic liver disease and later on to hepatocellular carcinoma.

Acquired immune deficiency syndrome (AIDS) is caused by human immunodeficiency virus (HIV). This has a window period of 6–8 weeks during which the antibody cannot be detected after donor infection. It is very rare for a blood product bag (1 : 4 000 000) to pass undetected.

Others such as cytomegalovirus and Epstein–Barr virus illnesses, Creutzfeldt–Jakob disease, bacterial, malaria and other parasitic infections can also occur.

Adverse effects from massive blood transfusion

Coagulopathy

Coagulopathy results from the dilution and consumption of platelets and clotting factors. It is important to regularly check clotting as well as the platelet count during massive blood transfusion. The thromboelastograph may be useful in this situation to give information about clot formation and lysis. 1 : 1 : 1 of red cell : FFP : platelet regimens, as used by the military, are useful in preventing coagulopathy in patients requiring massive transfusion.

Hypothermia

If cold blood is given too quickly and not warmed, this may lead to severe metabolic changes, arrhythmias and a worsening of coagulopathy. It also shifts the oxygen dissociation curve (ODC) to the left with increased affinity for oxygen and therefore less oxygen unloading to the tissues.

Citrate toxicity

Citrate anticoagulant found in blood units can bind to calcium and lead to hypocalcaemia. This is more pronounced in the presence of hypothermia and hepatic dysfunction. Citrate is converted to bicarbonate eventually and this may lead to a metabolic alkalosis, with a left shift of the ODC.

Hyperkalaemia

The longer blood is stored, the higher the extracellular concentration of potassium, and with high infusion rates this can lead to hyperkalaemia.

Transfusion-related acute lung injury (TRALI)

This is a severe respiratory disorder following transfusion of blood or blood products. It is more common with transfusion containing high volumes of plasma. The clinical presentation is very similar to acute lung injury (ALI) and cardiogenic pulmonary oedema. Hypoxia and pulmonary infiltrates are present but without a raised CVP, high JVP or gallop rhythm as in cardiogenic pulmonary oedema. It usually occurs within 1–6 hours after blood transfusion. Management is supportive using lung protective strategies.

Transfusion-associated circulatory overload (TACO)

This is more likely in patients with preexisting cardiac disease.

Key implications

- Rhesus immunisation – if a rhesus negative mother is given rhesus positive blood, then the mother can develop IgG antibodies. During this and subsequent pregnancies the antibodies are able to cross the placenta into the baby and will destroy the red blood cells of her rhesus positive baby.
- Transfusion reactions can increase the risk of infections due to immunomodulation.
- Reactions can be fatal to mother and baby if severe.

Key pointers

- In the majority of cases, acute haemolytic reactions due to ABO incompatibility are caused by misidentification of the patient, patient's blood specimen or the transfusion blood product bag.
- Poor screening of donors by medical history and investigations can lead to disease transmission.

Massive transfusion reaction

Key diagnostic signs

- Acute haemolytic reactions: chills, fever, chest and flank pain, tachycardia, hypotension, haemoglobinuria, and generalised oozing. Disseminated intravascular coagulation (DIC) may develop rapidly.
- Delayed haemolytic reactions: malaise, jaundice and fever.
- Febrile reactions: fever.
- Urticarial reactions: urticarial rash – pale red raised itchy areas, also called hives and look like nettle stings.
- Anaphylactic reactions are discussed later in this chapter.
- Others due to massive transfusion are outlined above.

Key sctions

For acute haemolytic reactions, stop the blood transfusion, recheck the blood product bag against the blood slip or patient's blood number and the patient's identity bracelet (or using local blood-checking protocols). Pretransfusion and post-transfusion tests may have to be repeated. Supportive therapy should be instituted for hypotension, bleeding, shock, renal failure.

Febrile reactions can be prevented by using leukocyte-poor components.

Urticarial reactions can be managed by slowing the transfusion and using antihistamines.

Anaphylactic reactions are discussed later in this chapter.

Key pitfalls

- Failure to fill out request forms and label tubes properly can lead to delays/incompatibility issues. Be diligent with checks when filling out forms and tubes.
- Delays in calling for help in an emergency setting. Calling for help early can save lives.

Key pearls

- Try to ensure cross matching of patients is done in advance if possible, as cross-matching of blood components under time-pressured situations may lead to errors.

- Errors often arise in labelling sample tubes and/or request forms or from inadequate checks at the time of transfusion. Always ask the patient to state their name and date of birth if they are conscious and able to do so.
- A meticulous surgical technique will help to avoid unnecessary blood loss.
- Ensure individuals administering blood components are competent and trained to do so.
- Avoid unnecessary transfusion. Always correlate the clinical picture with blood results. A single unit transfusion is now acceptable practice.
- Check baseline vitals prior to starting a blood component transfusion and then check vitals again in 15 minutes, and then at most 1 hour after the transfusion.
- Regular visual checks during the transfusion.
- Adverse reactions may occur within 24 hours after discharge therefore patients should be given a contact number and advised to call or return if they have any concerns after discharge.

Anaphylactic reactions

Key facts

- Definition: Anaphylaxis is a life-threatening, generalised hypersensitivity reaction.

Types:

- Allergic anaphylaxis.
- Non-allergic anaphylaxis.

Allergic anaphylaxis and non-allergic anaphylaxis are usually indistinguishable clinically. Allergic anaphylaxis applies only when the reaction is mediated by an immunological mechanism such as immunoglobulins E and G or complement activation by immune complexes and non-allergic applies when there are direct mast cell-releasing agents or agents that presumably alter arachidonic acid metabolism. 'Anaphylactoid' was previously used to describe non-IgE-mediated reactions but the European Academy of Allergy and Clinical Immunology has chosen to use the classification of allergic vs non-allergic reactions.

Examples of allergic anaphylaxis include reactions to penicillin, latex and suxamethonium. Examples of non-allergic anaphylaxis include reactions to atracurium, opiates and NSAIDS. Allergic reactions usually require prior exposure to an agent whereas a non-allergic reaction does not require prior exposure. The most common cause of anaphylaxis encountered in a hospital setting appears to be parenteral antibiotics, latex and intravenous contrast drugs. Anaphylaxis associated with anaesthesia and surgery includes reactions to the neuromuscular blocking agents listed above followed by latex, antibiotics, hypnotics and colloids.

The incidence of anaphylaxis varies globally but has been estimated at between 1 in 10 000 and 20 000.

Key implications

Anaphylaxis in obstetrics may be life threatening not only for the pregnant mother but also for the fetus. If anaphylaxis occurs at the time of a caesarean section, then the diagnosis may be difficult to make. There might be some confusion identifying the offending agent because several drugs are administered at the same time. Clinical features are usually exacerbated by the physiological changes of pregnancy including aortocaval compression and the effects of anaesthesia.

Key pointers

Unfortunately, it is difficult to predict when these reactions will occur in someone who is not previously known to have an allergic reaction. Previous exposure to an agent is necessary for allergic type reactions to be predicted. A history of atopy has not been shown to be a predisposing factor. It is important to highlight when someone has had a previous anaphylactic reaction in the case notes and drug chart. The patient should wear an alert bracelet at all times and a letter should be given to the patient and GP about the reaction.

Key diagnostic signs

Anaphylaxis usually occurs within minutes of exposure to the offending agent. The main clinical features in the order in which they appear to occur most frequently include cardiovascular collapse (commonest feature), erythema, rash, urticaria, bronchospasm and angioedema. All of the signs do not have to be present to make the diagnosis, they may occur in isolation or there may be different combinations of signs.

Key actions

In anaphylaxis, early recognition is very important. First-line treatment should include discontinuing the offending or suspected agent. The management should commence with using an ABC (**A**irway, **B**reathing and **C**irculation) approach.

First of all ensure the patient's airway is patent and the patient is breathing, administer high-flow oxygen, check the circulation, give adrenaline and start intravenous fluids simultaneously. Intravenous fluids should be commenced at about 20 ml/kg, and then reassess the patient. Adrenaline should be given intramuscularly 0.5 mg initially and repeat in 5–10 minutes if necessary. Adrenaline works by increasing the systemic vascular resistance and will treat the hypotension. It also produces bronchodilation by acting on the B_2 receptors and this will treat bronchospasm. Left lateral tilt should be instituted to avoid aortocaval compression in the pregnant mother of greater than 20 weeks' gestation. Intravenous hydrocortisone 200 mg and chlorpheniramine 10 mg are second-line drugs recommended for reducing further inflammatory response. Bronchodilators may also be required.

Take blood samples at 1, 6 and 24 hours for tryptase (the enzyme normally present in mast cells) levels. The normal tryptase levels are 1–15 ng/ml. In systemic anaphylaxis, a level greater than 15 ng/ml is significant. Refer the patient to an allergist for testing 4–6 weeks after the reaction.

Key pitfalls

- Failure to suspect anaphylaxis especially under general anaesthesia. Have a high index of suspicion. Cutaneous signs may not be present in about 30% of cases and there may be isolated cardiovascular or respiratory signs or symptoms.
- Delays in calling for help early. Communicate clearly that this is a life-threatening situation.
- Failure to give adrenaline early. Give adrenaline intramuscularly, initially 0.5 mg and repeat this in 5 minutes if necessary.
- Do not give intravenous adrenaline unless patient is in a cardiac arrest state. Intravenous adrenaline can be given in a peri-arrest state i.e. where the patient is severely cardiovascularly compromised, but should only be used in a setting where there is cardiac monitoring and should ideally by given by anaesthetists and/or intensivists.

Key pearls

- This is an emergency. Call for help early. An anaesthetist should be called as the patient may require intubation to secure the airway especially in the presence of severe angioedema. Give adrenaline intramuscularly early.

- Always follow ABCDE (**A**irway, **B**reathing, **C**irculation, **D**isability, **E**xposure) approach and keep reassessing the patient.
- Patient may require to be transferred to a high-dependency unit or intensive care unit. In 5–20% of cases there may be a further episode in 6–12 hours, another reason for close monitoring post-event.
- A yellow form should be filled out. This can be done online, at the Medicines and Healthcare Products Regulatory Agency (MHRA) site and is governed by the Commission on Human Medicines (CHM).
- Refer the patient for testing 4–6 weeks later. Skin testing and a radioallergoabsorbent (RAST) test may be necessary. The RAST test is a blood test used to determine specific IgE antibodies to suspected antigens.
- The patient should wear a medic alert bracelet and a copy of the test results should be sent to their general practitioner.

Drug reactions

Key facts

- Definition: The World Health Organization (WHO) defines an adverse dug reaction as 'a response to a drug that is noxious and unintended and occurs at doses normally used in man for the prophylaxis, diagnosis or therapy of disease, or for the modification of physiological function'.

Most reactions occur either due to an exaggeration of the predicted pharmacological effect or unpredictably and unrelated to a drug's main pharmacological action [5]. Adverse drug reactions can be classified into six types. However, it is not always possible to place each drug reaction into one of these categories. Classification:

- Dose-related (**A**ugmented) e.g. cyclizine and anticholinergic effect.
- Non-dose-related (**B**izarre) e.g. suxamethonium and malignant hyperthermia.
- Dose-related and time-related (**C**hronic) e.g. steroids and adrenal suppression.
- Time-related (**D**elayed) e.g. nitrous oxide and agranulocytosis.

- Withdrawal (**E**nd of use) e.g. opiate withdrawal syndrome.
- Failure of therapy (**F**ailure) e.g. oral contraceptive pill used in combination with barbiturates.

It is difficult to quote an overall incidence for drug reactions but it has been shown that the greater the number of drugs used, the greater the chances of having an associated drug reaction.

Key implications

The key point to note here is that if a pregnant woman has a drug reaction that affects her organ systems, especially in cases of cardiovascular and respiratory dysfunction, there can be a direct effect on her baby [6].

Key pointers

The rate at which some drugs are injected and the dose of agent given should be carefully considered as this can further precipitate an unwanted effect.

Key diagnostic signs

Examples of drug reactions that may occur in the obstetric setting:

- Cyclizine: Rapid intravenous administration may cause severe tachycardia [7].
- Oxytocin: Rapid intravenous administration and a dose greater than 5 IU may precipitate severe hypotension with reflex tachycardia. In some cases it may cause severe coronary spasm with ECG changes (ST depression) and chest pain. In the CEMACH (The Confidential Enquiry into Maternal and Child Health) 1997–9 report in the UK [8], the recommended dose of oxytocin postdelivery by caesarean section was reduced from 10 IU to 5 IU, to be given as a slow intravenous bolus to minimise the effects above.
- Carboprost: This is a synthetic analogue of prostaglandin F_2, and is usually given by deep intramuscular injection as a 250 µg dose. It may precipitate bronchospasm, pulmonary oedema or hypertension especially in women who are asthmatic or who have preeclampsia.
- Atracurium: Rapid intravenous administration may lead to exaggerated hypotension especially in patients who are already cardiovascularly compromised. This results from histamine release.

Key actions

Slow the rate of injection (cyclizine and atracurium) if there is a suspicion that a drug reaction/side effect/undesirable effect may be related to rate of injection.

Reduce the amount of drug (oxytocin) if there is a suspicion that a drug reaction may be dose related. Consider using a vasopressor to counteract the effects of hypotension.

Consider avoiding the drug in the future (e.g. carboprost if severe bronchospasm or hypertension occurs).

Key pitfalls

- Failure to use accurate doses of commonly used drugs and to appreciate their side effects.
- Review on a regular basis the side effects of drugs that are used and the specific routes of administration, as well as rate of injection.
- When it becomes necessary to use an unfamiliar drug, read about it or talk to a colleague who knows it.

Key pearls

- An unwanted side effect in one patient may be of benefit to another patient. Have a high index of suspicion when you see an unexpected response in a patient as it may be drug-related.
- Unpredictable drug reactions should be reported to the National Committee on Safety of Medicines in the UK or similar organisation [9].

Management of reactions in low-resource settings

Reactions may range from mild to severe. Management is mostly supportive and the ABCDE approach is useful. If applicable, stop infusing the offending blood component or drug and transfer to a centre with facilities for ventilation after providing emergency treatment for anaphylaxis.

References

1. Association of Anaesthetists of Great Britain & Ireland. *Blood Transfusion and the Anaesthetist – Red Cell Transfusion 2*. The Association of Anaesthetists of Great Britain & Ireland Safety Guideline. London: AAGBI, 2008.

2. Association of Anaesthetists of Great Britain & Ireland. *Blood Transfusion and the Anaesthetist – Management of Massive Haemorrhage*. The Association of Anaesthetists of Great Britain & Ireland Safety Guideline. London: AAGBI, 2010.

3. Association of Anaesthetists of Great Britain & Ireland. *Suspected Anaphylactic Reactions Associated with Anaesthesia*. The Association of Anaesthetists of Great Britain & Ireland Safety Guideline. London: AAGBI, 2009.

4. Resuscitation Council (UK). *Emergency Treatment of Anaphylactic Reactions. Guidelines for Healthcare Providers*. London: Resuscitation Council (UK), 2008.

5. Edwards R, Aronson JK. Adverse drug reaction: definitions, diagnosis, and management. *Lancet* 2000; 356: 1255–1259.

6. Wooten JM. Adverse drug reactions: Part 1. *Southern Med J* 2010; 103: 1025–1028.

7. Wooten JM. Adverse drug reactions: Part 2. *Southern Med J* 2010; 103: 1138–1147.

8. Lewis G, Drife J; The Confidential Enquiry into Maternal and Child Health (CEMACH). *Why Mothers Die 1997–1999: the Fifth Report of the Confidential Enquiries into Maternal Deaths in the United Kingdom*. London: RCOG, 2001.

9. McClelland DBL (Ed.) *UK Blood Transfusion and Tissue Transplantation Services Handbook of Transfusion Medicine*. Fourth edition. London: The Stationery Office, 2007.

Chapter

34

Major trauma including road traffic accidents

Kirsty Crocker and Tim Patel

Key facts

Trauma is a leading cause of non-obstetric maternal death in the developed world, complicating up to 7% of all pregnancies. The leading cause is road traffic accidents (RTAs) followed by domestic abuse of the obstetric patient [1, 2].

The core principles of trauma management are similar for both pregnant and non-pregnant patients. However, anatomical and physiological changes in the pregnant patient must be appreciated as they can pose significant challenges for the attending physicians. Physiological changes can mask normal findings in the trauma patient leading to inaccurate interpretation of vital signs, whilst anatomical changes can not only cause differing injury patterns depending on gestational age, but also can cause difficulties with intubation.

Mechanism of injury

Blunt trauma

Blunt trauma is the commonest type of trauma in pregnancy, being caused mainly by road traffic accidents. Differing mechanisms of injury give rise to differing injury patterns. Blunt forces commonly cause compression injuries, particularly laceration or fracture of solid organs. Sudden deceleration and consequent shearing forces cause avulsion of peritoneal attachments or arteries. Rapid increase in abdominal pressure, for example from a seat belt, can result in hollow viscus rupture, rib or pelvic fractures and cause laceration injuries.

Pregnancy-specific injuries include:

- Preterm labour
- Preterm prelabour rupture of membranes.
- Abruption.
- Direct uterine injury.
- Uterine rupture.
- Direct fetal injury.
- Pelvic fractures, fetal mortality 25%.

Although splenic injury is the most common significant injury in pregnancy secondary to trauma [3], it is not the commonest cause of maternal death. Maternal shock is the commonest cause of death [4] followed by abruption and uterine rupture [5, 6].

Penetrating trauma

Penetrating trauma, in particular gunshot and knife wounds, accounts for up to 10% of cases and causes a quarter of maternal deaths [7]. Maternal visceral injury is less common than direct fetal injury, 38% vs 70% during the third trimester [8]. During early pregnancy, the increased uterine density and uterine pelvic position protect the fetus. As the uterus becomes intra-abdominal from 13 weeks' gestation, it displaces bowel and abdominal viscera superiorly. It becomes increasingly vulnerable to direct injury with potential to cause catastrophic haemorrhage when injured. Although the uterus confers some protection to the maternal viscera, upper abdominal wounds can result in significant injury with a higher likelihood of multiple organ injury.

Obstetric and Intrapartum Emergencies, ed. Edwin Chandraharan and Sabaratnam Arulkumaran. Published by Cambridge University Press. © Cambridge University Press 2012.

Issues relating to blunt and penetrating trauma

Abdominal examination can be unreliable due to the peritoneal distension of pregnancy and neural desensitisation. This can result in anything from atypical pain referral to increased peritoneal pain threshold. Therefore it is essential to maintain a high index of suspicion. Abdominal pain with shoulder tip referral should be regarded as a potential liver injury until proven otherwise. It is essential to understand the consequences of organ displacement in the parturient. Haematuria should always be evaluated fully as the displaced bladder makes it more susceptible to injury and a palpable liver is always deemed abnormal until proven otherwise as the liver moves superiorly by approximately 4 cm in the full-term mother.

The decision to proceed to laparotomy depends on several factors:

- Gestation.
- Site of injury.
- Mechanism of injury.
- Maternal shock.
- Fetal distress.

Evidence of intraperitoneal haemorrhage secondary to blunt trauma is treated similarly in both pregnant and non-pregnant patients. Gunshot injury almost always requires an exploratory laparotomy. Conversely, laparotomy in patients with stab wounds is reserved for patients exhibiting signs of shock, radiographic evidence of organ injury or peritoneal injury, bearing in mind that the risk of peritoneal injury increases with increasing abdominal distention of pregnancy. Laparoscopy may be used for lower abdominal penetrating trauma in which both mother and fetus are stable, however exploratory laparotomy is recommended for upper abdominal trauma [9, 10]. Other investigations include performing a fistulogram or amniocentesis. A fistulogram can determine whether the peritoneum has been injured thus indicating the need for laparoscopy or laparotomy and amniocentesis can demonstrate a potential uterine injury. However the presence of bacteria or blood is not an absolute indication for delivery.

Laparotomy is not an indication for caesarean section. Provided that maternal injury can be correctly identified and safely managed, the gravid uterus should be undisturbed and the pregnancy allowed to proceed to term. However, a caesarean section should be considered if the uterus interferes with treatment of the mother. Other indications for a caesarean section include near term, irreparable uterine damage, maternal shock, unstable thoracolumbar injury and maternal death.

Key pitfalls

- Massive haemorrhage. Uterine blood flow increases from 60 ml/minnute to 750 ml/minute with resultant massive haemorrhage in blunt or penetrating trauma.
- Unreliable abdominal examination. Peritoneal distension of pregnancy and neural desensitisation leads to atypical pain referral and an increased peritoneal pain threshold.
- Burns: Maternal outcome with respect to burn injury is not affected by the pregnancy, however fetal survival parallels the percentage of burns with spontaneous abortion being more common in the first trimester. This is due to septicaemia, hypoxia and the intensely catabolic state of the burns victim [11, 12]. It is generally accepted that delivery is urgent if the patient has more than 50% burns in the second or third trimester. Treatment priorities are the same as for the non-pregnant woman but attention should be paid to fluid resuscitation and airway management.
- Fetal mortality is as high as 70% with electrical burns due to the fetus sitting in a bag of low-resistance fluid and fetal monitoring is essential even when the injury appears minor.

Key pearls

- Increase fluid requirements. Fluid volumes are greater than in the non-pregnant patient.
- Intubate early. Airway oedema can make a difficult pregnant airway extremely challenging.

Key actions

A multidisciplinary approach involving ED physicians, obstetricians, neonatologists, anaesthetists and surgeons is essential. The initial management approach for the parturient remains the same as for the non-pregnant patient, remembering that fetal outcomes are intimately dependent on adequate resuscitation of the mother prior to early fetal assessment. The initial sequence of trauma resuscitation follows the standard ABCDE approach to trauma [13]. The most recognisable additions are early left lateral tilt and fetal assessment. During the primary survey, life-threatening injuries are identified and managed simultaneously. The primary survey includes:

- Airway maintenance with cervical spine protection.
- Breathing and ventilation.
- Circulation with haemorrhage control.
- Disability: neurological status.
- Exposure and environmental control.

Airway with cervical spine control

If a cervical spine injury is suspected, the neck should be immobilised with three-point immobilisation, which should include a well-fitting cervical collar, blocks and tape. All patients should receive high-flow oxygen through a non-rebreather mask. Any airway compromise should give rise to early consideration of securing the airway with a definitive airway. The potential for a difficult intubation secondary to anatomical changes, airway oedema and delayed gastric emptying related to pregnancy should be anticipated. Therefore gastric prophylaxis and rapid sequence induction are essential if a general anaesthetic is required, however regional anaesthesia is always preferable. It is essential to aim for normal physiological parameters to reduce any chance of fetal hypoxia and acidosis. A 'light anaesthetic' causes increased catecholamine release, reducing placental flow, therefore ensure adequate anaesthetic doses during a general anaesthetic. The greater risk of failed intubation in the pregnant patient mandates the immediate availability of appropriate difficult-airway equipment.

Key pitfall

- Increased risk of difficult intubation and gastric aspiration.

Breathing and ventilation

Attention should be given to the physiological respiratory changes that can affect assessment and management in trauma. Respiratory changes are secondary to the effects of progesterone on the respiratory centre, compounded by the raised diaphragm compressing the lungs. This results in a physiological dyspnoea, increased metabolic demands and oxygen consumption and therefore a decreased respiratory reserve.

These changes can result in rapid oxygen desaturation if ventilation is impaired, hence all patients must receive high-flow oxygen through a non-rebreather mask. Tidal volumes are increased, resulting in a slightly lower $PaCO_2$ of 4 kPa. 'Normal' $PaCO_2$ levels should raise concerns, indicating possible ventilatory compromise. The diaphragm is raised by up to 4 cm therefore thoracostomy should be placed 1–2 intercostal spaces higher.

Key pitfalls

- Decreased FRC and increased oxygen consumption can lead to rapid desaturation; therefore oxygenate all patients.
- Thoracostomy placement should be 1–2 spaces higher.

Circulation and haemorrhage control

Insert two large-bore cannulae, take blood for FBC, coagulation studies, X-Match, Rh status, Kleihauer–Betke test for fetal cells and U & Es. Evidence of cardiovascular compromise may be masked or mimicked by both cardiac and vascular changes of normal pregnancy. The physiological increase in intravascular volume means that pregnant patients can lose a significant volume of blood before exhibiting any signs of hypovolaemia. Thus fetal hypoperfusion and distress can manifest well in advance of maternal compromise becoming apparent. Aggressive fluid replacement with warm crystalloid and type-specific blood is recommended even in normotensive patients until sources of haemorrhage have been located and controlled or excluded. Focused abdominal sonography for trauma (FAST) is excellent at identifying intraperitoneal fluid in patients with blunt trauma. During transfusion of blood, early consideration of additional blood products should be given to prevent a dilutional coagulopathy. Vasopressors will contribute further to fetal hypoxia by reducing uterine blood flow and should only be used to support maternal blood pressure if absolutely necessary, for example to maintain blood pressure in spinal shock. Other physiological changes to be mindful of include a reduction in systolic and diastolic blood pressure of 10–20 mmHg and a 10–20 beat per minute rise in heart rate. These changes are at their 'peak' at 28 weeks' gestation, returning to pre-pregnancy levels at term. Arrhythmias or palpitations are also common as are ECG changes such as nonspecific ST changes and inferior Q waves.

From 20 weeks' gestation the uterus can compress the inferior vena cava and aorta causing a significant reduction in cardiac output, exacerbating a potential shock state. Early displacement of the uterus to the left either manually or via tilting the patient to 15–30 degrees with a pillow or wedge is essential. If a spinal injury is suspected, the patient should be immobilised on a spinal board and the whole board should be tilted. Left lateral tilt should be maintained at all times, including during transport, as failure to do so may result in a fall in cardiac output of up to 30%.

Key pitfalls

- Physiological increase in circulating volume can mask signs of blood loss and hypovolaemia.
- Aortocaval compression can reduce maternal cardiac output by up to 30%, therefore perform left lateral tilt as early as possible.
- Consider physiological anaemia when transfusing blood as over-transfusion may increase blood viscosity causing fetal harm or increasing the risk of thrombosis [14].

Disability: neurological status

The assessment of the Glasgow Coma Score in the pregnant trauma patient is as for the non-pregnant patient. However, it must be remembered that seizures or alteration in mental status may be a consequence of eclampsia rather than traumatic head injury. Management of traumatic head injury is the same as for all patients, whilst remembering that the normal $PaCO_2$ in the parturient is lower. Hence, if intubation and ventilation is required the $PaCO_2$ must be maintained at the parturient's lower level.

Cardiac arrest is managed according to the Adult Life Support guidelines [15], ensuring that at least a 15–30 degree left lateral tilt position is maintained. If initial resuscitative attempts fail, then emergency caesarean section with delivery of the fetus may improve the chances of both maternal and fetal survival. The UK Resuscitation Council Guidelines recommend delivery within 5 minutes of cardiac arrest for those with a gestational age of more than 20 weeks. However, fetal survival before 23 weeks is unlikely.

Fetal assessment

Fetal injury can occur as a result of direct injury, e.g. secondary to pelvic fractures, or from indirect injury, e.g. placental abruption, uterine rupture or uterine contractions and preterm labour. Fetal assessment should commence as soon as the primary survey has been completed and immediate life-threatening injuries managed. Assessment involves palpating for fetal movements, and listening for fetal heart rate and heart sounds, using either a Pinard stethoscope or Doppler probe. Ultrasound examination should be performed to assess fetal viability. CTG monitoring should commence as soon as is practical. It is advisable that all patients who sustain abdominal trauma in the second half of pregnancy should be monitored with CTG.

Placental abruption occurs in up to 60% of major abdominal trauma following RTAs [16] and is responsible for approximately 70% of all fetal losses during trauma [17]. The majority of placental abruptions are nevertheless due to minor trauma. The diagnosis of placental abruption is largely clinical, relying on the identification of fetal heart rate abnormalities and patient symptoms such as abdominal or uterine tenderness, vaginal bleeding, ruptured membranes or shock. Ultrasound can miss up to 80% of abruptions [18] but is still used alongside measurements of platelet and fibrinogen levels to assist in diagnosis.

The ACOG currently recommends monitoring for a minimum of 4 hours post-trauma. It is generally accepted that monitoring can be stopped after 4 hours if the following are present [19]:

- A normal CTG.
- A normal ultrasound.
- Fewer than six contractions per hour.
- No abdominal pain.
- No vaginal bleeding.

The secondary survey

This involves a head-to-toe examination and is performed once the patient is stable, which may be several hours after presentation. The examination follows the same approach as for a non-pregnant patient but should also carefully look for any signs of pelvic or uterine injury such as vaginal bleeding, uterine tenderness and for signs of fetal compromise such as contractions and abnormalities in heart rate and rhythm. An obstetric history is essential as a past medical history of preterm labour or placental abruption would potentially necessitate a period of extended monitoring.

It is essential that all mothers should be immunised for tetanus in the event of a penetrating injury. Antibiotics should be administered as required and thromboprophylaxis in the immobile, prothrombotic mother is essential when all sources of bleeding have stopped.

Imaging modalities

There is often anxiety generated amongst physicians when diagnostic imaging is required, due to the perceived harmful effects of ionising radiation on the fetus. However, it is essential that there is no delay in obtaining time-critical imaging, remembering that maternal well-being is paramount to fetal well-being. Knowledge of the risks involved with various diagnostic modalities can allay or reduce most concerns.

Ultrasound is always preferred as a result of its recognised safety profile. In the context of trauma, it is very sensitive in detecting intraperitoneal free fluid and can also assess gestation, size, position, placenta etc. Although it is useful in the diagnosis of placental abruption, its sensitivity is poor.

The risk of ionising radiation depends on gestation and exposure intensity, which in turn depends on the number of rads used and the number of times a procedure is performed. A typical chest X-ray will produce a dosage of 0.005 rad whereas an abdominal CT can produce up to 9 rad. Total exposure can be reduced with lead shielding, use of spiral CT and changes in CT-slice thickness.

It has been shown that there is no significant increase in fetal anomalies or pregnancy loss when exposure to radiation is less than 5 rad [20, 21]. However, that is not to say there is no risk and timing of the radiation is important. The lethal effects of radiation are more likely prior to implantation of the fetus however at this early stage teratogenesis is unlikely. During the period of organogenesis (weeks 2–7) teratogenicity and neoplastic and growth retardation are more likely. After 20 weeks' gestation radiation is deemed to be safe [4] however CNS dysfunction and growth retardation have been shown. The 'trauma series' of radiographs, cervical spine, chest and pelvis, should not be delayed if they are deemed necessary. Interpretation of chest and pelvic radiographs requires knowledge of pregnancy-related changes. A heart which is rotated to the left, showing relative fluid overload, can give rise to the appearance of mild cardiomegaly, a widened mediastinum and increased vascular markings, whilst widened sacroiliac joints and symphysis pubis must not be mistaken for a pelvic injury.

As abdominal CT carries the most risk of teratogenesis during the first trimester, diagnostic peritoneal lavage should be considered. It can be performed in any trimester (although it becomes progressively more difficult as pregnancy advances), can be used for unstable patients when USS is not available or results are equivocal, is safe if a supra-umbilical open technique is used and is 100% sensitive for intra-abdominal bleeding [22].

Key pearls

- Exposure to ionising radiation is additive.
- Do not allow concerns over fetus to hinder maternal evaluation.
- Interpret all investigations in context of pregnancy-related changes.

Fetal maternal haemorrhage

Fetal maternal haemorrhage (FMH) occurs in up to 30% of obstetric trauma patients [23]. An anterior placenta is a risk factor for FMH [24] and can lead to fetal anaemia and exsanguination as well as arrhythmias and fetal death. The transfer of rhesus positive fetal blood into a rhesus negative maternal circulation can lead to alloimmunisation of the mother. The Kleihauer–Betke (KB) test or flow cytometry can be used to estimate the volume of blood transferred from the fetal to the maternal circulation. Volumes of 1 ml can lead to sensitisation and the development of rhesus antibodies. To prevent erythroblastosis fetalis in subsequent pregnancies all Rh-negative patients should be given 300 µg Anti D immunoglobulin within 72 hours of exposure to cover 15 ml FMH. In the event of a massive haemorrhage an additional 300 µg/30 ml of fetal blood should be administered. It is controversial as to whether the KB test should be routinely performed after abdominal trauma as it has not been shown to be predictive of fetal complications. However an association between preterm contractions and a positive KB test has been shown, indicating the need for prolonged fetal monitoring with a positive test.

Key pitfall

- Anti D administration can interfere with rhesus typing of the newborn if given close to delivery.

Table 34.1 Management of trauma in a low-resource setting.

Issues	Examples	Solutions
Limited skill mix	Lack of: Obstetricians Surgeons Anaesthetists Haematologists	*Protocols/Algorithms/Simulators* Practise skills that may not be done routinely *No haematologists* Simple X match technique: Drops of different blood on a smooth white surface may show major incompatibilities
Limited staff numbers		*Protocols/Simulators* Ensure an organised and efficient approach
Limited time	War zone	*WHO checklist* Decreases errors when time limited
Limited transport	Air travel	E.g. If unable to transfer patient do not perform a perimortem caesarean section in a 23-week gestation woman Unlikely to improve maternal outcome Baby unlikely to survive without specialist care
Limited supplies	Cannulae Central access lines Fluids Blood Laryngoscopes Oxygen Saturation probes	Outdated/suboptimal equipment can be used for another purpose *No central lines*: Use an NG tube with a cut-down technique. *No Pinard stethoscope*: Ear to abdomen to estimate fetal heart beat. *No saturation probe*: Very close observation patient's colour. *No laryngoscope*: Digital manipulation of tracheal tube into trachea. *No blood*: Permissive hypotension. Do not give blood to a patient who is unlikely to survive.
Diagnostic challenges	Diagnosing/locating haemorrhage without sphygmomanometer and CT scanner	*Clinical signs* e.g. palpate artery to estimate BP • Carotid only – 40 mmHg • Carotid and femoral – 50 mmHg • Carotid/femoral/peripheral > 70 mmHg [30] *Increase use of DPL*

Prevention

Despite advances in trauma management, education has been shown to be one of the most effective techniques in decreasing mortality. Education must focus on seatbelt use, domestic violence and drug and alcohol abuse.

A pregnant woman is twice as likely to lose a fetus in an RTA if she does not wear a seatbelt, but very few women wear seatbelts and even fewer wear them properly for fear of damaging the fetus [18]. Fears over the use of airbags and placental abruption have led to them being disarmed, but these fears are unfounded and airbags are life saving.

Antenatal education regarding the proper technique of the three-point seatbelt has been shown to be invaluable [25]. With the lap belt placed as low as possible under the 'bump' and the shoulder belt placed to the side of the uterus between the breasts and over the clavicle the force of transmission of energy through the uterus decreases [26]. It is also essential that the women should be at least 10 inches away from the dashboard/steering wheel containing the airbag [27].

Domestic violence is three times more common in pregnancy and is associated with recreational drug use [28, 29]. It is essential to screen all pregnant women for signs of domestic violence. It should preferably be done at their first antenatal visit and without their partner. It has been shown that the warning signs are almost always present but not acted upon [29]. A simple acronym to use when assessing the mother is 'SAFE':

S: Does the patient feel safe at home/work/school?
A: Has the patient been abused/felt afraid?
F: Friends/family support network?
E: Emergency/escape plan?

Key pearl

• Always have a high index of suspicion.

Management in a 'limited-resource' setting

A limited-resource setting is one where equipment, staff or experience are limited for the diagnosis and treatment of a pregnant patient with trauma. For example:

- Medical setting in a low resource or a developing country.
- War zone.
- Environmental disaster e.g. earthquake.

It can be a challenging and stressful situation where one has to make the best of what is available which often means that common sense is more important than knowledge. Table 34.1 highlights some examples.

Key pearls

- Left lateral tilt – costs nothing but saves lives.

Conclusion

Trauma is a leading cause of non-obstetric maternal death. The keys to success, particularly in the limited-resource setting are:

- Prevention.
- Preemption.
- Planning.
- Preparation.

A multidisciplinary approach is essential and it must always be remembered that fetal outcome is dependent on adequate resuscitation of the mother.

References

1. Connolly AM, Katz VL, Bash KL, McMahon MJ, Hansen WF. Trauma and pregnancy. *Am J Perinatol* 1997; 14 (6): 331–336.

2. Centre for Maternal and Child Enquiries (CMACE). *Saving Mothers' Lives: Reviewing Maternal Deaths to make Motherhood Safer – 2006–2008. The Eighth Report on Confidential Enquiries into Maternal Deaths in the United Kingdom. Br J Obstet Gynaecol* 2011; 118 (Suppl. 1): 1–208.

3. Davis JJ, Cohn I. Diagnosis and management of blunt abdominal trauma. *Ann Surgery* 1976; 183: 672.

4. Shah AJ, Kilcline BA. Trauma in pregnancy. *Emerg Med Clin N Am* 2003; 21 (3): 615–629.

5. Esposito TJ, Gens DR, Smith LG, Scorpio R. Evaluation of blunt abdominal trauma occurring during pregnancy. *J Trauma* 1989; 29 (12): 1628–1632.

6. Rothenberger D, Quattlebaum FW, Perry JF Jr, Zabel J, Fischer RP. Blunt maternal trauma: review of 103 cases. *J Trauma* 1978; 18 (3): 173–179.

7. Werman HA, Falcone RE. Trauma in pregnancy. *Emergency Medicine Reports and Pediatric Emergency Medicine Reports* 2008; 9 (4, supplement).

8. Buchsbaum H (Ed.) Penetrating injury of the abdomen. In *Trauma in Pregnancy*. Philadelphia, PA: WB Saunders, 1979, pp. 82–100.

9. Awwad JT, Azar GB, Seoud MA, Mroueh AM, Karam KS. High velocity penetrating wounds of the gravid uterus: review of 16 years of civil war. *Obstet Gynecol* 1994; 83: 259–264.

10. Meunch MV, Canterino JC. Trauma in pregnancy. *Obstet Gynecol Clin N Am* 2007; 34 (3): 555–583.

11. Matthews RM. Obstetric implications of burns in pregnancy. *Br J Obstet Gynecol* 1982; 89: 603–609.

12. Akhtar MA, Mulawakar PM, Kulkarni HR. Burns in pregnancy: effect on maternal and foetal outcomes. *Burns* 1994; 20: 351–355.

13. Howell C, Grady K, Cox C. *Managing Obstetric Emergencies and Trauma – the MOET Course Manual*. Second edition. London: RCOG, 2007.

14. Stephansson O, Dickman PW, Johansson A, Cnattingius S. Maternal hemoglobin concentration during pregnancy and risk of still birth. *J Am Med Assoc* 2000; 284: 2611–2617.

15. Resuscitation Council (UK). *Adult Advanced Life Support Guidelines – UK Resuscitation Guidelines* 2010. http://www.resus.org.uk/pages/guide.htm

16. Eposito TJ. Trauma during pregnancy. *Emerg Med Clin N Am* 1994; 12: 167–199.

17. Pearlman MD, Tintinalli JE. Evaluation and treatment of the gravida and fetus following trauma during pregnancy. *Obstet Gynecol N Am* 1991: 18: 371–381.

18. Incerpi M. Trauma in pregnancy. In Murphy Goodwin T, Montoro MN, Muderspach L, Paulson R, Roy S (Eds.), *Management of Common Problems in Obstetrics and Gynecology*. Fifth Edition. Chichester: Wiley-Blackwell, 2010, pp. 156–159.

19. American College of Obstetricians and Gynaecologists. ACOG Technical Bulletin Number 161. Trauma during pregnancy. November 1991. *Int J Gynaecol Obstet* 1993; 40 (2): 165–170.

20. American College of Obstetricians and Gynaecologists. *Guidelines for Diagnostic Imaging during Pregnancy*. Committee Opinion 158. September 1995.

21. Hall EJ. Scientific view of low radiation risks. *Radiographics* 1991; 11: 509–518.

22. Rothenberger DA, Quattlebaum FW, Zabel J, Fischer RP. Diagnostic peritoneal lavage in blunt trauma in pregnant women. *Am J Obset Gynecol* 1977; 129 (5): 479–481.

23. Chames MC, Pearlman MD. Trauma during pregnancy: outcomes and clinical management. *Clin Obstet Gynaecol* 2008; 51: 398–408.

24. Pearlman MD, Tintinalli JE, Lorenz RP. A prospective controlled study of outcome after trauma during pregnancy. *Am J Obstet Gynecol* 1990; 162: 1502–1507.

25. Pearlman MD, Phillips ME. Safety belt use in pregnancy. *Am J Obstet Gynecol* 1996; 88: 1026–1029.

26. Pearlman MD, Viano D. Automobile crash simulation with the first pregnant crash test dummy. *Am J Obstet Gynecol* 1996; 175: 977–981.

27. Schiff MA, Mack CD. The effect of airbags on pregnancy outcomes in Washington State 2002–2005. *Obstet Gynecol* 2010; 115 (1): 85–92.

28. McFarlane J, Campbell JC. Abuse during pregnancy and femicide: urgent implications for womens health. *Obstet Gynecol* 2002; 100 (1): 27–36.

29. The Confidential Enquiry into Maternal and Child Health (CEMACH). *Saving Mothers' Lives': Reviewing Maternal Deaths to make Motherhood Safer – 2003–2005. The Seventh Report on Confidential Enquiries into Maternal Deaths in the United Kingdom.* London: CEMACH, 2007.

30. Deakin CD, Low JL. Accuracy of the advanced trauma life support guidelines for predicting systolic blood pressure using carotid, femoral, and radial pulses: observational study. *Br Med J* 2000; 321 (7262): 673–674.

Chapter

35

Neonatal resuscitation and the management of immediate neonatal problems

Anay Kulkarni, Justin Richards, Nigel Kennea and Siromi Gunaratne

Introduction

Resuscitation of the newborn infant differs from that of any other age group. The newly born infant is small, wet and therefore prone to getting cold, and has lungs that contain lung fluid. The approach to resuscitation needs to be adapted to their needs.

Whilst the majority of infants will not require resuscitation at birth, approximately 3–5% of newborn infants may need some support [1]. Most of the time, the potential need for resuscitation may be anticipated from the maternal and obstetric history such as the presence of a congenital anomaly on the antenatal scans, preterm gestation, fetal distress (for example as indicated by abnormal fetal heart rate pattern or abnormal fetal scalp blood sample), or by the presence of meconium-stained liquor. In these cases trained members of the midwifery and/or neonatal team should be present prior to delivery. Very occasionally a newborn infant may be unexpectedly delivered in poor condition and resuscitation will need to be commenced whilst the neonatal team are being alerted. We therefore recommend that anyone who works in an environment where they may be required to resuscitate newborn babies should have training similar to the UK Newborn Life Support course (NLS) or the American Neonatal Advanced Life Support course (NALS).

Physiology

The primary reason for resuscitation in the newborn infant differs from that in adults. Whilst the majority of adults requiring resuscitation will have had a primary cardiac event, the newborn infant's heart is healthy and it will usually be a hypoxic or ischaemic event initially that will have compromised the infant. Particular attention to management of the airway and breathing is therefore imperative.

In normal circumstances, during the first few minutes of life the newborn baby will displace lung fluid and fill its lungs with air and establish resting lung volume. During this time, pneumocytes will change from actively secreting fluid to actively absorbing fluid under the influence of maternal hormones. Approximately 30 ml/kg of fluid (on average approximately 100 ml for the average term infant) is absorbed through the alveoli with a further 30 ml or so being present in the oropharynx and cleared more slowly. Routine use of suction removes an insignificant amount of fluid from the oropharynx. It cannot remove fluid from the alveoli. Routine suctioning of infants at birth may result in bradycardia and apnoea, as a result of vagal stimulation, and is therefore not recommended [2].

In order to initiate resuscitation at birth it is vital to have an understanding of the pathophysiological consequences of hypoxia during birth. Such information has been derived from the work of physiologists in the 1960s such as Cross, Dawes and Godfrey that demonstrated the physiological responses of animals subjected to a hypoxic stress at birth [3, 4, 5]. The results of their experiments have been used to guide the teaching of a logical and effective approach to resuscitation now known as the ABC(D) of resuscitation.

These experiments demonstrated that, when subjected to acute hypoxia by interrupting cord blood flow, the first response of the fetus is to breathe more deeply and rapidly. Within a few minutes of hypoxia, activity of the respiratory centre switches off and the fetus stops breathing. This is known as primary

Obstetric and Intrapartum Emergencies, ed. Edwin Chandraharan and Sabaratnam Arulkumaran. Published by Cambridge University Press. © Cambridge University Press 2012.

apnoea. The carbon dioxide level in the fetal blood (pCO_2) then starts to rise followed by a decrease in heart rate to about half the normal rate. The heart continues to beat slowly, rather than stop, because of the presence of glycogen in the cardiac muscle, which provides an energy source via anaerobic metabolism. This anaerobic metabolism subsequently contributes to lactic acidosis and in turn leads to peripheral vasoconstriction resulting in a clinically pale baby.

If the insult continues the fetus begins to gasp as a result of primitive spinal reflexes. These gasps are shuddering whole-body breathing movements that occur several times a minute. The effect of gasping may be enough for the infant to 'resuscitate itself' or if given resuscitation in the form of airway management the infant should respond quickly. Cardiac output continues and blood pressure is maintained but if these gasps fail to aerate the lungs they fade away, hypoxia and acidosis become increasingly severe, all vital functions cease and terminal apnoea supervenes. In the newborn human baby, this process probably takes about 20 minutes [6].

A baby who is not breathing could be in primary apnoea, about to gasp, or in terminal apnoea. Unfortunately, it is not possible to tell at the time but it is reassuring to know that almost all babies respond very rapidly once the lungs have been aerated.

Equipment needed

The items mentioned are not an exhaustive list and when faced with the delivery of the newborn infant out of the hospital setting making a note of the time, drying the infant and providing a warm environment with skin-to-skin contact between the infant and mother may be all that is needed.

In a planned delivery at home, midwives will take with them a bag–valve–mask device with suitable face masks, oropharyngeal airways, a laryngoscope, an oxygen supply and portable suction with large-bore catheters. They should also have cord clamps, scissors and disposable gloves.

In the hospital setting, all of this equipment should be more easily available including a resuscitaire to provide a flat surface, which is also able to provide warmth through radiant heat, a clock, pressure limited delivery of air/oxygen and suction. In addition a range of face masks, oropharyngeal airways, laryngoscopes with blades and endotracheal tubes should be available. Equipment for placement of an umbilical venous

catheter should also be available if required and emergency resuscitation drugs if needed.

Preparation for early management of a newborn infant should include a review of the obstetric notes and discussion with colleagues regarding any foreseeable complications at delivery. It is also important to ensure good communication with the parents before birth and during resuscitation if at all possible.

Initial assessment

After delivery the first step is to dry and assess the baby. Start the clock or note the time of birth. After drying and wrapping the baby in a fresh warm towel one should begin with assessment.

Initial assessment includes:

- Colour.
- Tone.
- Breathing.
- Heart rate.

- Colour: Colour is useful for assessing the initial condition of the baby at birth. Babies in difficulties often appear pale at birth. Well babies appear blue initially and turn pink soon after birth. Colour is not as good a means of assessing oxygenation as often thought previously.
- Tone: Well babies appear well flexed with good tone soon after birth. The floppy babies are often in significant difficulties. The tone can be easily assessed by handling the baby.
- Breathing: Breathing usually starts spontaneously after birth. The baby may show normal regular breaths, irregular breaths, gasping or breathing may be absent (apnoea).
- Heart rate: In healthy term babies the heart rate is usually greater than 100 beats/minute by 2 minutes of age but can be still below 100 beats/minute in about 10%.

Methods of assessment

Palpation of the apical cardiac impulse, umbilical or peripheral pulsation can be unreliable.

- Stethoscope: A stethoscope is used when first assessing the heart rate. The cardiac impulse can often be felt at the base of umbilicus, however it cannot always be felt and rate judged by cord pulsation may not reflect true heart rate.

Table 35.1 Reference range for oxygen saturation for infants after birth [24].

Time of birth	Acceptable (25th centile) right arm saturation (%)
2 minutes	60
3 minutes	70
4 minutes	80
5 minutes	85
10 minutes	90

It is not necessary to count the heart rate with complete accuracy as it is usually clear whether the heart rate is very slow (< 60/minute), slow (60–100/minute) or fast (> 100/minute).

Pulse oximetry

Using a pulse oximeter will allow accurate assessment of heart rate and oxygen saturation within about 2 minutes of application. Saturation levels in healthy babies in the first few minutes of life may be considerably lower than other times.

The values quoted in Table 35.1 are the oxygen saturation values measured on the right arm (preductal values). These data came from a study involving 450 healthy babies who received no resuscitation or supplemental oxygen within a few minutes after birth. The saturation levels listed in this table are considered 'acceptable' which means that babies with these saturations probably do not need supplemental oxygen.

Priorities

Clamping the cord

Unless the baby is clearly in need of immediate resuscitation, we recommend waiting for at least 1 minute from complete delivery of the baby before clamping the cord [7].

Warmth

Maintaining temperature is imperative, as hypothermia is associated with increased morbidity and mortality [8]. A wet baby can rapidly lose heat, and a small baby can become dangerously hypothermic. Babies subjected to cold stress immediately after birth have increased metabolic acidosis and lower oxygen tension respectively [9, 10]. Therefore, when present at the delivery of any newborn, irrespective of its need or not for resuscitation, drying the infant, disposing of the wet towels, and wrapping the infant with a dry warm towel are necessary before further steps are taken. After drying and wrapping, the infant should be immediately assessed (see above).

Airway

Newborn infants have a large occiput and when placed onto the resuscitaire or a hard surface there is the tendency for their head to flex forward thereby obstructing the airway. To overcome this, place the head in the neutral position by extending the neck very slightly (Figure 35.1). This will result in the plane between the nose and mouth being parallel to the plane of the ceiling. This is different from adults where you tilt the head and apply a chin lift. Sometimes this simple manoeuvre is all that is needed in order to assist the newborn's respiratory effort although there are further airway manoeuvres one can apply.

If, having placed the head in the 'neutral position', the baby's respiratory effort remains poor or absent, with a heart rate that is slow (< 100 beats per minute) the infant should be given 5 inflation breaths. The idea of inflation breaths is to establish a residual volume and displace lung fluid. Therefore these breaths are given with pressures set at 30 cm H_2O each lasting 2–3 seconds, given using a bag and mask, or preferably a pressure-limited T piece, 'Tom Thumb' or other ventilation device. The reason for 5 breaths is that the initial 2 or 3 breaths may only help in pushing lung liquid out of the alveoli and not expand the lungs with air. Watch for chest wall movement as the inflation breaths are given. In order to give these breaths effectively, the right sized mask should be used which covers the nose and mouth but does not go over the end of the chin or encroach onto the eyes. Once these 5 inflation breaths are given further assessment is necessary to see if this has aided the infant. Whilst assessing tone, colour and respiratory effort the most important sign of effective inflation breaths is a rise in the heart rate. If there is no rise in the heart rate and the chest was not seen to move whilst giving 5 inflation breaths it is likely that the lungs have not been inflated. Other airway manoeuvres in order to open the airway and ensure the infant receives the inflation breaths need to be considered.

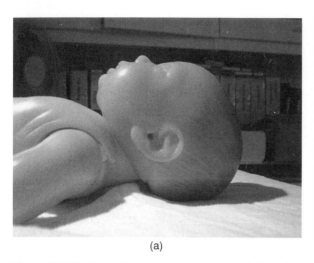
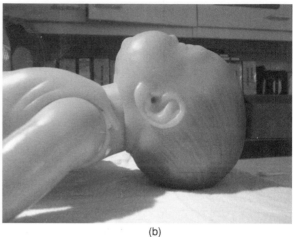

(a) (b)

Figure 35.1 Newborn infants have a large occiput and when placed onto the resuscitaire or a hard surface there is the tendency for the head to flex forward thereby obstructing the airway (a). Placing the infant's head in the 'neutral position' opens the airway (b). Care must be taken not to over-extend the head.

These airway manoeuvres include a single-handed jaw thrust; one places the third or fourth finger of the hand used to keep the face mask on the infant behind the angle of jaw and pushes it upward. This will aid opening the airway by bringing the lower jaw in line with the upper jaw and will help to lift the tongue, which may have dropped backwards obstructing the airway, out of the way. Having performed this manoeuvre 5 further inflation breaths should be given again. If this does not result in a rise in heart rate or chest wall movement, and if help is available, a two person jaw thrust can be attempted to open the airway. In this manoeuvre, one person applies the jaw thrust behind both jaw angles and holds the face mask in place whilst the other person gives the inflation breaths.

If this does not work or there is no help available, if competent, one should directly visualise the larynx and vocal cords using a laryngoscope placed in the left hand and perform suction if an obstruction such as a blood clot, vernix or meconium is seen. Alternatively, if there is no obstruction, placing an appropriately sized oropharyngeal airway using the laryngoscope or a tongue depressor should be performed. To size an oropharyngeal airway, hold it along the line of the lower jaw with the flange in the middle of the lips, immediately below the tip of the nose and the end of the airway should be level with the angle of the jaw. The airway is inserted in the anatomical position you want

it to be, i.e. it is not rotated in the mouth due to the fragile palate.

Following these manoeuvres, 5 inflation breaths should again be given. One can only feel reassured if there is an increase in heart rate or chest wall movement is seen. If, using these manoeuvres, the chest wall moves with the inflation breaths but there is no rise in heart rate one then needs to undertake chest compressions. One may at any of these points intubate the baby using an appropriately sized endotracheal tube if trained and skilled to do so. The advantage of being able to insert an endotracheal tube is that the airway is secured and in an extended resuscitation the hands can be freed to concentrate on circulatory resuscitation.

Breathing

If the chest wall has moved with the inflation breaths with a rise in heart rate but the newborn continues not to breathe or has poor respiratory effort, ventilation breaths should be given. These breaths are to 'breathe for the baby' and therefore given with shorter inspiratory times, and given quicker at a rate of 30 breaths per minute. Having overcome the initial stiffness of the lungs and dispersed some of the lung liquid, the inspiratory pressure given should also be reduced to a pressure sufficient to achieve adequate chest wall movement (normally around 20–25 cmH$_2$O).

If after 30 seconds of ventilation breaths the infant is still not breathing effectively, consider admission of the infant to the neonatal unit for continued ventilatory support and further management. Gasping suggests that the baby was in terminal apnoea.

Evidence from both animal and human studies has demonstrated that resuscitation of infants with room air is as effective as 100% oxygen. There is growing evidence that 100% oxygen can cause tissue damage via liberation of free radicals. While we recommend commencing resuscitation with room air, supplementary oxygen should be available as a back-up [11]; the need for supplemental oxygen is judged by clinical response and saturation monitoring. International guidelines on neonatal resuscitation recommend using room air to start resuscitation [7, 12, 13]. Additional oxygen is rarely needed. If it is thought to be necessary it should be given via an air/oxygen blender and the effect monitored using pulse oximetry.

Some devices are now available where one can set positive end expiratory pressure (PEEP) as well as a peak inspiratory pressure, such as the Neopuff®. There is a theoretical benefit to the infant when using PEEP as this establishes and maintains functional residual capacity. Whilst there have been several papers showing the benefit particularly in preterm infants where there is an association between absence of functional residual capacity and subsequent respiratory distress syndrome in those requiring ventilation [14], a Cochrane review undertaken in 2003 and recently updated in 2008 concluded that there was insufficient evidence to determine the efficacy and safety of PEEP in ventilation breaths given during resuscitation of the newborn infant and that further randomised clinical trials were needed [15].

Circulation

The baby who does not respond to lung inflation at birth is rare and the most likely reason for an inadequate rise in the heart rate is inadequate lung inflation. If despite good chest wall movement with inflation breaths, there is no rise in heart rate, chest compressions must be given. The aim of these chest compressions is to move oxygenated blood from the lungs to the coronary arteries. *You are only trying to move a few teaspoons of oxygenated blood from the pulmonary veins to coronary arteries – a distance of about 5 cm.* The best method for administering chest compressions is to encircle the whole of the infant's chest with both

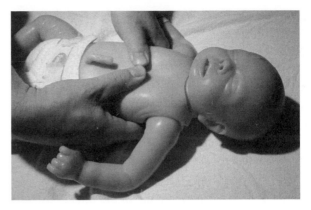

Figure 35.2 Position of hands for cardiac compression in a newborn infant.

hands and place the tips of your thumbs just below an imaginary inter-nipple line (Figure 35.2).

The chest compressions should ideally compress the chest by one-third to safely achieve maximum effectiveness and are given at a ratio of one ventilation breath to three chest compressions [16]. After approximately 15 cycles or 30 seconds, one needs to assess the infant with regards to colour, tone, respiration and heart rate. If the heart rate has improved (>60/minute) then chest compressions can be stopped and depending on the respiratory effort ventilation breaths may or may not need to continue.

If however despite good airway management with chest movement and chest compressions the heart rate does not increase, drugs should be considered.

Drugs

Emergency resuscitation drugs are very rarely required in the neonate. If you need to obtain vascular access and give drugs, the outcome for this newborn infant is likely to be poor. The drugs used in resuscitation are 4.2% sodium bicarbonate (1–2 mmol/kg), adrenaline (10 µg/kg) and 10% dextrose (2.5 ml/kg). Occasionally volume replacement (0.9% sodium chloride or O rhesus negative blood) can be given particularly if there is an obvious history of blood loss. As babies who require resuscitation often have poor peripheral circulation, the best method of administering drugs is via central access. This, in the newborn infant, will be by way of a catheter that has been inserted into the umbilical vein of the cord. Alternatively an intra-osseous needle may be used.

If central venous access is difficult the only drug that can be given via an endotracheal tube is adrenaline but due to variable absorption the efficacy of this route is questionable and therefore it is not recommended [17].

Preterm infants

Infants that are born prematurely are even more vulnerable to heat loss and therefore attention to temperature control is important. Hypothermia not only increases the risk of death in very low birthweight babies [18] but also significantly increases morbidity [19]. For those born at 30 weeks' gestation or less, immediately placing the body of the infant (without prior drying) into a plastic bag/wrap and subsequently under a radiant heater has been shown to improve maintenance of normothermia [20]. Preterm infants are more likely to require stabilisation rather than resuscitation. The approach to resuscitation is exactly the same as the approach to that of a term newborn.

Due to fragility of their lungs, the pressures required to inflate their lungs and move the chest wall will be less and if inflation breaths are required, starting with pressures of 20 cmH$_2$O should be adequate. Having given inflation breaths, prematurity may cause their respiratory effort to be insufficient and hence intubation by a trained and skilled member of the team may need to be undertaken. One may also consider using a device which is able to provide PEEP when delivering ventilation breaths. If intubation is required, administration of surfactant at this time via the endotracheal tube should be considered. Having stabilised the infant, it should be transferred to the neonatal unit for ongoing assessment and management.

Meconium aspiration

Most babies that pass meconium in utero are either term or post-term. Its presence could be an indicator of fetal stress. The fetus must be gasping in order to aspirate meconium.

If a newborn cries at delivery, despite the presence of meconium, it will imply that the infant has an open airway and therefore no action is required. If however the infant is born with no respiratory effort (i.e. apnoeic), there may have been a period of gasping in utero and this infant is at risk of meconium aspiration. Therefore it is important, having firstly paid attention to keeping the infant warm, to directly visualise the larynx and vocal cords in order to suction any large plugs of meconium which may be present using a large-bore suction catheter. Having directly visualised

the cords and either assessed that there is no obstruction or removed the obstruction one can then continue with the normal approach to newborn resuscitation [21]. There is no evidence to suggest that upper airway suctioning during delivery reduces the number of babies with meconium aspiration syndrome.

Known congenital problems

Many antenatal problems, such as oesophageal atresia with a tracheo-oesophageal fistula or a congenital diaphragmatic hernia, that could alter the approach to resuscitation, can be picked up antenatally and these babies should be delivered at an appropriate tertiary centre. However, potential congenital problems with the airway, such as Pierre–Robin sequence or Goldenhar syndrome, can be difficult to pick up on an antenatal scan and therefore the use of adjunct airways may be required if an infant needing resuscitation fails to inflate their chest with airway positioning and jaw thrust. Insertion of an appropriately sized oropharyngeal or nasopharyngeal airway can aid the maintenance of a patent airway by preventing the tongue, which is large in relation to the size of the oral cavity, flopping backwards and occluding the larynx.

Stopping resuscitation

The Resuscitation Council (UK) has suggested that if there are no signs of life after 10 minutes of continuous and adequate resuscitation then discontinuation of resuscitation may be justified [13]. This is supported with data published in 2004 which looked at outcome of term newborn infants who had resuscitation beyond 10 minutes. Of the 29 babies included in the observation study 20 died before leaving hospital. Of the nine that were discharged alive, eight had severe disability and one had moderate disability [22].

Summary

Newborn resuscitation follows a systematic stepwise approach with emphasis placed on temperature control, airway and breathing. The majority of newborn infants will not need resuscitation but should they do so, the vast majority will respond when airway and breathing are managed adequately. It is estimated that more aggressive resuscitation will be required in 1 : 2000 deliveries [23]. In the small minority who

Newborn Life Support

Figure 35.3 An algorithm for newborn resuscitation [13].

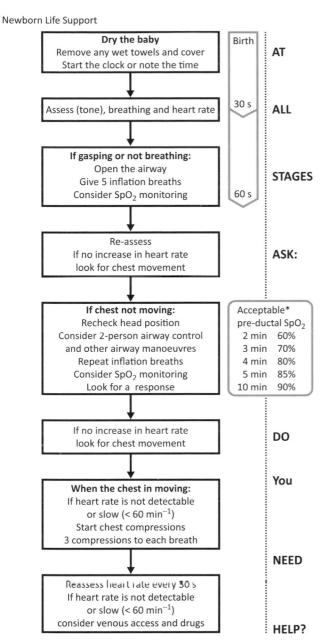

need further resuscitative measures the outcome of resuscitation is likely to be poor and good documentation of the times from birth to resuscitation steps including intubation, cardiac compressions, administration of drugs and subsequent responses will help with further management and the counselling of parents. An approach to newborn resuscitation is summarised by the algorithm provided by the Resuscitation Council (Figure 35.3) [13]. The importance of clear communication and documentation during and following resuscitation cannot be over-emphasised.

Management in low-resource settings

Each year approximately 10 million babies do not breathe immediately at birth, of which about 6 million require basic neonatal resuscitation [25, 26]. Between 5 and 10% of all babies born in facilities need some degree of resuscitation, such as tactile stimulation or airway clearing or positioning, and approximately 3–6% require basic neonatal resuscitation, consisting of these simple initial steps and assisted ventilation. The need for neonatal resuscitation is most urgent in low-resource settings, where access to intrapartum obstetric care is not consistent. In such settings, the incidence, mortality and burden of long-term impairment from intrapartum-related events is highest. Therefore the training of junior doctors and birth attendants in neonatal resuscitation is a vital component which could lead to reduction in neonatal morbidity and mortality.

The WHO guide recommends a simple, more feasible clinical criterion based on assessment of breathing alone: all babies who do not cry, do not breathe at all, or who are gasping 30 seconds after birth should be resuscitated with bag-and-mask ventilation. The key equipment for neonatal resuscitation is a self-inflating bag-and-mask. While the typical self-inflating bag-and-mask devices used in high-income countries are expensive there are affordable versions now available in many low-income settings. Key considerations are that the bag-and-mask device is designed to be reusable and easily cleaned for safe reuse.

The WHO guide does not include chest compressions in basic resuscitation unless the baby has persistent bradycardia 'despite adequate ventilation', and as long as two trained providers are present and the heart rate has been 'assessed correctly'. With the priority being ventilation, followed by chest compressions, drugs should probably not be considered, except in circumstances where three trained providers are available: a person to continue ventilation, a person to perform compressions, and a third person to administer drugs. Thus, there is probably no role for drugs in low-income settings except in advanced resuscitation in referral facilities.

Key pitfalls

- Inadequate preparation.
- Incorrect assessment of baby.
- Failure to keep baby warm.
- Incorrect position of the baby.
- Use of incorrect sized face mask.
- Incorrect technique of holding face mask.
- Not checking for chest expansion and ventilating despite no chest expansion.

- Starting chest compressions without proper lung inflation.
- Failing to call for help.

Key pearls

- Anticipation, preparation, good communication, call for help.
- Keep baby warm.
- Assessment.
- Airway…neutral position of head…jaw thrust.
- Use correct size mask and hold it correctly.
- Never proceed to chest compressions unless good chest expansion.
- Good record keeping.
- Communicate with parents.

References

1. Saugstad OD. Practical aspects of resuscitating newborn infants. *Eur J Pediatr* 1998; 157: S11–S15.
2. Richmond S. ILCOR and neonatal resuscitation 2005. *Archiv Dis Childh Fetal Neonatal Ed* 2007; 92: F163–F165.
3. Cross KW. Resuscitation of the asphyxiated infant. *Br Med Bull* 1966; 22: 73–78.
4. Dawes G. 1968. *Fetal and Neonatal Physiology*. Chicago: Year Book Publisher, 1968, pp. 141–159.
5. Godfrey S. Blood gases during asphyxia and resuscitation of fetal and newborn rabbits. *Respir Physiol* 1968; 4: 309–321.
6. Hey E, Kelly J. Gaseous exchange during endotracheal ventilation for asphyxia at birth. *J Obstet Gynaecol Br Commonw* 1968; 75: 414–423.
7. Richmond S, Wyllie J. European Resuscitation Council Guidelines for Resuscitation 2010 Section 7. Resuscitation of babies at birth. *Resuscitation* 2010; 81: 1389–1399.
8. Bhatt DR, White R, Martin G *et al.* Transitional hypothermia in preterm newborns. *J Perinatol* 2007; 27: S45–S47.
9. Gandy GM, Adamsons K, Jr., Cunningham N, Silverman WA, James LS. The thermal environment and acid–base homeostasis in human infants in first few hours of life. *J Clin Invest* 1964; 43: 751–758.
10. Stephenson JM, Du JN, Oliver TK. The effect of cooling on blood gas tension in newborn infants. *J Pediatr* 1970; 76: 848–851.
11. Tan A, Schulze A, O'Donnell CPF, Davis PG. Air versus oxygen for resuscitation of infants at birth. *Cochrane Database Syst Rev* 2005; 2: CD002273.

12. Perlman JM *et al.*; on behalf of the Neonatal Resuscitation Chapter Collaborators. Part 11: Neonatal resuscitation: 2010 International Consensus on Cardiopulmonary Resuscitation and Emergency Cardiovascular Care Science with Treatment Recommendations. *Circulation* 2010; 122 (suppl. 2): S516–S538.

13. Resuscitation Council (UK). http://www.resus.org.uk/pages/guide.htm

14. Upton CJ, Milner AD. Endotracheal resuscitation of neonates using rebreathing bag. *Archiv Dis Childhood* 1991; 66: 39–42.

15. O'Donnell C, Davis P, Morley C. Positive end-expiratory pressure for resuscitation of newborn infants at birth. *Cochrane Database System Rev* 2008; 2.

16. Meyer A, Nadkarni V, Pollock A *et al.* Evaluation of the Neonatal Resuscitation Program's recommended chest compression depth using computerized tomography imaging. *Resuscitation* 2010; 81 (5): 544–548.

17. Barber CA, Wyckoff MH. Use and efficacy of endotracheal versus intravenous epinephrine during neonatal cardiopulmonary resuscitation in the delivery room. *Paediatrics* 2006; 118: 1028–1034.

18. Stanley FJ, Alberman ED. Infants of very low birth weight. 1. Factors affecting survival. *Develop Med Child Neurol* 1978; 20: 300–312.

19. Merritt TA, Farrell PM. Diminished pulmonary lecithin synthesis in acidosis: experimental findings as related to the respiratory distress syndrome. *Pediatrics* 1976; 57: 32–40.

20. Soll RF. Heat loss prevention in neonates. *J Perinatol* 2008; 28: S57–S59.

21. National Institute of Health and Clinical Excellence. Intrapartum care: management and delivery of care to women in labour. *Clinical Guidelines* (UK) 2007, p. 42.

22. Patel H, Beeby PJ. Resuscitation beyond 10 minutes of term babies born without signs of life. *J Paediatr Child Health* 2004; 40: 136–138.

23. Morley CJ, Davis PG. Advances in neonatal resuscitation: supporting transition. *Archiv Dis Childhood Fetal Neonatal Ed* 2008; 93: F334–F336.

24. Dawson JA, Kamlin COF, Vento M *et al.* Defining the reference range for oxygen saturation for infants after birth. *Pediatrics* 2010; 125 (6): e1340–e1347.

25. Kattwinkel J. *Textbook of Neonatal Resuscitation*. Fifth Edition. Elk Grove Village, IL: American Academy of Pediatrics, 2005.

26. World Health Organization. *Basic Newborn Resuscitation: A Practical Guide*. Geneva: WHO, 1997. Available at: http://www.who.int/reproductivehealth/publications/maternal_perinatal_health/MSM_98_1/en/index.html.

Chapter 36

Morbidly adherent placenta

Nilesh Agarwal, Richard Hartopp and Edwin Chandraharan

Key facts

- Definition: Morbidly adherent placenta is a condition involving an abnormally deep attachment of the placenta, through the uterine decidua endometrium and into the myometrium. This is believed to be due to the deficiency of deciduas basalis that normally prevents placental invasion into the deeper myometrial layer. There are three types of placenta accreta, distinguishable by the depth of penetration.

  · Accreta – the placenta attaches to the muscle of the uterine wall (78% of cases).
  · Increta – the placenta extends into the muscles of the uterus (17% of cases).
  · Percreta – the placenta extends through the entire wall of the uterus (5% of cases).

- Incidence: There has been increasing incidence from 1 in 2500 deliveries to 1 in 533 deliveries [1]. It is believed that this increasing incidence is related to increasing caesarean section rates.

Key implications

- Maternal: Severe maternal morbidity and maternal mortality (7–10%), massive bleeding at delivery or postpartum and psychological sequelae secondary to traumatic birth experience.
- Fetal: neonatal admission for preterm delivery.

Key pointers

- Placenta praevia.
- Advanced maternal age.
- Previous placenta accreta.
- Previous uterine surgery like caesarean section, or myomectomy.

Key diagnostic signs

- The definitive diagnosis can be made only at surgery.
- Ultrasound examination with colour Doppler and MRI scans may aid diagnosis.
- First trimester: Vascular lacunae may be seen within the placental mass. Placenta percreta can be suspected in an early pregnancy when there is free fluid in the abdomen, which may indicate that the patient is at risk of placenta percreta.
- Second and third trimester: Vascular lacunae which are long and thin rather than round (sensitivity of 93% and a positive predictive value of 93%). Thinning or absence of the clear zone thought to be the decidua basalis, between the placenta and myometrium, is suggestive of a morbidly adherent placenta.
- Colour flow Doppler ultrasonography may be performed in women with placenta praevia to diagnose a morbidly adherent placenta in the antenatal period. Diffuse lacunae with increased blood flow (peak systolic velocity > 15 cm/s) and increased vascularity in the serosal–bladder interphase are suggestive of morbidly adherent placenta (Figure 36.1). If colour Doppler is not

Obstetric and Intrapartum Emergencies, ed. Edwin Chandraharan and Sabaratnam Arulkumaran. Published by Cambridge University Press. © Cambridge University Press 2012.

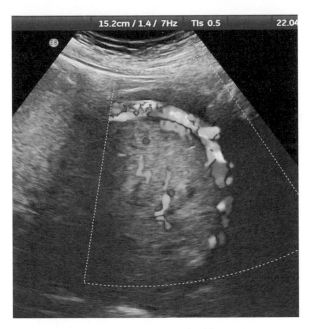

Figure 36.1 Vascular lacunae and increased flow in the serosal/bladder interphase.

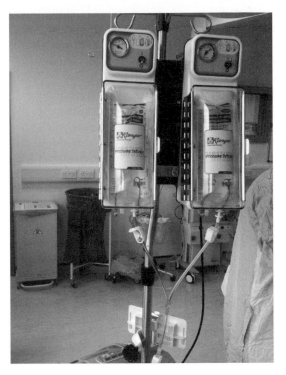

Figure 36.2 Cell saver.

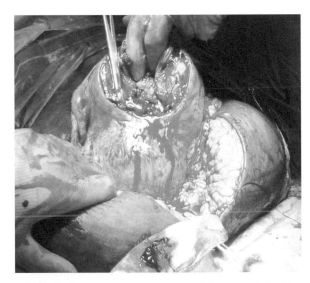

Figure 36.3 Conservative management of placenta with fundal uterine incision.

available locally, patients should be managed as per the findings of the greyscale ultrasound scan.

- The exact role of MRI has not yet been defined, but it may be of use in posterior placenta or when there is suspicion of lateral extension into the broad ligament.

Key actions

- Antenatal diagnosis should be made to ensure optimum outcome.
- A dedicated multidisciplinary team – midwives, obstetricians, anaesthetists, interventional radiologists, haematologists and others (urologists and neonatologists).
- Develop a local care bundle based on recommendation by the National Patient Safety Agency (NPSA).
- Blood and blood products should be made available at the time of surgery (i.e. if diagnosis was suspected). Facilities for cell salvage (Figure 36.2) should be used if available [2]. A clear multidisciplinary care plan should be made for women who refuse blood and blood products.

Antepartum management

- Care should be tailored to the individual needs, including the desire to retain future fertility. The different risks and treatment options should be discussed and a plan agreed, including the anticipated skin and uterine incisions, tubal sterilisation or hysterectomy [3].

- For women with placenta percreta, management options include conservative management of the placenta (intentional retention of placenta or IRP) (Figure 36.3), elective caesarean hysterectomy with or without bladder resection or uretetric implantation or the 'Triple P Procedure'. For women with suspected placenta accreta or increta, a range of conservative surgical options such as myometrial excision, multiple haemostatic sutures, uterine balloon tamponade or uterine compression sutures may be used.

- All women who are at increased risk of massive obstetric haemorrhage should be counselled regarding cell salvage and interventional radiology (prophylactic uterine artery balloon placement with or without pelvic arterial embolisation). Prevention and treatment of anaemia during the antenatal period should be optimised.

- Women should be counselled about the risks of preterm delivery and implications of massive obstetric haemorrhage such as multiple blood transfusion, admission to intensive treatment unit, needs for additional surgical procedures and emergency peripartum hysterectomy.

- If women are managed at home, they should be advised to attend immediately if they experience any bleeding, contractions or pain (including vague supra-pubic period-like aches). Prolonged inpatient care is not required (except if there is evidence of placenta percreta and the threat of uterine rupture or perforation) and can be associated with an increased risk of thromboembolism.

- If a woman is suspected of having placenta accreta, it is recommended that she be transferred to a unit with facilities for cell salvage, blood bank/haematology services and a round-the-clock interventional radiology service.

Conservative management – leaving the placenta *in situ*

- This should be considered when the preservation of fertility is desired or if placenta percreta has been diagnosed to invade vital structures. This may necessitate an extensive surgical procedure

(e.g. peripartum hysterectomy with bladder resection, ureteric implantation) that may be associated with increased maternal morbidity and mortality.

- Interventional radiologist should be involved in the care plan and a pre-operative prophylactic uterine balloon catheter placement should be considered. Therapeutic pelvic artery embolisation or surgical internal iliac artery ligation can be attempted if massive obstetric haemorrhage is encountered during surgery.

- A midline supra-umbilical incision should be considered and the uterine incision should be preferably made in the uterine fundus to avoid incising the placental bed. Fetus should be delivered through the uterine fundus and the umbilical cord should be cut clamped and ligated very close to the placental surface (approximately 4 cm).

- Patient should be prescribed antibiotics for 10 days post-surgery and inflammatory parameters should be carefully monitored. Serum beta HCG should be performed on the day of the surgery and weekly for 2 weeks.

- Methotrexate should be considered to aid placental absorption if there is a persistence of serum beta HCG for 2 weeks. However, if the serum beta HCG levels demonstrate a consistent fall in levels, methotrexate should be withheld. This is because of its effect on breastfeeding and bone marrow suppression that may aggravate anaemia and predispose to infection of retained placenta. Moreover, as methotrexate acts on rapidly dividing cells, a term placenta with falling serum beta HCG levels is unlikely to respond to it.

- Conservative management may be complicated by delayed haemorrhage or infection postoperatively that may necessitate a hysterectomy.

- Coagulopathy due to release of thromboplastins may also occur. Hence, coagulation profile should be monitored weekly.

Radical surgical management

This involves total abdominal hysterectomy with or without bladder resection for placenta percreta. If placental tissue invades the broad ligament and ureters, ureteric resection and re-implantation may be

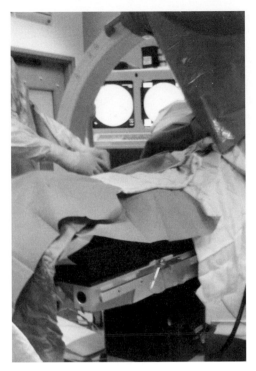

Figure 36.4 Emergency pelvic arterial embolisation with image intensifier.

required. An experienced obstetrician and gynaecologist should undertake or directly supervise this procedure and multidisciplinary input should be sought, if appropriate (e.g. urologist).

Planned caesarean hysterectomy

If antenatal diagnosis of placenta percreta has been made, prophylactic uterine artery balloon catheters may be placed and an elective caesarean hysterectomy may be performed.

Emergency caesarean hysterectomy

This procedure may become essential if placenta percreta is encountered during surgery (i.e. not diagnosed in the antenatal period) or when the attempt at conservative surgery fails and the clinician encounters massive obstetric haemorrhage. Emergency pelvic arterial embolisation also may be carried out as an adjuvant to achieve haemostasis (Figure 36.4).

Conservative surgical procedure: 'The Triple P Procedure'

This is indicated in cases of infiltration of urinary bladder wall by placental tissue and when a woman makes an informed decision to avoid a peripartum hysterectomy, after counselling [4]. It is based on avoidance of separating the morbidly adherent placenta from its underlying uterine myometrium and consists of the following three steps:

Step 1. <u>P</u>eri-operative placental localisation and delivery of the fetus through an incision placed above the upper border of the placenta.

A uterine incision is made above the upper border of the placenta to avoid incising the placental bed. As the upper border of the placenta is not always obvious after opening the abdomen, a pre-operative abdominal ultrasound scan is recommended on the operating table to identify the upper margin of the placenta. Once the abdomen is opened, direct visualisation of the anterior uterine wall should be carried out and the myometrium should be incised transversely, two finger breadths above the predetermined upper border of the placenta.

A transverse 'high' uterine incision is made above the upper border of the placenta without cutting through the placenta. In practice, as placenta percreta is commonly associated with previous caesarean section (i.e. placenta praevia), such transverse incision need not be 'too high' as the upper border of the placenta is at a lower level on the uterine wall. Hence, it could be easily accessed through a supra-pubic transverse incision.

Step 2. <u>P</u>elvic devascularisation.

After the fetus is delivered, uterus should be devascularised to avoid massive obstetric haemorrhage during myometrial excision. This could be achieved by placement of occlusion balloon catheters with their tips in the anterior division of the internal iliac arteries in the interventional radiology suite prior to caesarean section. Their position is checked prior to commencing caesarean section and the balloons are inflated with a predetermined volume to occlude flow, as assessed in the radiology suite (usually 2 ml of a contrast medium/saline mixture) immediately after the delivery of the fetus. Inflation of occlusion balloons significantly reduces the amount of bleeding from the myometrial edges during the next step. If facilities for interventional radiology are not available, systematic pelvic devascularisation could be carried out by

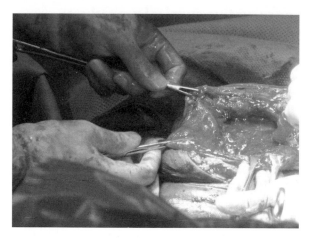

Figure 36.5 Myometrial excision: note the morbidly adherent placenta with its underlying myometrial bed has been excised.

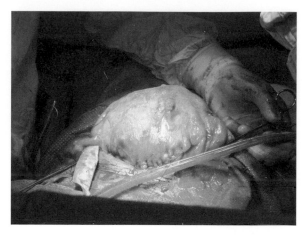

Figure 36.6 Uterus after reconstruction of the myometrial defect.

ligation of the uterine arteries or quadruple ligation or ligation of internal iliac arteries.

Step 3. 'Placental non-separation' with myometrial excision.

The entire anterior wall of the uterus (myometrium) is excised using a pair of scissors along with the deeply adherent placenta (Figure 36.5). The lateral border of the excision extends to the angles of the uterine incision. The upper border can be excised free of trophoblastic tissue. Inferiorly, the myometrium is excised up to a horizontal line drawn approximately 2 cm above the bladder reflection (upper border of the bladder) to ensure that sufficient myometrium is available to aid closure. As there has been no separation of the placenta from the myometrial wall and the blood supply to the uterus has been significantly reduced by Step 2, the bleeding is often very minimal during this procedure. Once the myometrium is excised with the bulk of the placenta, the lower lip of the incision can be everted to expose the line of invasion of the trophoblastic tissue into the posterior wall of the bladder. Placenta can be removed piecemeal from the inferior edge of the uterine incision and multiple haemostatic sutures can be directly applied to this area to prevent bleeding. Uterus is then closed in two layers as in caesarean section without any difficulty (Figure 36.6). Uterine artery balloon catheters are deflated 4 hours post-delivery if there is no bleeding. If bleeding continues postoperatively, pelvic arterial embolisation is carried out to control bleeding, by the interventional radiology team. Women should be followed up at 6 weeks and a transvaginal scan is recommended to confirm normal involution.

Postoperative care

- Patients should be managed in obstetric high dependency unit or ITU to recognise and manage complications.
- Prophylactic uterine artery balloon catheters should be deflated in 4 hours after the caesarean section, if there is no further bleeding. If the patient continues to bleed, uterine artery embolisation should be considered.
- Prophylactic antibiotics should be continued for 5 days and serum beta HCG is recommended for 2 weeks after the Triple P Procedure to ensure complete trophoblastic resorption.
- In the postnatal period, immobility, massive haemorrhage and operative delivery are independent risk factors for thromboembolism and hence thromboprophylaxis should be instituted, if there is no vaginal bleeding.
- Clinical incident reporting should be carried out for all cases of massive haemorrhage, any peripartum hysterectomy and any unexpected admission to the neonatal intensive care unit.
- Postnatal follow-up should include debriefing with an explanation of the procedures and complications, if any, and any implications for future pregnancy or fertility.

Key pitfalls

- Failure to diagnose morbidly adherent placenta antenatally.
- Failure to formulate a multidisciplinary care plan.
- Failure to counsel pre-operatively regarding management options based on clinical circumstances.
- Repeated attempts to manually remove a morbidly adherent placenta during caesarean section may produce severe haemorrhage.
- Failure to communicate clearly and effectively in an emergency.
- Failure to anticipate postpartum haemorrhage (PPH).

Key pearls

- Placenta accreta should be managed by a dedicated multidisciplinary team.
- In intentional retention of placenta (conservative management) care should be taken to avoid incising through the placenta and the umbilical cord should be cut close to the placenta.
- Ensure patient compliance prior to embarking on conservative management as delay in treatment for secondary haemorrhage or sepsis may increase maternal morbidity and mortality.

- Discuss possible complications (blood transfusion, hysterectomy and ITU admission) and involve the patient and her family in all discussions, if appropriate.
- If a woman declines blood and blood products, a multidisciplinary care plan should also involve an 'advance directive'.
- It is important to discuss sterilisation and implications on future pregnancies antenatally.

References

1. Wu S, Kocherginsky M, Hibbard JU. Abnormal placentation: twenty-year analysis. *Am J Obstet Gynecol* 2005; 192 (5): 1458–1461.

2. Royal College of Obstetricians and Gynaecologists. *Placenta Praevia, Placenta Praevia Accreta and Vasa Praevia: Diagnosis and Management.* Green-top Guideline No. 27. London: RCOG, 2011.

3. Doumouchtsis SK, Arulkumaran S. The morbidly adherent placenta: an overview of management options. *Acta Obstet Gynecol Scand* 2010; 89 (9): 1126–1133.

4. Chandraharan E, Rao S, Belli AM, Arulkumaran S. The Triple-P procedure as a conservative surgical alternative to peripartum hysterectomy for placenta percreta. *Int J Gynaecol Obstet* 2012; 117 (2): 191–194.

Chapter

37

Peri- and postmortem caesarean section

Priyantha Kandanearachchi and Edwin Chandraharan

Key facts

Perimortem caesarean section refers to caesarean delivery in an event of cardiac arrest after the initiation of cardiopulmonary resuscitation.

It is widely believed that caesarean section initially started as a postmortem procedure as a result of 'Lex Caesarea' issued by the Roman Emperor Numa Pomphillus in 715 BC. He decreed 'if a woman died whilst pregnant, the child must be cut out of her abdomen'. There are numerous historical accounts relating to postmortem caesarean sections performed with varying success but the fetal survival had been generally very low [1, 2].

The main emphasis is focused on perimortem caesarean section in view of maternal and fetal survival in modern-day obstetrics.

Perimortem caesarean section: practice points

- Cardiac arrest is a rare event in pregnancy – incidence is about 1/30 000 pregnancies [3, 4].
- Rising maternal age and associated increased incidence of medical conditions may increase risk of cardiac arrest during pregnancy [5].
- Although chest compressions in the event of a cardiac arrest in pregnancy can produce 30% of normal cardiac output, this is dependent on the woman being in a supine position. In advanced pregnancy, aorto-caval compression by the gravid uterus hinders this process and cardiac output obtained is only around 10%.

- Hence, chest compressions should be carried out with the woman in lateral tilt position which decompresses aorto-caval vessels to optimise cardiac output [6].
- Further, delivery of the fetus can, theoretically, facilitate effective cardiopulmonary resuscitation and is believed to increase cardiac output by another 60–80% which in turn may improve maternal survival. In addition to relieving mechanical difficulties and pressure on the great vessels, delivery of the fetus increases the functional residual capacity (FRC) of the maternal lungs and hence improves oxygenation. Moreover, there is a concomitant reduction of oxygen demand by the feto-placental unit, aiding further maternal oxygenation [7].
- Since the 1980s, many cases of unexpected maternal recovery following perimortem caesarean section have been reported. The evidence does seem to suggest that perimortem caesarean section will enhance maternal survival and may increase the likelihood of the birth of a viable fetus [8].
- However, the primary aim is to increase the likelihood of maternal survival by facilitating cardiopulmonary resuscitation [9].

Key implications

- Perimortem caesarean section is performed under a stressful, unfamiliar situation – with a collapsed mother, without any analgesia, with ongoing cardiac compressions and usually in an unfamiliar environment (A&E department or a labour room) without recourse to appropriate equipment and support.

Obstetric and Intrapartum Emergencies, ed. Edwin Chandraharan and Sabaratnam Arulkumaran. Published by Cambridge University Press. © Cambridge University Press 2012.

- The most senior obstetrician on the floor should demonstrate leadership and undertake this procedure in conjunction with the anaesthetist and the cardiac arrest team. The primary intention is to save the life of the mother and it should be anticipated that the fetus may be neurologically compromised due to prolonged circulatory collapse – hence, the neonatal team should be informed.
- The timing of the caesarean section is the key factor in successful neonatal outcome and evidence so far suggests that if the baby survives the early neonatal period, the chances of long-term sequelae are low [10].
- Obtaining an informed consent for the procedure is not necessary as the clinician is acting in the best interest of the woman to save her life, unless she has signed an advanced directive. The decision to do perimortem caesarean section should be taken by a senior member of medical staff and preferably involve the next of kin. However, the circumstances can vary widely and the common law doctrine of necessity may become applicable and the doctor is required to do what is necessary to preserve life.

Key pointers

The outcome of a resuscitation attempt in cardiac arrest depends on the underlying cause of the arrest and the effectiveness of initial resuscitation [10]. The same causes of cardiac arrest in non-pregnant women can occur during pregnancy.

Trauma and road traffic accidents occur in 6–7% of all pregnancies and are an important cause of co-incidental maternal deaths. However, the important pregnancy-specific causes are as follows:

- Venous thromboembolism.
- Eclampsia.
- Sepsis.
- Amniotic fluid embolism.
- Massive obstetric haemorrhage.
- Heart disease.
- Vasovagal attack (e.g. uterine rupture).
- Poisoning (e.g. organophosphates or yellow oleander).
- Iatrogenic causes such as magnesium sulphate toxicity and anaesthetic complications (e.g. total spinal).

Key actions

- 'The 4-minute rule' is the recommended approach [11]. The patient should be resuscitated in the left lateral position and any treatable cause such as magnesium sulphate toxicity or poisoning should be addressed at the same time.
- The caesarean section should be carried out after 4 minutes of arrest and should be completed in 1 minute. This is because if CPR does not restore circulation within 4 minutes, further intervention becomes necessary at this stage to prevent maternal neurological damage resulting from inadequate cerebral perfusion. There are no specific technical recommendations that exist to deliver the baby in a speedy manner via perimortem caesarean section. The 'midline approach' is often advocated because of the likelihood of a quick extraction. However, it is recognised that the current generation of obstetricians are competent in delivering via supra-pubic transverse incisions equally rapidly in extreme emergencies [12].
- The most senior obstetrician should carry out the procedure though this may not always be feasible, especially outside the labour ward setting. Caesarean can be performed with a scalpel and strict aseptic precautions may/may not be adhered to in these circumstances. However, care should be taken to avoid bowel or bladder injury and resuscitation efforts should not be interrupted during the delivery [13].
- If maternal recovery seems a likely possibility, careful closure of the incision is required as the patient may start bleeding once the circulation is restored. Generally, no anaesthesia is needed for perimortem caesarean section. However some anaesthesia or analgesia is required if the patient recovers from arrest. Timeliness of intervention is extremely important and time-consuming activities such as transportation to the operating theatre or fetal monitoring reduce the chances of maternal survival and should be avoided.
- Intra-uterine death should not prevent an obstetrician from performing perimortem caesarean section to facilitate maternal resuscitation [14].
- A place where the need for perimortem caesarean section could arise is the A&E department [15]. A protocol to deal with the event and preferably

staff capable of performing the operation are required.

- It is necessary to include this procedure in regular drills. Whether necessary training should be given to ambulance crew or paramedics who may find themselves in a situation requiring perimortem caesarean section outside the hospital setting is debatable [16].

Key pitfalls

- Due to the rarity of this procedure, all the above recommendations are based on case reports and expert opinions [17].
- The confounding factors such as differing causes of cardiac arrest, maternal comorbidities, the quality of resuscitation and the skills of the surgeon can give rise to difficulties when evaluating a complex clinical issue like this.
- There are ethical and medico-legal issues such as informed consent which cannot be taken due to the necessary rapidity of decision-making to perform perimortem caesarean section. However, there are no reports of court decisions against doctors performing perimortem caesarean section [6].
- Failure to undertake due care and follow standard surgical techniques may result in both recognised and unrecognised bowel or bladder injuries.
- Unfamiliarity of the situation and need for rapid delivery may result in unintended needle-stick and other injury to surgeon and staff.

Key pearls

- Clinicians should be aware of the situations which can potentially give rise to cardiorespiratory arrest in pregnancy.
- Regular mock drills in CPR in pregnancy and to include perimortem caesarean section in the training sessions – cardiac arrest trolleys should have a fixed scalpel and basic equipment (i.e. a suture set).
- Senior input to the decision-making in performing perimortem caesarean section.
- Dedicated perimortem caesarean packs to be located in labour suite and emergency departments which contain aseptic solution, disposable solution and packs for the uterus [18].

- For cardiorespiratory arrest following massive obstetric haemorrhage, a hysterectomy should be considered as a life-saving procedure during perimortem caesarean section if bleeding persists despite measures to achieve haemostasis.
- Clinicians should be aware of the very rare but potential locations in which women may have cardiac arrest such as the supermarket. In this case use of alcoholic drinks to clean the abdomen and use of knives from the 'kitchen section' may help expedite delivery within 4 minutes of cardiac arrest, whilst awaiting help.
- Continuous learning and dissemination of lessons learned is very valuable as there is limited scientific literature in this subject.
- The patient, her partner and her family should be debriefed by a senior clinician.
- All staff involved in perimortem caesarean section should have a de-briefing as this is a stressful and traumatic incident.

References

1. Lanoix R, Akkapeddi V, Goldfeder B. Perimortem cesarean section: case reports and recommendations. *Acad Emerg Med* 1995; 2: 1063.

2. Katz VL, Dotters DJ, Droegemueller W. Perimortem cesarean delivery.*Obstet Gynecol* 1986; 68: 571–576.

3. Bowers W, Wagner C. Field perimortem cesarean section. *Air Med J* 2001; 20: 10–11.

4. Marx GF. Cardiopulmonary resuscitation of late-pregnant women. *Anesthesiology* 1982; 56: 156.

5. The Confidential Enquiry into Maternal and Child Health (CEMACH). *Saving Mothers' Lives': Reviewing Maternal Deaths to make Motherhood Safer – 2003–2005. The Seventh Report on Confidential Enquiries into Maternal Deaths in the United Kingdom.* London: CEMACH, 2007.

6. Howell C, Grady K, Cox C. *Managing Obstetric Emergencies and Trauma – the MOET Course Manual.* Second edition. London: RCOG, 2007.

7. Whitten M, Montgomery L. Post-mortem and perimortem caesarean section: what are the indications? *J Royal Soc Med* 2000; 93: 6–9.

8. Capobianco G, Balata A, Mannazzu MC *et al.* Perimortem cesarean delivery 30 min after a laboring patient jumped from a fourth-floor window: baby survives and is normal at age 4 years. *Am J Obstet Gynecol* 2008; 198: e15–e16.

9. Oates S, Williams GL, Rees GAD. Cardiopulmonary resuscitation in late pregnancy. *Br Med J* 1988; 297: 404–405.

10. O'Connor RL, Sevarino FB. Cardiopulmonary arrest in the pregnant patient: a report of a successful resuscitation. *J Clin Anesth* 1994; 6: 66–68.

11. Page-Rodriguez A, Gonzalez-Sanchez JA. Perimortem caesarean section of a twin pregnancy: case report and review of the literature. *Acad Emerg Med* 1999; 6: 1072–1074.

12. Parker J, Balis N, Chester S, Adey D. Cardiopulmonary arrest in pregnancy: successful resuscitation of mother and infant following immediate cesarean section in labour ward. *Aust N Z J Obstet Gynaecol* 1996; 36: 207–210.

13. Yeomans ER, Gilstrap LC. Physiologic changes in pregnancy and their impact on critical care. *Crit Care Med* 2005; 33 (10): S256–S258.

14. Dijkman A, Huisman C, Smit M *et al.* Cardiac arrest in pregnancy: increasing use of perimortem caesarean section due to emergency skills training? *Br J Obstet Gynaecol* 2010; 117: 282–287.

15. Warraich Q, Esen U. For perimortem caesarean section, the surgical knife is the most important instrument. *Br J Obstet Gynaecol* 2010; 117: 768.

16. Katz V, Balderston K, DeFreest M. Perimortem cesarean delivery: were our assumptions correct? *Am J Obstet Gynecol* 2005; 192: 1916–1920.

17. American Heart Association. The American Heart Association Guidelines 2005 for cardiopulmonary resuscitation and emergency cardiovascular Care. Part 10.8: cardiac arrest associated with pregnancy. *Circulation* 2005; 112: IV150–IV153.

18. Mallampalli A, Powner DJ, Gardner MO. Cardiopulmonary resuscitation and somatic support of the pregnant patient. *Crit Care Clin* 2004; 20: 747–761.

38

Setting up and running labour ward fire drills

Karolina Afors and Edwin Chandraharan

Definition

'Labour Ward Fire Drills' refers to the use of simulation of obstetric emergencies within the labour ward to ensure effective communication, multidisciplinary and multiprofessional team working in order to promote good practice as well as to identify and rectify individual and system factors so as to optimise the clinical outcome.

Key facts

- Substandard care accounts for over half of maternal and perinatal deaths in the UK.
- Failures in effective communication, team working and leadership during emergencies contribute to poor outcome.
- Obstetric emergencies cannot always be anticipated, but the impact of these adverse events can be decreased with the use of training through simulation.
- Simulation refers to the recreating of real-life clinical scenarios.
- 'Fire drill' programmes using simulation of patients and clinical scenarios are useful for training doctors, midwives and allied staff to manage critical emergencies effectively.

Key areas where labour ward fire drills may be used

- Umbilical cord prolapse, shoulder dystocia, obstetric haemorrhage, eclampsia and undiagnosed vaginal breech.
- Sudden postpartum maternal collapse, unexpected poor neonatal outcome.

Key implications

- Fire drills were initially advocated in the 1999 'Confidential Enquiry into Maternal Deaths' for use in obstetric emergencies.
- The most recent centre for maternal and child health enquiries (CEMACE report, 2006–2008) reiterated and emphasised the use of high-fidelity simulation training in maternity care [1].
- The use of simulation training in other medical fields has shown to lead to improved performance.
- Studies exploring the use of simulation as a training tool within obstetrics have been encouraging. Improved clinical outcome has been demonstrated where simulation training was used in the management of shoulder dystocia [2].
- 'Fire drills' provide a relaxed stress-free environment in which trainees and clinicians can learn and develop hands-on skills.
- Regular fire drills and simulation training can also be applied as a means of improving patient safety aimed at reducing medical errors and adverse events.

Key pointers to setting up labour ward fire drills

Planning

- Get the required equipment for the 'planned simulation' of the given obstetric emergency (e.g. manikin, postpartum haemorrhage (PPH) trolley) (Figures 38.1–38.4).

Obstetric and Intrapartum Emergencies, ed. Edwin Chandraharan and Sabaratnam Arulkumaran. Published by Cambridge University Press. © Cambridge University Press 2012.

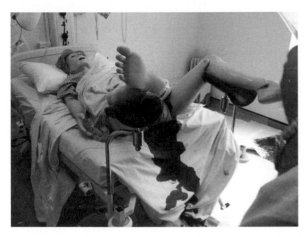

Figure 38.1 Postpartum haemorrhage (to estimate blood loss and to initiate appropriate actions).

- Identify a suitable location within the labour ward (e.g. a vacant delivery room).
- Develop a structured process for each obstetric emergency and clearly define roles for all team members involved in the fire drill.
- Assigned roles include that for the anaesthetist, obstetrician, senior midwife, junior midwife, healthcare assistant and midwifery student.
- Prior to commencing the fire drill, inform labour ward matron to ensure maximum participation of clinicians.
- Ensure that the fire drill is conducted at a time when there is no ongoing obstetric emergency in the labour ward to maximise participation and learning.

Implementation

- As staff enter the room, inform them that it is a fire drill and that staff are expected to participate.
- Provide required clinical information and encourage questions and clarifications.
- Assign specific roles to team members. Deep immersion simulation involving life-like manikins and monitoring devices may also be used, if available.
- Individual drills may be videotaped and immediately reviewed, if facilities are available.
- Assign one team member to lead the critique and facilitate discussion.

Evaluation

- Assess response times, leadership, delegation of tasks and cross-checking that assigned tasks have been performed.
- Interventions and documentation of fire drill e.g. shoulder dystocia is revised and mnemonics revisited.
- Ensure that specific manoeuvres e.g. McRobert's and correct positioning for supra-pubic pressure is demonstrated on a manikin.
- Pendleton's Rules may be used in providing group feedback, by asking the following questions:
  - How did the scenario go?
  - What went right?
  - Were there areas of difficulty?
  - What would the individual/team do differently next time?
- Identify any system/organisational factors (e.g. PPH trolley not available? Guidelines ambiguous?).

Learning from the experience

- Fire drill sessions provide an environment where algorithms and management guidelines can be discussed, revised and improved.
- Fire drills may help the team to revise and update the dosages and routes of administration of drugs used in obstetric emergencies.
- Fire drills represent an informal way of assessing clinical performance.
- Fire drills may help identify training needs for individuals as well as the team.
- Fire drills enable clinicians to develop communication skills in an emergency.
- Helps in developing leadership in an emergency.

Key actions

Equipment needed

- Simulated patient – either manikin or role playing.
- Other key members of medical team i.e. anaesthetist, obstetrician, senior midwife, junior midwife and healthcare assistant.
- Pelvic models to revise practical procedures e.g. vaginal breech, internal manoeuvres for management of shoulder dystocia.

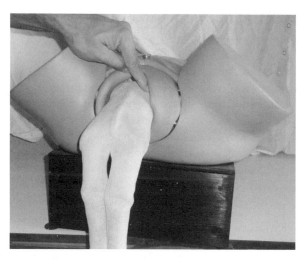

Figure 38.2 Assisted vaginal breech delivery (if inferior angle does not become visible – the need to initiate Løvset's manoeuvre).

- Monitoring equipment for assessment of pulse, blood pressure, pulse oximetry.
- Intravenous drugs and associated instrument sets, syringes to practise drawing-up drugs e.g. for eclampsia, PPH.
- Early-warning system for recording observations. Pen and paper or proforma for documentation.

Example of a labour ward fire drill in an 'all-resource' setting

Scenario: Shoulder dystocia

- Suspected by midwife – 'head bobbing', 'Turtle neck sign'.

Assess whether the following occurred during simulation:

- Call activated for 'help' – obstetrician, anaesthetist, neonatologist and senior midwife. Ensure scribe assigned role and 30-second time intervals called out.
- Explanation and reassurance was provided to the woman by the senior clinician entering the room.
- Positioning – whether the clinician instructed the midwives to draw woman to edge of bed.
- Clear instruction was provided as to how to perform a McRobert's manoeuvre – hyperflexion of hips, abduction and external rotation of the thighs.

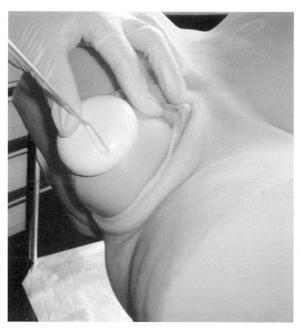

Figure 38.3 Cord prolapse in second stage of labour – emergency ventouse delivery.

- Fetal position was assessed prior to requesting supra-pubic pressure plus moderate traction.
- If the above measures failed, did the clinician assess the need for episiotomy?
- Performance of secondary manoeuvres.
- Rotational manoeuvres (Wood's screw/reverse Wood's screw or delivery posterior arm and shoulder).
- Management options were discussed if above measures failed.
- Moved patient on to all fours/repeated manoeuvres again.
- Cephalic replacement and caesarean section (Zavanelli manoeuvre), symphysiotomy or cleidotomy.
- Examination of genital tract was performed and whether there was recognition of increased risk of PPH.
- Documentation and postdelivery actions were completed – use 'Shoulder Dystocia proforma', record of umbilical cord gases, timings and which shoulder was anterior. Incident reporting. Debriefing the woman and her partner. Arranging follow-up if complications occurred.

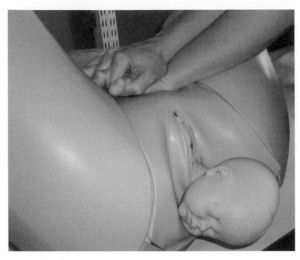

Figure 38.4 Shoulder dystocia – legs abducted and in McRobert's position plus directed supra-pubic pressure.

Debriefing and feedback

Pendleton's principles provide a structured interactive approach of giving feedback. It consists of a step-by-step model.

(1) Trainee performs skills activity.
(2) Questions on points of clarification are allowed.
(3) Trainee leads on what they thought was done well.
(4) Assessor discusses what went well.
(5) Trainee identifies what didn't go well.
(6) Assessor discusses what didn't go well.
(7) The trainee identifies elements that can be improved upon.
(8) Assessor discusses how improvements can be implemented.

Key pitfalls

- High-fidelity simulation manikins can be expensive and drill scenarios can be time consuming.
- Ensuring availability of clinical staff is often difficult to accommodate, especially if the labour ward is busy.
- Lack of constructive structured feedback that may impact on the trainees' learning experience.

Key pearls

- Fire drills promote multidisciplinary, multiprofessional teamwork.
- Simulation of obstetric emergencies allows trainees to develop clinical skills without exposing patients to suboptimal care.
- Fire drill sessions provide an environment in which protocols and guidelines can be reviewed and revised.
- Fire drills help identify and rectify organisational or system factors that may contribute to poor outcome during an obstetric emergency.

References

1. Centre for Maternal and Child Enquiries (CMACE). *Saving Mothers' Lives: Reviewing Maternal Deaths to make Motherhood Safer – 2006–2008. The Eighth Report on Confidential Enquiries into Maternal Deaths in the United Kingdom. Br J Obstet Gynaecol* 2011; 118 (Suppl. 1): 1–208.

2. Crofts JF, Bartlett C, Ellis D *et al.* Training for shoulder dystocia: a trial of simulation using low-fidelity and high-fidelity mannequins. *Am J Obstet Gynecol* 2006; 108 (6): 1477–1485.

Chapter

39

Simulation training

Emma Evans and Polly Hughes

Key facts

Simulation training is an educational tool that incorporates exposure/exploration of human factors/situational awareness/team working and communication in 'real life' scenarios i.e. non-technical skills as well as technical actual clinical management of a patient.

Types of simulation training

- Low fidelity: This includes the use of patient actors to play simulated patients with an emphasis on role-play and lifeless 'resus' style manikins or models.
- Hybrid: This incorporates both simulated patients and part-task trainers in combination to allow emphasis on communication while completing a skilled task e.g. delivering a baby using a PROMPT trainer. This has been evaluated and found to improve the attainment of skills training [1].
- Medium fidelity: This style of simulation training incorporates human patient simulators that have trainer-controlled electronic physiology in-built with monitors that can be read during simulated emergencies. They are designed to allow abnormal physiology to be found on examination and to be acted on in real time by candidates.
- High fidelity: The most highly technical of all human patient simulators, these manikins have the ability to respond to the actions of candidates

within scenarios via physiologically modelled software. As such they are the most costly of all and require technical expertise to use effectively.

The concept of fidelity does not only relate to the complexity and realism of the manikin. Fidelity can also be thought of as the potential to allow participants to suspend disbelief and to engage in simulation as if it were a real clinical scenario. For example, one can increase psychological and environmental fidelity by using part-task trainers or manikins within a clinical environment and utilising real members of an obstetric team, rather than in a simulation laboratory; this has been shown to increase learning.

Role of simulation training

- To introduce and explore the concept of human factors.
- To allow development of technical and non-technical skills [2].
- For individual and team training, especially to explore communication across specialities.
- To emphasise the role of feedback to enhance performance [3].
- To allow rehearsal of rare events, for example maternal cardiac arrest.
- To recreate critical incidents within a unit to allow for system error recognition as part of a combined risk reduction/education strategy.
- To allow testing of new protocols and guidelines.
- To facilitate medical device training.

Obstetric and Intrapartum Emergencies, ed. Edwin Chandraharan and Sabaratnam Arulkumaran. Published by Cambridge University Press. © Cambridge University Press 2012.

Key implications

- Maternal: Aimed at increasing exposure to rare events which can reduce poor outcomes and ultimately improve maternal care and patient experience.
- Fetal/neonatal: Outcome improvement has been seen through several strategies using simulation within UK obstetric units, particularly in relation to hypoxic ischaemic encephalopathy (HIE) and brachial plexus injury relating to shoulder dystocia [4, 5].
- Medico-legal: Clinical negligence claims may be reduced due to improved communication, team working and as a result of changing systems through regular evaluation of performance and ergonomics of the clinical environment to minimise the impact of system error on medical care. Ultimately the end result should be improved patient care.

Key pointers

- Useful for trainees to reduce the impact of European Working Time Directive (EWTD) and subsequent reduction in hours of training (Templeton review) that may reduce their exposure to rare events [6].
- Risk management – may help to address communication and team working.
- Clinical environment – additional sphere/parameter to work with and enhance reality.
- To help teams to learn from CEMACH recommendations/guidelines/revalidation/good medical practice.

Key actions

Simulation training personnel

- The background of personnel delivering simulation training can be extremely varied and represents the skill mix required specifically for the complexity of manikin used or whether the training involves a full immersion simulation laboratory or a clinical environment, uses video debrief or team evaluation, for example.
- Many will be very familiar with low-fidelity simulation. Identifying the training needs of faculty is as important to allow all members to contribute effectively in scenario design and evaluation.

Time

- Time should be scheduled within the job plans of trainers involved in order to develop and deliver training aligned with learning needs and clinical outcome improvement strategies.
- Time to deliver training can be in the form of mandatory study days where staff are released from clinical duties and/or as part of 'fire-drills' where training occurs on wards using real teams in carrying out clinical duties [7]. Both have their relative merits and both require a set-up, delivery and debrief time allowance; drills always carry the possibility that clinical areas may be too busy and that training will present too great a pressure, so rescheduling may be necessary.

Teaching skills

- All clinical teaching operates around principles of evaluation of learning needs, design of training aligned with educational outcomes and evaluation of learning and feedback, though historically on a more informal basis. These can be developed easily in those without formal teaching experience who have the time, enthusiasm and drive to deliver simulation through appropriately designed 'Train the Trainers' programmes and are generic skills relevant to all clinical teaching.

Multidisciplinary input, including ancillary staff

- The key to success is the involvement of a multiprofessional training team, from midwifery through to obstetric, anaesthetic, theatre and ancillary (e.g. portering, laboratory) staff in order to represent the key professionals that will benefit most from recreating a clinical situation. Each professional group has their own valuable contribution and perspectives on the limiting steps within clinical scenarios.

Report writing and actions with feedback

- Disseminating the learning outcomes from this form of training is paramount to sharing the experience with a whole unit. Simulation is time and labour intensive and clinical workload itself often prohibits optimum frequency of delivery of training. In addition due to working patterns it is often not possible to encompass all staff. Reports allow for shared learning and for staff to discover where working environment or system difficulties have been revealed through training exercises, and improvements put in place as a result. Dissemination of this information can be as part of a risk newsletter, poster and/or presentation at clinical governance forums.
- Incorporate into regular clinical environment so non-threatening and minimising cost implications.
- Familiarisation of staff with simulation can be easily achieved by training on the unit itself but may need to be introduced in a step-wise fashion in order to be accepted as a valuable resource to a unit. From a psychological perspective simulation is more realistic in the workplace, and as such its learning potential has been found to be greater. This approach gradually reduces the dependence on dedicated simulation centres and staff that can be very costly.

Integration of teamwork principles

- Simulation training provides an invaluable platform on which to develop non-technical skills and to improve team working. Literature suggests that its benefits exceed that of traditional lecture-based teamwork theory training. Bringing together teams that work together, particularly in their own clinical environment, has powerful learning transfer.

Use of actors and real training tools/equipment

- Use patient actors and anatomical models alongside more complex manikins. The priority is achieving learning and high fidelity may be unnecessary or detrimental in certain scenarios e.g. recreating eclampsia or conducting a birthing pool evacuation. This has enormous implications for low-resource settings and has been the basis for development of the PROMPT programme [8].

Conducting an obstetric simulation training exercise – the three Es

Examine – what happened during training?

- What was the clinical situation?
- What did the management of the patient involve (mother/fetus if relevant)?
- Who did what? For example who took the role of the leader/scribe?
- Were there any difficulties/ways to do things differently?

Explore – issues arising from the training

- Were there any difficulties communicating with team members?
- Were there any issues about obtaining key equipment/drugs when needed?
- What happened about care of other women?
- How effectively did the team function?

Escalate – risk issues highlighted and how to action them

- How to communicate more efficiently – for example, use of Situation–Awareness–Background–Recommendation (SBAR) format, use of emergency bell.
- Delegation of staff i.e. appropriate use of other personnel – for example healthcare assistant to call the lift for transfer.
- Development of emergency scribing proforma/availability of haemorrhage box or emergency box in other clinical areas, not just the labour ward.
- Uncover and address latent safety threats in the clinical setting.

Key pitfalls

- Do not assess individuals on their clinical skills.
- Failure to engage whole team i.e. make simulation training multidisciplinary to allow wide range of factors to be explored, for example

communication with theatre staff, logistics of retrieving blood products.

Outcomes from simulation training: scientific evidence

Ideally simulation training should ultimately lead to improved clinical outcomes for the women and their babies by reducing preventable harm. Current proven benefits of training include increased confidence in managing obstetric emergencies and better team working.

The Simulation and Fire-drill Evaluation (SaFE) Study demonstrated that multiprofessional obstetric emergency training:

- Improves knowledge of both midwives and doctors of all experience levels.
- Significantly improves the proportion of maternity staff who can competently manage a simulation of shoulder dystocia, with retention of skills.
- Significantly improves the completeness and efficiency of the management of simulated eclampsia.
- Improves the patient-actor's perception of care.

This important study did not find additional improvement by conducting the training in a simulation centre compared with the local hospital and also suggests that training using actors rather than computerised manikins may improve care further, in particular with respect to safety and communication [9].

In addition, there is now research evidence available detailing measureable improvements in quantifiable important outcomes. In one UK unit, the introduction of multiprofessional obstetric emergency training was associated with:

- 50% reduction in Apgar score < 7 at 5 minutes in term infants.
- 50% reduction in the incidence of HIE in term infants [4].
- 70% reduction in brachial plexus injuries after shoulder dystocia [5].
- 40% reduction in median decision-to-delivery time in cases of cord prolapse [7].

Key pearls

- All staff providing intrapartum and emergency obstetric care should undergo annual skills and

drills training to include multidisciplinary simulation training.

- Regular simulation training should be conducted in the clinical areas as this allows realistic situational awareness to be explored and acted upon as well as increasing multiprofessional input.
- Lessons learned from simulation training should feed into the risk-management system i.e. primary prevention and vice versa: risk management highlighting areas of care that simulation training can address (secondary prevention). In addition the use of 'maternity dashboards' may also identify areas to direct the focus of this type of training within a unit.
- All staff should be encouraged to give feedback.
- Reports of simulation training exercises and resultant actions/improvements in the service should be disseminated to the entire team by newsletters and governance seminars.
- There is increasing evidence that multidisciplinary training in obstetric emergencies improves outcome.

References

1. Crofts JF, Bartlett C, Ellis D *et al.* Training for shoulder dystocia: a trial of simulation using low-fidelity and high-fidelity mannequins. *Obstet Gynecol* 2006; 108 (6): 1477–1185.

2. Crofts JF, Ellis D, Draycott TJ *et al.* Change in knowledge of midwives and obstetricians following obstetric emergency training: a randomised controlled trial of local hospital, simulation centre and teamwork training. *Br J Obstet Gynaecol* 2007; 114 (12): 1534–1541.

3. Crofts JF, Bartlett C, Ellis D *et al.* Patient-actor perception of care: a comparison of obstetric emergency training using manikins and patient-actors. *Quality Safety Health Care* 2008; 17 (1): 20–24.

4. Draycott T, Sibanda T, Owen L *et al.* Does training in obstetric emergencies improve neonatal outcome? *Br J Obstet Gynaecol* 2006; 113 (2): 177–182.

5. Draycott TJ, Crofts JF, Ash JP *et al.* Improving neonatal outcome through practical shoulder dystocia training. *Obstet Gynecol* 2008; 112 (1): 14–20.

6. Ellis D, Crofts JF, Hunt LP *et al.* Hospital, simulation center, and teamwork training for eclampsia management: a randomized controlled trial. *Obstet Gynecol* 2008; 111 (3): 723–733.

7. Siassakos D, Hasafa Z, Sibanda T *et al*. Retrospective cohort study of diagnosis–delivery interval with umbilical cord prolapse: the effect of team training. *Br J Obstet Gynaecol* 2009; 116 (8): 1089–1096.

8. Draycott T, Winter C, Crofts J, Barnfield S (Eds.) *PROMPT. Practical Obstetric Multiprofessional Training: Course Manual*. London: RCOG, 2008; pp. 3–10 and 69–85.

9. Siassakos D, Crofts J, Winter C, Draycott T. Multiprofessional 'fire-drill' training in the labour ward. *Obstet Gynaecologist* 2009; 11: 55–60.

Chapter

40

Risk management (emergency obstetric and intrapartum care)

Jessica Moore

Key facts

There are high expectations for a good outcome for mother and baby in pregnancy. With advances in healthcare the expectations are also increasing for so-called high-risk pregnancies.

Labour is a risky business where the clinical situation can change very quickly and without warning. Therefore obstetric emergencies require prompt action by the right clinicians with the required expertise and equipment to deal with the problem effectively. During such emergencies this critical decision-making and intervention can mean the difference between a good and bad outcome for mother and baby.

What is risk management?

Risk management is a systematic approach to reducing the risk of harm to a patient.

The concept of patient safety is not new; it has always been the goal of clinicians to achieve the best outcome for a patient. However, the formal process of risk management is a relatively new and evolving aspect of healthcare. A key publication by the Department of Health in the UK in 2000 highlighted the need to learn from clinical errors [1]. As a consequence recommendations were made for a new system of national reporting and analysis of adverse healthcare events bringing risk management to the fore. In the UK subsequent documents aimed at the standards for safer childbirth have spelled out the need for robust risk management procedures to ensure quality care [2, 3].

The process of risk management arose from the response to rising litigation in obstetrics. However, the key aim now is patient safety with a reduction in litigation as a result of this.

The process of providing the best care for patients by regular monitoring of performance and a constant striving to improve performance is known as clinical governance. Risk management is one of the cornerstones of clinical governance and encompasses many of the other pillars of clinical governance including audit, education and training and the resolution of complaints.

The importance of risk management

There is an increasing awareness of patient safety and the fact that patient safety is everyone's responsibility. Hence it is essential that all clinicians at every level are aware of the processes and function of risk management. It is wrong to think that risk management is just the concern of managers or the risk management team and not all clinicians. It is also wrong to think that risk management is just about blaming individuals when there is an adverse outcome. Although individuals may play a part in an adverse outcome risk management is about looking at the systems behind individuals' actions. By embracing the risk management process and making it a part of the everyday practice of all clinicians both patients and the clinician will benefit. Although the aims of risk management are to prevent adverse outcomes for the mother and baby it also provides a vital role in ensuring safe practice by clinicians. Clinicians involved in cases with poor outcomes are likely themselves to be affected psychologically which may impact on their working practice and general well-being.

The other important impact of good risk management is a financial gain by the reduction

Obstetric and Intrapartum Emergencies, ed. Edwin Chandraharan and Sabaratnam Arulkumaran. Published by Cambridge University Press. © Cambridge University Press 2012.

of litigation claims. Although mistakes do not occur more frequently in obstetric practice than other areas of medicine the litigation costs associated with adverse outcomes are high. Hence obstetric claims make up the biggest financial outlay for most health services [4].

Risk management is important in the local context of each maternity department but also as part of regional and national risk management.

What are the risks in emergency and intrapartum care?

Obstetric emergencies can result in maternal and perinatal morbidity and mortality. Even the best maternity departments will experience adverse outcomes, some of which were anticipated, others not. Very often risk-management cases looking at obstetric emergencies may identify factors earlier in pregnancy or labour which contributed to the outcome.

Some emergencies are frequently encountered on a maternity unit, such as postpartum haemorrhage. Such emergencies will be familiar to the healthcare professionals working on the delivery suite and there may well be protocols and guidelines to help with their management and other tools such as proformas to ensure good documentation during these emergencies. However, even with such emergencies which are familiar and may be anticipated, it is still important to incorporate them into the risk management process to ensure the best possible outcome.

In addition to the well-recognised complications in obstetrics there are rare emergencies and complications during the intrapartum period which may occur, such as cardiac arrest in labour. Such adverse events may not be anticipated and have potential for a major adverse outcome. These cases are most likely to be investigated after the event has occurred.

The potential for risk events in intrapartum care may be obvious in high-risk pregnancy such as a twin pregnancy. In other cases risk events may occur unexpectedly in low-risk pregnancy such as a shoulder dystocia at a home delivery.

The incidence of risk events

It is difficult to provide data on the incidence of risk events in obstetric and intrapartum emergencies since this is lacking. This is exacerbated by lack of clear definitions of risk-management incidents and poor reporting, especially of near misses. However, some evidence points to around 8% of deliveries resulting in a suboptimal outcome [5].

It is important for individuals to have an appreciation of the incidence of risk events in their department. Such information should be made readily available by the departmental risk-management team through risk meetings, monthly newsletters and the maternity dashboard [6].

It is also useful to know how these incidents compare with other similar departments.

Finally, there are national audits such as the audit on maternal mortality by the Centre for Maternal and Child Enquiries (CEMACE) which collect data on maternal deaths in the UK so lessons can be learned and changes implemented. Such national audits are useful on an international scale too and may allow similar countries to compare themselves. In the most recent triennial report [7] the assessors felt that a degree of substandard care contributed to 70% of direct deaths and 55% of indirect deaths.

Key pointers

- Risk management is the concern of every clinician working in the maternity department. Individuals have a responsibility to participate and embrace the risk management process.
- Risk management is a multidisciplinary process. A risk-management team for obstetric incidents would most likely include a senior obstetrician, midwife, anaesthetist, neonatologist and service manager. It is also very important to include trainees to ensure representation from trainees and to instil risk management in the curriculum.
- Risk management involves both prospective and retrospective analysis of risk events. Potential risks are examined to minimise the chance of them occurring and where mistakes have been made lessons are learned to prevent recurrence.
- Good risk management looks at systems failures and not individual failures contributing to an adverse outcome to promote a fair-blame culture.
- Successful risk management arises from good leadership to embed risk management into everyday practice.
- Risk management is important at local, regional and national levels.

Key implications

Adverse outcomes from obstetric emergencies can affect:

- Mother and baby.
- Partner and family.
- Healthcare professionals – those directly and indirectly involved.
- Departmental managers.
- Hospital reputation.

The effects may be:

- Physical in terms of morbidity and mortality.
- Psychological.
- Financial.

Key implications of risk management

- The safety of patients – mother and baby.
- To ensure good evidence-based practice by staff.
- To look at systems and not individuals which contribute to an adverse outcome.
- To learn from mistakes and avoid repeating them.

There is evidence that good risk management can make a difference in terms of safer patient care. In the UK the largest maternity unit has achieved an 11% reduction in the number of clinical incidents where there was felt to be a degree of substandard care following the introduction of a comprehensive risk-management strategy [8].

Key actions

The risk-management process

When looking at the risk-management process it is useful to remember that risk events may be investigated in two ways:

- Retrospectively or reactively – the investigation of an adverse incident after the event has occurred.
- Prospectively or proactively – anticipation of risk events.

It is very important to be aware that risk management is not just about investigating cases with an adverse outcome.

The steps in the risk-management process

There are four key steps in the risk process [9]:

- Identification of risk event.
- Analysis of risk event.
- Treatment of risk events.
- Measures to control risk events.

Identification of risk

The identification of risk events may come from local sources within a department or external sources such as national audits.

Proactive risk

- Risk assessment conducted on delivery suite.
- Staff consultation – workshops, surveys.
- Fire drills.
- National confidential enquiries into maternal and perinatal mortality and morbidity.
- National guidelines on risk management, for example Clinical Negligence Scheme for Trusts guidelines.
- National college guidelines and care bundles.
- Advice for organisations devoted to patient safety, for example National Patient Safety Agency alerts in the UK.

With regard to obstetric emergencies much can be done with prospective identification of risk. For example staff consultation in workshops or surveys may highlight risk events when managing obstetric emergencies that were not reported as the outcome was good but could in a subsequent emergency result in a poor outcome. In addition there may be potential risks identified in the department with the use of fire drills on the delivery suite.

In the UK the Centre for Maternal and Child Enquiries (CEMACE) carries out the Confidential Enquiry into Maternal and Child Health with a national audit of maternal deaths. The reports are published triennially with recommendations on improving care from the lessons learned as a result of the maternal deaths reviewed. The last triennial report [7] highlighted 10 key recommendations aimed at improving patient care which should be implemented in every maternity department. One of these recommendations related to the standard of investigation and reporting following a serious incident. As maternal deaths are rare in countries like the UK attention has turned to looking at severe morbidity and the lessons which can be learned. The UK Obstetric Surveillance System is collecting data on near-miss maternal morbidity in the UK such as amniotic fluid embolism and septic shock to make recommendations for best practice and improve outcomes for women.

Organisations such as the National Patient Safety Agency (NPSA) in the UK exist with the aims to lead and contribute to improved, safe patient care by informing, supporting and influencing individuals and organisations working in the health sector. The NPSA analyses reports on patient safety nationally and identifies risks and recommends actions to reduce risks [10].

National colleges such as the Royal College of Obstetricians and Gynaecologists (RCOG) in the UK provide guidance on clinical practice to reduce risks. More recently the concept of care bundles is being developed to improve safety in clinical practice. A care bundle is a set of three to five practices or precautionary steps developed in a clear and straightforward manner with the focus being on delivering the best care [11]. The RCOG also provides guidance on clinical governance including risk management [9]. Other national bodies such as the National Institute for Health and Clinical Excellence (NICE) produce evidence-based guidelines for use in England and Wales. One such guideline exists on intrapartum care [12].

There may be national schemes to ensure quality care such as those standards imposed in the UK by the NHS Litigation Authority (NHSLA) which deals with litigation claims and works to improve risk-management practice in the UK. There is a set of clinical risk management standards for NHS maternity services known as the Clinical Negligence Scheme for Trusts (CNST) standards [13]. The CNST is a central pool of funds which deals with litigation claims for trusts with each trust contributing a proportion of its turnover. The amount paid by a trust is reflected by the rating achieved by assessing the performance and the extent of risk management employed in a department. Higher-performing trusts achieve a greater reduction in cost in the premium they are required to pay, effectively a financial reward for providing high-quality care.

Reactive risk

- Incident reporting.
- Complaints and claims to legal department.
- Clinical audit.

Most maternity units will have a trigger list of certain risk events which require reporting and possible further investigation. The majority of these triggers will be obstetric emergencies and intrapartum events. These triggers may rely on individuals completing a risk form either manually or electronically. Increasingly the data from maternity units are captured on a hospital database and in doing so automatic risk forms can be filled for events on the trigger list. Although trigger lists will capture the majority of risk events it is important that any perceived risk event can be reported by maternity staff.

In addition to trigger lists for risk events there may be a separate list of risk events which are deemed more serious and require a full investigation. Such a trigger list is the equivalent of using a risk matrix to grade risk events according to their severity and likelihood of recurrence. Such events may be known as Serious Incidents (SI) or Serious Untoward Incidents (SUI). These lists may be devised by the local department or there may be a separate body which oversees all the hospitals in a geographical area.

Analysis of risk event

Retrospective analysis

Once a risk event has been flagged up it is important that it is analysed. The question that needs to be asked is:

'Why did this even happen to this patient at this time?'

Once this is established there must be an assessment of the likelihood of the risk event recurring and actions taken to prevent this.

It is important to adopt a systematic approach to the investigation and root cause analysis (RCA) is a widely accepted tool to use. The steps of an RCA include:

- Gathering and mapping of information.
- Identifying service and care-delivery problems.
- Analysing the information and identifying contributory factors and root causes.
- Generating recommendations and solutions.
- Implementing solutions.
- Writing report.

Root cause analysis is a time-consuming process. There are tools for use in the RCA process on the NPSA website [10].

Although RCA is an accepted tool for investigating incidents it has been criticised for oversimplifying the process by assuming there is only one root cause. An adapted approach is that of 'systems analysis' [14] which is a broader examination of all the aspects of the healthcare system in question.

To help with the evaluation of a risk event a risk score may be used. Such a score arises from a risk score matrix to assess the likely frequency of a risk occurring and the likely severity of the risk. Such a score can help risk management teams prioritise cases for investigation. They are also a useful tool for the staff members completing risk forms to assess the risk incident.

A risk register is a live document held by a maternity unit to aid the risk process. It should contain up-to-date information on risk events identified by trigger lists plus risk identified proactively. The register may also contain information on the risk score plus actions arising during the investigation.

A further tool which can be employed is a maternity dashboard, a practical way of implementing clinical governance. It can provide contemporary information about clinical activity, risk management issues, resources and user views [5]. The principle of the dashboard is to set locally agreed standards against which the current practice is compared to flag up problems as they start to appear, rather than waiting for crisis point. With regard to obstetric emergencies the dashboard may collect data on the number of unexpected intensive treatment units (ITU) admissions or massive postpartum haemorrhages.

Prospective analysis

Risks may be identified prospectively such as those highlighted as a result of a fire drill or as a result of a staff risk workshop. These also benefit from a structured tool to analyse them further. One such tool is Failure Mode and Effects Analysis (FMEA) [8]. This looks at the process in detail and identifies what can go wrong at each step, the so-called 'failure modes', and then looks at the contributory factors for these steps going wrong. The contributory factors can be assessed in terms of how frequently they occur and the likely severity of their outcome. A further analysis of any existing controls in place to prevent the risk allows the risks to be rated and a decision on which risks are unacceptable and need to be treated. This should conclude with a clear action plan on how to implement any changes.

Treatment of risk events

Risk treatment looks at what can be done to minimise the chance of something happening again. This process is closely linked in with the risk control. It may also look at ways to limit the damage as a result of a risk event which has already occurred.

Control of risk events

The control of risk events is the process of learning lessons and sharing these findings. This may be done at a local departmental level or at a national level. It is vital to the risk management process that lessons are learned from an adverse outcome to prevent recurrence. It is not only important for all the hospital staff involved in the case to learn but also for these findings to be shared with other members of staff. In addition these findings often help the patient and their family to understand why an adverse outcome occurred. Many patients want reassurance that what happened to them is not going to happen to another patient.

The feedback after an adverse incident investigation will take many forms, from individual feedback to group discussion; however it is important to keep staff motivated and interested in the process. The manner in which feedback is done is important to establish a fair-blame culture. Individual feedback may be given either verbally or in written form. It is important that the involvement of an individual is looked at as part of a system in order for an individual not to feel victimised and resentful of the risk-management investigation.

Sharing the lessons learned with a department may take the form of a monthly newsletter and interactive risk meetings where cases are discussed.

As well as the feedback it is vital for a department to be seen to be imposing the recommendations from the investigation. After all, there is no point in going to the lengths of a full investigation if the advised actions to prevent the event occurring again are not implemented.

Key pearls

For successful risk management:

- Engage and motivate all staff.
- Ensure it is a multidisciplinary process.
- Ensure good leadership of the risk-management team.

- Avoid apportioning blame to individuals, look at the systems instead.
- Make risk management part of the day-to-day working on the delivery suite.
- Ensure findings from risk-management investigations are disseminated to staff on a regular basis, ideally in forums which allow discussion.
- Address risk events which are repeated.

Key pitfalls

- For staff to see risk management as a threat.
- For individuals to think that they will never be involved in risk cases.
- To fail to learn from mistakes.
- To fail to implement guidance from national audits.

Risk management in low-resource settings

All the principles of risk management described in this chapter are applicable in any clinical setting. However they require time and personnel to execute them. The concept of risk management may be new and daunting to staff, so education will be the key. Ideally the risk management coordinator will have the time and resources to set up risk reporting and the investigation of adverse outcomes.

References

1. Department of Health. *An Organisation with a Memory: Report of an Expert Advisory Group on Learning from Adverse Events in the NHS.* London: The Stationery Office, 2000.

2. Royal College of Obstetricians and Gynaecologists, Royal College of Anaesthetists, Royal College of Midwives and Royal College of Paediatrics and Child Health. *Safer Childbirth: Minimum Standards for the Organisation and Delivery of Care in Labour.* London: RCOG, 2007.

3. Royal College of Anaesthetists, Royal College of Midwives, Royal College of Obstetricians and Gynaecologists, Royal College of Paediatrics and Child Health. *Standards for Maternity Care. Report of a Working Party.* London: RCOG Press, 2008.

4. The NHS Litigation Authority. *Factsheet 3: Information on Claims.* http://www.nhsla.com/claims

5. Neilson PE, Goldman MB, Mann S *et al.* Effects of teamwork training on adverse outcomes and process of care in labour and delivery: a randomised control trial. *Obstet Gynecol* 2007; 109: 48–55.

6. Royal College of Obstetricians and Gynaecologists. *Maternity Dashboard: Clinical Performance and Governance Scorecard.* Good Practice No. 7. London: RCOG, 2008.

7. Centre for Maternal and Child Enquiries (CMACE). *Saving Mothers' Lives: Reviewing Maternal Deaths to make Motherhood Safer – 2006–2008. The Eighth Report on Confidential Enquiries into Maternal Deaths in the United Kingdom. Br J Obstet Gynaecol* 2011; 118 (Suppl. 1): 1–208.

8. Schofield H. Embedding quality improvement and patient safety at Liverpool Women's NHS Foundation Trust. *Best Pract Res Clin Obstet Gynaecol* 2007; 21 (4): 593–607.

9. Royal College of Obstetricians and Gynaecologists. *Improving Patient Safety: Risk Management for Maternity and Gynaecology.* Clinical Governance Advice No. 2. London: RCOG, 2009.

10. National Patient Safety Agency. www.npsa.nhs.uk

11. Royal College of Obstetricians and Gynaecologists, Royal College of Midwives, National Patient Safety Agency. *Safer Practice in Intrapartum Care Project Care Bundles.* London: RCOG, 2010.

12. National Institute for Health and Clinical Excellence. *Intrapartum Care: Management and Delivery of Care to Women in Labour.* Clinical Guideline No. 55. London: NICE, 2007.

13. NHS Litigation Authority. *Clinical Negligence Scheme for Trusts: Maternity Clinical Risk Management Standards Version 1.* 2010/11

14. Taylor-Adams S, Vincent C. Systems analysis of clinical incidents: the London protocol. *Clin Risk* 2004; 10: 211–220.

Index